You Code It! Abstracting Case Studies Practicum

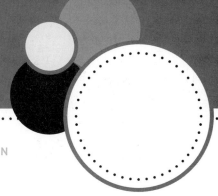

SECOND EDITION

Shelley C. Safian

MAOM/HSM, CCS-P, CPC-H, CPC-I, CHA
AHIMA-Approved ICD-10-CM/PCS Trainer

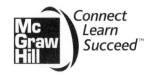

Connect
Learn
Succeed™

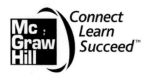

YOU CODE IT! ABSTRACTING CASE STUDIES PRACTICUM
Published by McGraw-Hill, a business unit of The McGraw-Hill Companies, Inc., 1221 Avenue
of the Americas, New York, NY, 10020. Copyright © 2012 by The McGraw-Hill Companies, Inc.
All rights reserved. Previous edition © 2009. No part of this publication may be reproduced or
distributed in any form or by any means, or stored in a database or retrieval system, without the
prior written consent of The McGraw-Hill Companies, Inc., including, but not limited to, in any
network or other electronic storage or transmission, or broadcast for distance learning.
Some ancillaries, including electronic and print components, may not be available to customers
outside the United States.
This book is printed on acid-free paper.

1 2 3 4 5 6 7 8 9 0 QDB/QDB 1 0 9 8 7 6 5 4 3 2 1

ISBN   978-0-07-337452-9
MHID   0-07-337452-0

Vice president/Editor in chief: *Elizabeth Haefele*
Vice president/Director of marketing: *Alice Harra*
Publisher: *Kenneth S. Kasee Jr.*
Senior sponsoring editor: *Natalie J. Ruffatto*
Development editor: *Raisa Priebe Kreek*
Executive marketing manager: *Roxan Kinsey*
Lead digital product manager: *Damian Moshak*
Director, Editing/Design/Production: *Jess Ann Kosic*
Project manager: *Jean R. Starr*
Buyer: *Susan Culbertson*
Senior designer: *Marianna Kinigakis*
Lead photo research coordinator: *Carrie K. Burger*
Digital production coordinator: *Brent dela Cruz*
Cover design: Alexa Viscius
Typeface: *10.5/13 Melior*
Compositor: *Aptara, Inc.*
Printer: *Quad/Graphics*
Credits: The credits section for this book begins on page 519 and is considered an extension of the
copyright page.

www.mhhe.com

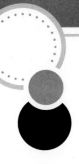

About the Author

Shelley C. Safian has been teaching medical coding and health information management for more than a decade, at both on ground and online campuses. In addition to her regular teaching responsibilities at Herzing University, Berkeley College Online, and Dover Business College, she often presents seminars sponsored by AHIMA, AAPC, and Kaplan University, writes regularly about coding for the *Just Coding* newsletter, and has written articles published in AAPC *Coding Edge, SurgiStrategies,* and *HFM* (Healthcare Financial Management) magazine. Safian is the course author for several AHIMA distance education courses on various coding topics including ICD-10-CM, ICD-10-PCS, and HCPCS Level II coding.

Safian is a Certified Coding Specialist-Physician-based (CCS-P) from the American Health Information Management Association and a Certified Professional Coder-Hospital (CPC-H) and a Certified Professional Coding Instructor (CPC-I) from the American Academy of Professional Coders. She is also a Certified HIPAA Administrator (CHA), and has earned the designation of AHIMA-Approved ICD-10-CM/PCS Trainer.

Safian completed her Graduate Certificate in Health Care Management in June 2005 at Keller Graduate School of Management. The University of Phoenix awarded her Master of Arts/Organizational Management degree in 2002. She is currently working on the dissertation for her Ph.D. in Health Care Administration with a focus in Health Information Management.

Contents

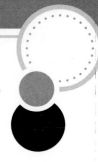

Preface vi

CHAPTER 1 How to Abstract Notes 1

CHAPTER 2 Allergy and Immunology Cases and Patient Records 24

CHAPTER 3 Cardiology and Cardiovascular Cases and Patient Records 38

CHAPTER 4 Dentistry Cases and Patient Records 59

CHAPTER 5 Dermatology and Burns Cases and Patient Records 80

CHAPTER 6 Emergency Services Cases and Patient Records 110

CHAPTER 7 Endocrinology Cases and Patient Records 133

CHAPTER 8 Family Practice Cases and Patient Records 153

CHAPTER 9 Gastroenterology Cases and Patient Records 173

CHAPTER 10 Gerontology Cases and Patient Records 201

CHAPTER 11 Neonatal and Pediatrics Cases and Patient Records 222

CHAPTER 12 Neurology Cases and Patient Records 244

CHAPTER 13 Obstetrics and Gynecology Cases and Patient Records 266

CHAPTER 14 Oncology Cases and Patient Records 287

CHAPTER 15 Ophthalmology Cases and Patient Records 312

CHAPTER 16 Orthopedics Cases and Patient Records 334

CHAPTER 17 Otolaryngology Cases and Patient Records 352

CHAPTER 18 Pathology and Laboratory Cases and Patient Records 368

CHAPTER 19   Plastic and Reconstructive Surgery Cases and Patient Records   388

CHAPTER 20   Podiatry Cases and Patient Records   399

CHAPTER 21   Psychiatric Cases and Patient Records   420

CHAPTER 22   Pulmonary and Respiratory Cases and Patient Records   437

CHAPTER 23   Radiology and Nuclear Medicine Cases and Patient Records   457

CHAPTER 24   Urology, Nephrology, and Men's Health Cases and Patient Records   483

CHAPTER 25   Alternative Medicine: Acupuncture, Chiropractics, and Physical Therapy Cases and Patient Records   502

CREDITS   519

Preface

Welcome to *You Code It!* This book is part of a three-book series that instructs students on how to become proficient in medical coding—a health care field that continues to be in high demand. The Bureau of Labor Statistics notes the demand for health information management professions (which includes coders) will continue to increase incredibly through 2018 and beyond.

This series of books was written to speak directly to the medical coding student using step-by-step instructions and conversational language to maximize understanding. Built into the structure of these texts are many opportunities for students to practice coding and apply what they have learned. Students will also have the chance to practice abstracting with real-world health professionals' documentation and accurately translating these facts into the best, most accurate codes.

TO THE STUDENT

Your medical coding classes introduce you to the skills you will need to work in the health information management field. A fundamental role of an insurance coding and medical billing specialist's job is to work with the insurance companies that will reimburse the health care facility for the services and treatments provided to patients. You may be employed by a hospital, clinic, doctor's office, health maintenance organization, mental health care facility, insurance company, government agency or long-term care facility. Your career will be challenging, interesting, and one of the top ten fastest-growing Allied Health professions.

Before you begin your adventure, here are some tips to help you succeed:

- First, take a deep breath. Coding is complex and is not like anything else you have tackled to learn before. Remember that you are learning a new skill! Give yourself some time to become proficient.

- Second, *never* code directly from the alphabetic index. *Always* look the code up in the tabular list before deciding on a code. If you remember this rule, you will always head in the right direction.

- Third, when you encounter a word or abbreviation that you don't understand, stop and look it up in your medical dictionary. Your instructor can recommend a medical dictionary for you, or you can purchase McGraw-Hill's *Medical Dictionary for Allied Health* (ISBN: 0-07-351096-3).

- Fourth, after you finish coding the case studies, scenarios, or whatever you are coding, put it all aside. Then, later or the next day, go back and do "back coding." In the tabular list, look up each code you came up with and match the code description carefully with the case study or scenario words. This is a very effective way to double-check your answers. Your fresh eyes will enable you see words and notations you may have missed before.

- Finally, re-evaluate your work by checking each and every question to make certain you understand how you found your answer. When you find you have gotten an exercise, test question, or other activity wrong, try to figure out what happened. Make sure you ask your instructor for help when you need it!

Good luck on your medical coding journey!

TO THE INSTRUCTOR

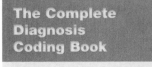

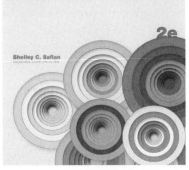

Shelley Safian's Medical Coding Series includes three books:

The Complete Diagnosis Coding Book (ISBN: 0-07-337451-2)

The Complete Procedure Coding Book (ISBN: 0-07-337450-4)

You Code It! (ISBN: 0-07-337452-0)

These books are designed to give your students the medical coding experience they need in order to pass their first medical coding certification exams, like the CCS/CCS-P or CPC/CPC-H. The books offer students a variety of practice opportunities by reinforcing the learning outcomes set forth in every chapter. The chapter materials are organized in short bursts of text followed by practice—keeping students active and coding throughout!

In order to provide your students with realistic practice before entering the coding field, this book contains actual physician's notes, hospital documents, and lab reports from virtually every medical specialty (with identifying information redacted). Using real-life notes allows your students to practice abstracting documentation written by many different health-care professionals, each of whom has his or her own documenting style. In almost all cases, this documentation has not been augmented, in order to provide you with more flexibility in using the book's many case studies.

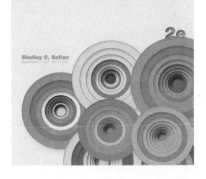

For more information about the resources available to help you plan your course, visit the Online Learning Center at **www.mhhe.com/safian2e.**

WHAT'S NEW IN OUR 2ND EDITION

You Code It!, second edition, has been revised to include a greater number of realistic scenarios and case studies for students to gain hands-on learning. These exercises make it easier for students to connect learning concepts and specific official guidelines to critical thinking.

The entire text has been updated using 2011 CPT, 2011 ICD-9-CM, and 2011 HCPCS Level II codes. The instructor's manual features a 2011-compliant answer key to all case studies in the book.

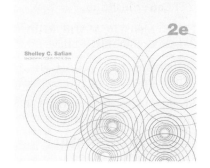

CODEITRIGHTONLINE™: YOUR ONLINE CODING TOOL

So that your students can gain experience with the use of an online coding tool, they will have access for a 14-day period to CodeitRight Online, produced by Contexo Media, a division of Access Intelligence.

CodeitRightOnline offers a comprehensive search function for CPT, HCPCS Level II, and ICD-9-CM codes, along with ICD-10-CM/PCS code sets. It includes helpful tools like search indexing for easy reference, and offers newsletter articles and other coding resources. For more information about the features of CodeitRightOnline and how to sign up for a trial, visit **www.mhhe.com/safian2e**.

ACKNOWLEDGMENTS

Book Reviews

Many instructors reviewed the first and second editions and provided valuable feedback that directly affected the books' development. Their contributions are greatly appreciated.

Bobette Anderson
MedVance Institute of Fort Lauderdale

Norma Bird, M.Ed., BS, CMA
Idaho State University

Mary M. Cantwell, RHIT, CPC, CPC-I, CPC-H, CPC-P
Metropolitan Community College

Adelia M. Cooley, BBA, MSHA, CPC
Baker College of Auburn Hills

Carol T. Courtney, MS, CPC, OCS
Clark Community College

Barbara Desch
San Joaquin Valley College, Visalia Campus

John Dingle, CMA
Sawyer School, Butler Business School

Pennie Eckard, MAOM, CPC, CMA (AAMA)
Davis College

Carolyn H. Greene
Virginia College at Birmingham

Debra S. Grieshop, RHIA, BS
Wright State University

Robin Kern, BSN
Moultrie Technical College

Naomi Kupfer, CMA
Heritage College

Fannie Sue Martin, CPC
YTI Career Institute

Norma Mercado, MAHS, RHIA
Austin Community College

Della Moon, RHIT, CCS, CTR
San Jacinto College

Rosemarie Scaringella, BA, CBCS
Hunter Business School

Gene Simon, RHIA, RMD
Florida Career College

Debra A. Slusarczyk, BHS, RHIT
Camden County College

Corinne Smith, MBA, RHIA, CCS
Montgomery College

Robyn Stambaugh, BS, RHIT
Central Carolina Technical College

Nona K. Stinemetz, LPN
Vatterott College

Jennifer L. Thorman, CPC, Master MOS
MedVance Institute of Fort Lauderdale

Jim Wallace, MHSA
Stars Behavioral Health Group

Carole Stemple Zeglin, MSEd, BSMT, RMA
Westmoreland County Community College

Technical Editing/Accuracy Panel

A panel of instructors completed a technical edit and review of all content in the book page proofs to verify its accuracy, along with the supplements.

Sue Butler, CPC, CIMC
Lansing Community College

Laurie Dennis, CBCS, CHI
Florida Career College

Pamela Fleming
Quinsigamond Community College

Betty Haar, BS, RHIA
Kirkwood Community College

LaWanda Hamilton, CCA, CPC
Remington College

Marsha Holtsberry, AA, CMA (AAMA), CPC-A
Ohio Business College

Cheryl Miller, MBA/HCM
Westmoreland County Community College

Kimberly S. Poag, MHA Ed., CMA, CPC
Baker College

Patricia Stich, M.Ed., CCS-P
Waubonsee Community College

Sheba Schlaikjer, BA, RHIT
Colorado Technical University

How to Abstract Notes

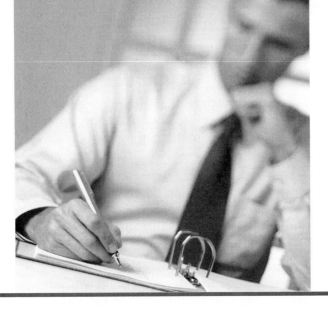

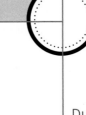

INTRODUCTION

The most efficient and effective way to code an encounter between a health care professional and a patient is to review the physician's notes, lab reports, and all documentation for that encounter (also referred to as a visit). When the coder can read exactly what the physician thought, heard, and observed in his or her own words, there is less confusion and miscommunication. The more accurate the communication between the providing professional and the professional coding specialist, the more accurate the codes will be—ensuring accurate and optimal reimbursement.

Many physicians' offices are specialized. So you will most likely end up working with a limited number of sections within the International Classification of Diseases, Ninth Revision, Clinical Modification (ICD-9-CM) and Current Procedural Terminology (CPT) books. This will not change when ICD-10-CM (International

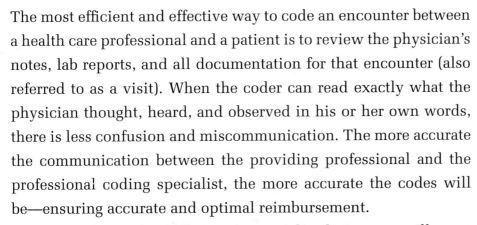

«« CODING TIP

Patient = *Who* came to see the provider for health care

Diagnosis = *Why* the provider is caring for this individual during this visit

In cases of injury or poisoning, E codes from the ICD-9-CM diagnosis book will report *how* and *where* the patient got hurt.

Procedure = *What* the provider did for the individual

Abstracting

The process of identifying the relevant words or phrases in health care documentation in order to determine the best, most appropriate code(s).

Query

To ask.

KEYS TO CODING »»

Is it a diagnosis or a procedure?

Do the key words tell you WHY or WHAT?

- A **diagnostic statement** will explain WHY the physician cared for the patient, saw the patient, and/or provided a service or treatment or performed a procedure.
- A **procedural statement** will explain WHAT the physician did for the patient or to the patient.

Look at the parts of the medical term. There are parts of medical terms, particularly the suffixes that are specific to a diagnosis or a procedure.

Examples:

A diagnostic term might have a suffix like

-itis means inflammation (a condition or something wrong)

-edema means swelling (a condition or something wrong)

whereas a procedural term might have a suffix like

-ectomy means to surgically remove (an action)

-scopy means to view or look (an action)

Classification of Diseases, Tenth Revision, Clinical Modification) and ICD-10-PCS (International Classification of Diseases, Tenth Revision, Procedural Coding System) are implemented in October 2013. The following chapters of this book are set up to align with types of health care specialties, so you can practice coding as if you were working for a specific health care facility.

Example

If you are working for a gastroenterologist you would rarely, if ever, use codes for mental disorders 290-319.

THE SEVEN STEPS OF CODING

There is a seven-step process for coding a health care encounter (also referred to as a visit) in the approved manner. As you gain experience, it will take less time. However, remember that time is not the number one consideration - —accuracy is the most important factor.

The steps are as follows:

1. Read through the superbill and the physician's notes for the encounter completely, from beginning to end. Make a copy of the pages relating to the visit so that you can write on the copy without marking the originals. Or, use some scratch paper alongside so that you can jot down details you want to remember.

2. Read through the physician's notes again, this time highlighting key words and phrases regarding diagnoses and procedures directly relating to this encounter. Pulling out the *key words* is known as **abstracting** physician's notes. You will need to evaluate the key words and distinguish between diagnostic statements and procedural statements.

3. Make a list of any questions you have regarding unclear or missing information necessary to code the encounter. **Query** the health care provider who wrote or dictated the notes. *Never assume.* Code only what you know from actual documentation. It is the law that you must have documentation to back up every code you submit on a claim form.

   Note: In class, your instructor is the person to query about anything you need to code an encounter properly.

Example

The documentation indicates that the physician performed a posterior vestibuloplasty on Marion Jones. You pull out the key words: *vestibuloplasty* and *posterior*. However, when you look up the procedure in the CPT book, you see that there are two codes to choose from:

    40842 Vestibuloplasty; posterior, unilateral

    40843 Vestibuloplasty; posterior, bilateral

»»

You must query the physician to find out whether the procedure was done unilaterally (one side) or bilaterally (both sides). Make certain the physician writes the answer down in the chart *and* initials it. Now, you know which code is the best, most appropriate code.

4. Code all diagnoses confirmed by the physician to be relevant during this encounter. Remember that coding, for both reimbursement and statistical purposes, will report only those conditions addressed by the provider during this encounter, not the patient's entire health history. When there is no confirmed diagnosis to provide medical necessity for a procedure, service, or treatment performed, code the patient's signs and/or symptoms that led to the physician's decision to perform that procedure. Use the best, most appropriate code or codes available based on the documentation.

Begin by dissecting the diagnostic statement. Take the statement apart and determine which word identifies the disease, illness, condition, or primary reason for the visit (also known as the "main term"). Separate this from any words that may simply describe the type of condition or the location of the condition (anatomical site/ body site). Ask yourself WHY is the physician caring for the patient? Specifically. When you look at these examples, you can see the reason the physician is seeing the patient for this visit.

EXAMPLES:

i. Herpes zoster . . . The disease is "herpes" and "zoster" is the type of herpes.

ii. Acute bronchospasm . . . The condition is "bronchospasm" and the term "acute" (which means severe) describes what type of broncho-spasm the patient has.

iii. Family history of lung cancer . . . The issue of concern is "history" — why the patient is being seen. The type of history is "family", and the secondary descriptor is "malignant neoplasm of the lung (lung cancer)" to explain "a history of what?"

iv. Myocardial infarction . . . The condition is "infarction" (area of dead tissue) and "myocardial" (heart muscle) is the anatomical site of the infarction.

v. Congenital Pneumothorax . . . The condition is "pneumothorax" (air in the chest cavity) and the term "congenital" (occurring in utero) describes the cause of the condition.

vi. Family history of renal failure . . . The issue of concern is "history" — why the patient is being seen. The type of history is "family", and the secondary descriptor is "renal failure" (loss of function of the kidneys) to explain "a history of what?"

Once you have determined the condition or issue ("main term"), find that term(s) in the ICD-9-CM alphabetic index (volume 2). If all the words in the diagnostic statement seem to have the same impact to you, just look up all the words, one at a time, in the ICD-9-CM alphabetic index. You will get to the correct "main term" and find the code. Write the suggested code down on a piece of scratch paper and move to the next step.

«« **CODING TIP**

Use a medical dictionary to learn the true meaning of a medical term. If you don't know what the term means, you will have a problem interpreting it into an accurate code.

«« **BRIDGE TO ICD-10-CM/PCS**

Additional specifics are going to become even more important as we move closer to the implementation of ICD-10-CM and ICD-10-PCS. Complete documentation with comprehensive details is critical to determining the correct code because ICD-10-CM and ICD-10-PCS code descriptions contain more specifics.

«« **CODING TIP**

Before using an unspecified diagnosis code, query the physician to gain the details needed to use a more specific code. Unspecified or NOS (not otherwise specified) codes should only be used as a last resort when the physician cannot be contacted.

«« **BRIDGE TO ICD-10-CM**

You will follow these samesteps when ICD-10-CM is implemented. This process will not change. Only the way the codes look will change.

Medical necessity

The assessment that the provider was acting according to standard practices in providing a procedure or service for an individual with a specific diagnosis.

Next, turn to the tabular list (volume 1) of ICD-9-CM to find the code suggested by the alphabetic index. This is a mandatory step. The tabular list of ICD-9-CM provides more detail for the code description, as well as additional notations such as INCLUDES and EXCLUDES notes and directives for the requirement of additional digits and codes. **NEVER, NEVER, NEVER code from the alphabetic index.**

5. Code the procedure(s) as stated in the notes describing what the provider did for the patient. Use the best, most appropriate code(s) available based on the documentation.

   Begin by dissecting the procedural statement. Identify the term that describes WHAT action was taken and the anatomical site that was treated.

   EXAMPLES:

   i. Cranial nerve neuroplasty . . . the procedure is a "neuroplasty" and the anatomical site is the "cranial nerve"

   ii. Pelvic ultrasound . . . the procedure is an "ultrasound" and the anatomical site is the "pelvis"

   iii. Coronary thrombolysis . . . the procedure is a "thrombolysis" and the anatomical site is the "heart" (coronary refers to the heart).

   Next, look for the "action" term in the CPT alphabetic index. The "action" term is the specific procedure (such as hysterectomy), the service (such as counseling), or the treatment (such as injection). If you are reporting procedures and services performed in a hospital for an inpatient, you may use the ICD-9-CM volume 3 code set. To report services provided by a physician at any type of facility or procedures and services provided at an outpatient facility, you will use the CPT code set.

   Now, find the code(s) suggested by the alphabetic index in the numeric listing of CPT or the tabular list of ICD-9-CM Volume 3. This is not a suggestion; it is a mandatory step. The section listing all the codes in numerical order provides additional detail for the code description, as well as additional notations and directives for the requirement of additional codes and/or modifiers.

   Often, the CPT alphabetic index will suggest several codes (12345, 12349, 25443) or a range of codes (12345-12357). You must look at ALL suggested codes in the numeric list (not just the first one), read the complete code descriptions and all notations, and *then* choose the most accurate. And, the correct code is NEVER a range.

   NEVER, NEVER, NEVER code from the alphabetic index.

6. Connect every procedure code to at least one diagnosis code for the same encounter to document **medical necessity.** This is known as linking; it is not only required on the claim form, but it is also an excellent way to confirm that all your procedure codes are supported by a diagnosis code.

7. Double-check your work by back coding. It means that you look up the code you have chosen in the tabular list, reread the code description, and compare it to the original notes to make certain they match. This will help you catch innocent typos, accidentally missing a fourth or fifth digit, or another relevant notation.

Chapter 1   How to Abstract Notes

Following these steps will help you code precisely, resulting in a greater number of your claims being paid quickly, at the highest earned reimbursement rate.

DIAGNOSIS AND MEDICAL NECESSITY _____

The International Classification of Diseases, ninth revision, Clinical Modification (ICD-9-CM) volumes 1 & 2 is a directory of every diagnosis, sign, symptom, or reason, why a health care provider would spend time with, and/or provide a service to, a patient. Diagnosis codes establish medical necessity. Every procedure code reported must be accompanied by a diagnosis code that justifies providing that specific procedure to the patient at the time he or she is seen by the provider. Some examples of diagnoses are a broken ankle, diabetes, or the flu.

Example

Jerri Cavanaugh, a 13-year-old female, is brought to the emergency department by her mother after she fell off her skateboard and hurt her ankle. Dr. Roberts orders x-rays that confirm Jerri's ankle is broken, and he applies a short leg (knee-to-toe) cast. The diagnosis of a broken ankle makes taking the x-ray and applying the cast good medical decisions. Dr. Roberts documented medical necessity for both services (x-ray and cast application).

Example

Morris Cruz, a 65-year-old male, went to see his physician, Dr. Bridges. Morris was complaining of pain upon urination. Dr. Bridges ordered an urinalysis. The results of the test showed that Morris had a urinary tract infection (UTI). Dr. Bridges was in a hurry and scribbled in his notes what looked like URI. The problem is that URI stands for upper respiratory infection (chest congestion). You can see that the diagnosis of an upper respiratory infection does not justify the urinalysis that was ordered. This will be looked at as either an error or very poor medical judgment. In either case, the claim will be denied for lack of medical necessity.

PROCEDURES (Services and Treatments) _____

During the process of translating procedures (services and treatments) in health care into codes, you might use any of the following code sets:

- CPT—Current Procedural Terminology
- HCPCS—Healthcare Common Procedure Coding System, Level II
- ICD-9-CM, volume 3—International Classifications of Diseases, ninth revision, Clinical Modification, Volume 3

Current Procedural Terminology (CPT) is used for reporting procedures, treatments, and services provided to outpatients—such as an x-ray, a vaccination, or the removal of a cyst—as well as physician's services provided almost anywhere.

The Healthcare Common Procedure Coding System, Level II (HCPCS, which is pronounced "hick-picks") lists codes used to identify the provision

⟪⟪ CODING TIP

A physical examination, ordering and/or performing a test, and writing a prescription are all ways that a physician might address a condition. *Only code those conditions that are relevant to this visit.*

⟪⟪ BRIDGE TO ICD-10-PCS

In ICD-10-PCS, the "action" is known as the *"root operation."* This is the term that clarifies the specific service or type of procedure. The anatomical site affected by the root operation, in ICD-10-PCS, may be categorized by the "body system" or specific "body part."

CPT & ICD-10-PCS: ICD-10-PCS will replace procedure codes from ICD-9-CM volume 3 used to report inpatient services and treatments. It is not planned to replace CPT codes. CPT codes will remain the code set to report physician services and outpatient facility services.

⟪⟪ BRIDGE TO ICD-10-CM

On October 1, 2013, ICD-10-CM will replace ICD-9-CM codes for reporting diagnoses, signs, and symptoms, in addition to other reasons individuals see a health care professional.

⟪⟪ BRIDGE TO ICD-10-PCS

On October 1, 2013, ICD-10-PCS will replace ICD-9-CM volume 3 codes for reporting procedures performed in acute care facilities (hospitals) on inpatients. CPT and HCPCS Level II codes will not be affected.

Durable medical equipment (DME)

Items that are used in the care and treatment of a patient that can either last a long time or can be used again and again.

of **durable medical equipment (DME),** medications, and certain other services not listed in the CPT book. Items coded from the HCPCS book might include a wheelchair, crutches, or a unit of blood for a transfusion.

International Classification of Diseases, ninth revision, Clinical Modification, volume 3 (ICD-9-CM vol. 3) is used to report procedures, treatments, and other services provided to an inpatient, one who has been admitted into a hospital and stays overnight in this acute care facility. Codes are used from this volume to reimburse the hospital for its expenses. The physician's, or surgeon's, services are typically reported from CPT, by the physician's office coder, even though the services were provided in a hospital.

ACCURACY

Each set of numbers and letters is a code that means something so specific that a code number just one digit off could mean something totally unrelated. Everyone can make an error occasionally transposing two numbers when writing, or typing, a sequence. You will be thinking 1-7-1, and accidentally write down 711. Instead of dialing the wrong phone number, that difference could cause the claim to be rejected, denied, or pulled for investigation, resulting in your office having to deal with delayed payment, or no payment at all, for the work it did. That is why it is critical to be careful and accurate when coding. *Always* double-check your codes.

Example

301.7 Antisocial personality disorder (a neurosis)

307.1 Anorexia nervosa (an eating disorder)

Example

30520 Septoplasty or submucous resection, with or without cartilage scoring, contouring or replacement with graft . . . *nose surgery*

50320 Donor nephrectomy (including cold preservation); open, from living donor . . . *the removal of a kidney from a live person to be transplanted into another*

THE CODING PROCESS

As you read in *The Seven Steps of Coding*, the best place to begin the coding process is with the physician's notes for the encounter. Abstract, or pull out, the key words relating to *why* the patient was treated by the physician during this encounter to determine accurate diagnosis codes and *what* the physician did for the patient to get accurate procedure codes.

Remember, the key words may be identified directly as the diagnosis, or you may need to find the patient's signs and symptoms (often called the patient's *chief complaint*). The procedure provided may be labeled as such, or you may need to read through the complete notes to identify everything that was done for the patient during the encounter.

Once you have identified the related key words abstracted from the notes, turn to the alphabetic index of the appropriate book: ICD-9-CM or CPT. You will use the alphabetic index to guide you to the correct page

Chapter 1   How to Abstract Notes

or category in the tabular list (volume 1). Then you need to carefully read the code descriptions, beginning at the top of the category, so you can make certain that you find the best code, to the highest level of specificity, according to the physician's notes for a particular encounter, and within the guidelines of the code set.

When you begin, you will find that looking for a diagnostic or procedural key word in the alphabetic index may be a snap!

Example

Dr. Kinner diagnoses Alvira Gomez with polyphagia. Turn to the alphabetic index in ICD-9-CM and find Polyphagia 783.6. Confirm this in the tabular list and you've got the correct code.

Sometimes, it is like looking for a contact lens on a carpet—you have to really look carefully and think about what the facts are.

Example

While washing the dishes, Darlene Samanski broke a drinking glass in her hand. She was pretty certain she got all the glass out and cleaned the wound well, but, two days later, it was still hurting. She went to Dr. Mahoney, who removed several tiny shards of glass from the wound.

You have to think about this and realize that the glass is actually a foreign body. In addition, you must figure out that the glass is not actually in Darlene's hand; it is in her soft tissue. Now, you will be able to find this in the alphabetic index:

Foreign Body, in, soft tissue (residual) 729.6

Other times, you may have to use alternate terms, or synonyms, from those used in the notes to find the correct listing. A medical dictionary will help you in these situations.

Example

Stephanie Lewis fell off of her bicycle and scraped her knee very badly, so she came to see Dr. Bartlett.

Scrape is not in the ICD-9-CM alphabetic index. Another term for scrape is *abrasion*. Turn to abrasion in the alphabetic index. It will direct you to *Injury, Superficial, by site,* and you find:

Injury, superficial, knee (and ankle, hip, leg, or thigh) 916

Remember that accuracy is the *most* important issue here. It is not a race. You need to be careful and meticulous.

<<< **CODING TIP**

Never, never, never code *only* from the alphabetic index in any of your coding books. *Always check* the code in the tabular list and read the entire code description and all notations before deciding on the code. You may feel this is slowing you down or frustrating, but, honestly, your coding will be accurate when you read all the information available to you.

<<< **BRIDGE TO ICD-10-CM AND ICD-10-PCS**

The coding process, as reviewed previously, remains the same for ICD-10-CM/PCS. The only difference you will find is that the codes will look differently once you find them.

LET'S CODE IT! SCENARIO

Patient: Brackman, Nathan
Procedure: Steroid injection
Indications: Left shoulder subacromial bursitis

Procedure: Patient arrived at our office for the procedure as planned during his visit earlier in the week. After obtaining consent, the area of the left

Betadine

Antibacterial topical substance to assure that an injection does not penetrate the skin and permit bacteria in with it. Similar to the alcohol swipe one uses prior to giving a regular injection.

Lidocaine

A local anesthetic, to numb the area so the patient will not feel pain.

Kenalog

A steroid medication.

CODING TIP »»»

Even though the alphabetic index suggests code 726.19, it is wise to begin reviewing the code descriptions, notations, and symbols throughout the entire code category. You don't want to miss any information.

KEYS TO CODING »»»

WHAT did the physician do for Nathan? He gave him a steroid injection in the left shoulder. More specifically, there were two parts to this procedure:

The administration of the injection. This will be reported with a CPT code.

What was injected . . . in this case, the Kenalog. This will be reported with a HCPCS Level II code (starting with a J).

---

shoulder was prepped in the usual fashion with **betadine.** *6cc of 1%* **lidocaine** *with 10 mg of* **Kenalog** *was injected in the left subacromial bursa without difficulty. He tolerated the procedure well without immediate complications. There was moderate relief of pain afterward. He was advised to call me if he exhibits any signs of infection, such as fever, chills, erythema, or swelling. He agreed to call me in 3–4 days and tell me how he is doing.*

Let's Code It! The Diagnosis

Diagnosis codes report the medical rationale for providing the procedure, in this case, the injection.

WHY was it medically necessary to give Nathan this injection? Because he had *subacromial bursitis of his left shoulder.*

The condition = bursitis

What type of bursitis = subacromial

The anatomical site affected by this condition = shoulder, left

In the ICD-9-CM alphabetic index (volume 2), find the term "bursitis." In the list of terms indented beneath you must find the term that describes what type of bursitis the patient has . . . "subacromial." The alphabetic index suggests code 726.19.

Turn to volume 1, the ICD-9-CM tabular list, and find the 726 code category.

Begin reading at the three-digit code.

√4th 726 Peripheral enthesopathies and allied syndromes

There is a *note* and an *excludes* notation. You will notice that neither relate to our case, so keep reading down to review all the choices for that required 4th digit.

√5th 726.1 Rotator cuff syndrome of shoulder and allied disorders

There are four choices for the 5th digit and you will find that 726.19 fits the physician's diagnosis for this patient.

726.19 Other specified disorders of the shoulder, rotator cuff

You can see that having a medical dictionary would be very helpful because while the physician wrote 'bursitis' in his notes, and 'bursitis' was listed in the alphabetic index, the term 'bursitis' is not specifically shown here in the tabular list. The only way you can be certain this is the correct code is to know the meaning of the terms used in the description of the other codes listed in this code category, such as supraspinatus syndrome, calcifying tendinitis, and bicipital tenosynovitis. The only way you can know these codes are not correct for a dignosis of bursitis is to know what they mean.

Let's Code It! The Procedure

Ask yourself WHAT did the physician do for this patient? He INJECTED the patient. So, in the CPT alphabetic index, look up INJECTION.

You will see the indented list under the term INJECTION contains mostly anatomical sites. At what ANATOMICAL SITE did the physician INJECT the patient? You might begin with "shoulder." However, when you look at the term "shoulder" under Injection, you will see that it describes an arthrographic radiologic procedure. There is nothing in the notes about this type of procedure, so that can't be correct.

Go back to the notes . . . what other words do we have to describe the exact location where the injection was inserted? Do you see the term **bursa**?

Look for the term BURSA indented under the term INJECTION. This suggests codes 20600-20610.

Let's now go to the main portion of CPT to check these codes out.

> **20600** Arthrocentesis, aspiration and/or injection; small joint or bursa (e.g., Fingers, toes)
>
> **20605** Arthrocentesis, aspiration and/or injection; intermediate joint or bursa (e.g., Temporomandibular, acromioclavicular, wrist, elbow, or ankle, olecranon bursa)
>
> **20610** Arthrocentesis, aspiration and/or injection; major joint or bursa (e.g,, shoulder, hip, knee joint, subacromial bursa)

All of these code descriptions seem to include our key words: injection and bursa. However, only one code description includes the correct anatomical site for this patient . . . shoulder. Therefore, code 20610 is the correct code.

Let's Code It! The Medication

There is one more item that this physician provided to this patient for which he deserves to get reimbursed. As you read, code 20610 reports the administration of the injection. However, to tell the WHOLE story, you also need to report WHICH medication was injected into Nathan's bursa.

Drugs administered to a patient by a health care professional are reported by using codes from the HCPCS Level II code set. In this separate book of codes, you can look up this particular drug one of two ways: using the alphabetic index or the Table of Drugs in Appendix 1.

In the HCPCS Level II alphabetic index, look up the name of the medication injected into Nathan—Kenalog. You will see

> Kenalog [-10, -40], J3301

The Table of Drugs in Appendix 1 also lists drugs in alphabetic order. You will find the same reference to code J3301.

Find code J3301 in the alphanumerical listing of HCPCS Level II and confirm this is the correct code. You will see:

> **J3301** Injection, triamcinolone acetonide, not otherwise specified, 10 mg
>
> Use this code for Kenalog-10, Kenalog-40, Tri-Kort, Kenaject-40, Cenacort A-40, Triam-A, Trilog.

Bursa

A closed fluid-filled sac that functions to provide a gliding surface to reduce friction between tissues of the body.

««« CODING TIP

The CPT code for the injection administration will ensure the reimbursement of the provider for the knowledge and skill to give the injection, the cost of the sterilization of the injection site (e.g., alcohol swab, betadine), topical anesthetic, the syringe, and the bandage or sterile cover of the injection site.

««« CODING TIP

The betadine and the lidocaine are already included in the injection procedure because it would be wrong to inject the patient without these two elements. However, because all sorts of drugs can be injected into a patient, we must code the contents of the injection separately, in this case, the Kenalog.

When you put this all together, you have the accurate codes for Nathan's encounter.

Diagnosis code: 726.19

Procedure code: 20610

Medication code: J3301

DIFFERENT STYLES OF MEDICAL NOTES

SOAP Notes

No, SOAP notes do not have anything to do with the importance of washing your hands before seeing a patient. These notes are written in an outline format using four sections: subjective, objective, assessment, and plan. The term SOAP is an acronym for the four section titles.

Subjective is the first section and will include the reason for the patient's visit today (chief complaint), status regarding current medications and/or treatments, history (past, family, and/or social), and an itemization of any signs and/or symptoms.

Objective, the second section, will contain the results of any physical examination performed, including vital signs, height/weight, physician's observations, and the results of any diagnostic testing related to the concern at hand.

Assessment is the diagnosis, or the physician's conclusions. If there is no definitive diagnosis, the coder must reread the objective portion of the notes to look for positive test results (such as a statement reading, "X-ray showed lateral fracture of the tibia") for coding a diagnosis. If there is no confirmed diagnosis as a result of the testing, then the patient's signs and symptoms must be coded.

Plan, the last part of the notes, will document the physician's orders for the patient. These may include diagnostic tests to be done in the future, procedures to be performed ("Colonoscopy scheduled to be done in one week"), recommendations for lifestyle changes ("Patient is advised to quit drinking alcoholic beverages as soon as possible"), and follow-up care ("Recheck CBC in 2 weeks").

Many physicians like SOAP notes because they are more orderly and tend to be more thorough. With this format, they are reminded to address each portion, as they are dictating, or writing, to document all aspects of the encounter with the patient.

Figure 1-1 is an example of SOAP notes taken from a family practitioner. See if you can determine what each of the four terms mean by the content of each paragraph or section.

Narrative Notes

Some physicians prefer to dictate their notes using the narrative format, as shown in Figure 1-2. It means that they tell the story of the encounter with the patient, including all the details. This is typed and presented in paragraph format.

CODING TIP »»

It is important that the coder always read the entire document. Remember that you are permitted to code and report only procedures, services, and treatments that have been DONE by your staff. Just because the physician *ordered* a test or procedure is not a valid reason to report the code. It must have been provided, and provided by a professional for whom you are responsible to report codes.

Chapter 1   How to Abstract Notes

```
                              PROGRESS NOTE

        PT NAME:              YORK, MARY LOU
        DOB:                  05/27/88
        MRN:                  05015979

        DATE:                 03/03/11
```

S: This pt is an 18-year-old white female, G0, LMP 2/18, not sexually active, not on any birth control that presents today with two main complaints. The first complaint is she feels a lump in her right groin. The second complaint is a vaginal discharge, no odor or itching, just feels irritated.

O: Pelvic exam revealed the external genitalia to be within normal limits. The vagina was without lesions. Scant discharge seen. Wet mount neg for Trichomonas, clue cells or hyphae. Increased bacteria in the background noted. Inspection of the rt groin revealed no abnormality. The pt was asked to point out the area of abnormality and this felt to be dilated areas within one of the vessels in the groin. These were less than the size of a pea and did not feel like lymphadenopathy. Similar areas were felt on the lt side as well. The patient was reassured.

A: Possible nonspecific vaginitis

P: 1. Cleocin vaginal cream qhs times seven nights.
    2. Follow up in one month for reinspection of the rt groin
    3. Otherwise follow up with us prn. She verbalized understanding
    4. All questions were answered. She will follow up with us prn or for her yearly Pap smear.

_____

Harold Donnelson, M.D.

D: 03/03/11
T: 03/08/11 nk

Figure 1-1 Example of SOAP Notes

»»» **CODING TIP**

In Figure 1-1, an example of SOAP notes, you will notice the acronym MRN that stands for medical record number. At the bottom, under the physician's signature, you will see the date the notes were dictated (identified by the *D*), the date the notes were transcribed (identified by the *T*), and the initials of the medical transcriptionist (which in this case are *nk*).

Generally, it seems that family physicians, who may plan more time between appointments and have a wider scope of interest with regard to their patient's health (the whole body), tend to prefer SOAP notes, whereas specialists, who see their patients in sequenced appointments with more regularity and for a more singular focus (one particular part of the body and often one concern), tend to prefer the narrative notes format. This may be because specialists typically will not have vital signs taken and documented with each visit, unless they are applicable to the problem, as well as the fact that each consecutive visit with a specialist is a follow-up to the original concern.

However, it is the physician's personal preference. For the coder and biller in the office, the only difference will be that the SOAP notes outline format can make it easier and faster to find the diagnosis, whereas the narrative format would require a more thorough reading of the entire encounter.

PROGRESS NOTE

PT NAME: GROGANZI, ALFRED
DOB: 07/13/11
MRN: 06002795

Date: 09/08/10

[Office Visit] This patient is coming along well since his colonoscopy. He is having minimal problems. Examination reveals mild colitis. He was told I would not put him on any type of treatment at this time. The patient doesn't want to take steroids; he is not having enough problems to warrant steroids. We will see him again in 3 months. ks

Date: 12/18/10

[Office Visit] This patient is getting along exceptionally well. He was scoped up to 40 cm and has colitis up this far. However the worst of it is in the last 10 centimeters. The patient will be given another course of Flagyl to see if we can get this to resolve. We will check him in 3 weeks. ks

Date: 01/09/11

[Office Visit] This patient is in today and he still has his colitis. It is getting worse. We will start him on some Rowasa. We will give him one a night for 3 weeks. We will see him after that and see how he is getting along. He will probably have to take it for 6 weeks before we will see a difference. ks

Suzanne Esperanza, M.D.

Figure 1-2   Example of Narrative Notes

Procedure Notes

Procedure notes and operative reports, as shown in Figure 1-3, contain different types of information than standard office visit documentation. That is why these reports take on a different format.

For extensive procedures that need operative support, such as those usually done in same-day surgical centers, the attending physicians may use an indications, procedure, impression, and plan (IPIP) outline format for their reports. In these cases, time is not typically spent discussing things with the patient or any other evaluation and management services. Often, the patient comes in, the procedure is performed, and the patient goes home. Follow-up will be done when the patient sees the physician in the office for the next appointment. Take a look at Figure 1-3.

The sections on these reports include

Indications: A statement of the diagnosis that is the reason for the procedure

Procedure: A step-by-step accounting of what was done during the procedure

PROCEDURE NOTE

PT NAME:	CASSIDY, CAROLINE
DOB:	07/13/85
MRN:	06002711
Date:	07/29/11
Procedure Performed:	Colonoscopy
Physician:	Morris Samson, M.D.
Indications:	History of colitis

PROCEDURE: The patient was given no premedication at her request and the Olympus PCF-130 colonoscope was used. The mucosa of the rectum was essentially normal apart from some mild nonspecific edema. Photographs and biopsies were obtained. The remainder of the rectum was normal. The sigmoid was normal as was the descending colon, splenic flexure, transverse colon, hepatic flexure, right colon and cecum. No evidence of polyps, tumors, masses, or inflammation. The scope was then withdrawn, these findings confirmed. The procedure was terminated and the patient tolerated it well.

IMPRESSION: Normal colonic mucosa through the cecum.

PLAN: Await results of rectal biopsies.

Morris Samson, M.D.

Figure 1-3 Example of Physician's Procedure Notes

Impression: The physician's interpretation of the results or findings of the procedure

Plan: The action to be taken for the patient's continued treatment

Hospital operative reports are similar but will typically include a preoperative diagnosis and a postoperative diagnosis, along with a report of what was done during the procedure and what the findings were.

LET'S CODE IT!

Let's go over a couple of cases, and review the notes together.

Case 1. Maria Whitson

COMMUNITY HEALTH CENTER
A Complete Health Care Facility
159 CENTRAL AVENUE • SOMEWHERE, FL 32811 • 407-555-4321

PATIENT:	WHITSON, MARIA
ACCOUNT/EHR #:	WHITMA001
Date:	09/16/11
Attending Physician:	James I. Cipher, MD

S: This new Pt is a 23-year-old female who was involved in a 2-car MVA while driving on the job. She is complaining about some neck pain. She states that her right leg hurts when she walks. PMH is remarkable for kidney trouble. Past bronchoscopy, laparoscopy, and kidney stone surgery, otherwise noncontributory as per the medical history form completed by the patient and reviewed at this visit.

O: Ht 5'6" Wt. 179 lb. R 16. Pt presented limping on her right leg. She states that she has not had any prior injury to this area, and has no previous problems with her musculoskeletal system. On exam, HEENT: unremarkable. Neck muscles are taut, particularly on the left side. The left shoulder demonstrates full passive motion, with normal strength testing. No deformity is observable. Pt states there is some tenderness in the right posterior femoral area upon palpation. The reflexes are brisk and symmetric. X-rays of her C spine AP/LAT, taken here today, are relatively benign, as are x-rays of the right femur (two views).

A: Strain of sacroiliac ligament, right posterior

P: 1. Order MRI to rule/out torn ligament
    2. Rx Naprosyn.
    3. Referral to PT
    4. Referral to orthopedist.

James I. Cipher, MD
JIC/mg D: 9/16/11 09:50:16 T: 9/18/11 12:55:01

Let's begin by identifying the key words relating to the diagnosis or diagnoses: the reason *why* Maria Whitson came to see Dr. Cipher on September 16. Let's go through the notes and pull out the terms.

PATIENT:	WHITSON, MARIA
ACCOUNT/EHR #:	WHITMA001
Date:	09/16/11
Attending Physician:	James I. Cipher, MD

S: This new Pt is a 23-year-old female who was involved in a *2-car MVA* while *driving on the job*. She is complaining about some *neck pain*. She states that her *right leg hurts* when she walks. PMH is remarkable for kidney trouble. Past bronchoscopy, laparoscopy and kidney stone surgery, otherwise noncontributory as per the medical history form completed by the patient and reviewed at this visit.

O: Ht 5'6" Wt. 179 lb. R 16. Pt presented *limping on her right leg*. She states that she has not had any prior injury to this area, and has no previous problems with her musculoskeletal system. On exam, HEENT: unremarkable. Neck muscles are taut, particularly on the left side. The left shoulder demonstrates full passive motion, with normal strength testing. No deformity is observable. Pt. states there is some tenderness in the right posterior femoral area upon palpation. The reflexes are brisk and symmetric. X-rays of her C spine AP/LAT, taken here today, are relatively benign, as are x-rays of the right femur (two views).

Chapter 1   How to Abstract Notes

A: *Strain of sacroiliac ligament, right posterior*

P: 1. Order MRI to rule/out torn ligament
   2. Rx Naprosyn.
   3. Referral to PT
   4. Referral to orthopedist.

You can see from the notes that Ms. Whitson was involved in a *car accident* while on the job. This tells us *how* the patient was injured, leading us to the correct E code. The E code gives you the opportunity to report that she was in a motor vehicle collision.

E812.0 Other motor vehicle traffic accident involving collision with motor vehicle, driver of motor vehicle other than motorcycle, driver

On the basis of the notes, this is all the information you have about the accident. In the real world, you would need to query the patient to get more details about where the accident occurred so that you could determine whether the claim should be sent to the automobile insurance company or workers' compensation.

Key words and terms that identify *why* Dr. Cipher was caring for Ms. Whitson include:

Neck pain

Leg hurts

Strain of sacroiliac ligament, right posterior

Let's begin with the physician's confirmed diagnosis: Strain of sacroiliac ligament, right posterior. Go to the alphabetic index of the ICD-9-CM book and look up *strain.* You will find

Sprain, strain
Sacroiliac (region) 846.9
Chronic or old 724.6
Ligament 846.1
Specified site NEC 846.8

Which of these listings matches the physician's notes? Strain, sacroiliac, ligament matches exactly!

You know that you should *never, never, never* code from the alphabetic index, so let's go into the tabular list of the ICD-9-CM book and check the code suggested by the index.

√4th 846 Sprains and strains of sacroiliac region

Review all of the choices for the required fourth digit and find

846.1 Strain of sacroiliac ligament

The description matches our physician's notes.

So the codes we need to identify *why* Dr. Cipher cared for Maria Whitson during this encounter are:

846.1

E812.0.

Good job!

»» **CODING TIP**

E codes are never first-listed codes.

E codes are never permitted to stand alone.

E codes are reported only for the first health care encounter for the injury.

Now, let's go through the notes to determine the correct procedure codes. Read through the notes and choose the key words that identify *what* Dr. Cipher did for Ms. Whitson.

PATIENT: WHITSON, MARIA
ACCOUNT/EHR #:   WHITMA001

Date: 09/16/11

Attending Physician: James I. Cipher, MD

S: This *new Pt* is a 23-year-old female who was involved in a 2-car MVA while driving on the job. She is complaining about some neck pain. She states that her right leg hurts when she walks. *PMH* is remarkable for kidney trouble. Past bronchoscopy, laparoscopy and kidney stone surgery, otherwise noncontributory as per the *medical history form* completed by the patient and *reviewed at this visit.*

O: Ht 5'6" Wt. 179 lb. R 16. Pt presented limping on her right leg. She states that she has not had any prior injury to this area, and has no previous problems with her musculoskeletal system. *On exam, HEENT:* unremarkable. Neck muscles are taut, particularly on the left side. The left shoulder demonstrates full passive motion, with normal strength testing. No deformity is observable. Pt. states there is some tenderness in the right posterior femoral area upon palpation. The reflexes are brisk and symmetric. *X-rays of her C spine AP/LAT,* taken here today, are relatively benign, as are *x-rays of the right femur (two views).*

A: Strain of sacroiliac ligament, right posterior

P: 1. Order MRI to rule/out torn ligament
    2. Rx Naprosyn.
    3. Referral to PT
    4. Referral to orthopedist.

During the time that Dr. Cipher spent with Ms. Whitson during this *office visit,* he did the following:

- Took a *detailed history* (pertinent past, family, and/or social history directly related to the patient's problem).
- Examined her HEENT (head, eyes, ears, nose, throat), and neck.
- Examined her leg.

This information tells us that, during the office visit, Dr. Cipher examined three body areas (head, neck, and one extremity) and three organ systems (eyes; ears, nose, mouth, and throat; and musculoskeletal). As per the guidelines, this is a *detailed examination.*

- Dr. Cipher's medical decision-making was of a *low complexity.* The number of possible diagnoses are limited, based on his examination; there are not many treatment options from which to choose; and the complications and comorbidities involved are few to none.
- The notes also identify that Ms. Whitson is a *new patient.*

All these key components lead us directly to the E/M code *99203.*

In addition to the evaluation of Ms. Whitson's condition, the notes also indicate that x-rays were taken in the office. Each x-ray must be reported so Dr. Cipher and his facility can be reimbursed for these services.

Chapter 1 How to Abstract Notes

First, the notes indicate that "C spine AP/LAT" x-rays were taken:

»» **KEYS TO CODING**

C spine = cervical spine; AP = anterioroposterior; Lat = lateral

72040 Radiologic examination, spine, cervical; 2 or 3 views

Second, you need to code "X-rays of the femur, two views"

73550 Radiological examination, femur, 2 views

Therefore, our claim form for Maria Whitson's visit with Dr. Cipher on September 16 will show

Diagnosis codes:	**846.1**
	E812.0
Procedure codes:	**99203**
	72040
	73550

Wait a minute. Remember, that all procedures must be tied to at least one diagnosis code to document medical necessity. The diagnosis code for the Strain, sacroiliac ligament, right posterior provides support for the E/M code (99203) and the x-rays of the femur (73550). However, how could this diagnosis justify taking x-rays of the patient's cervical spine?

Dr. Cipher did have a valid medical reason for ordering those x-rays, so you must go back into the notes and find the reasons. The only confirmed diagnosis was the Strain, sacroiliac ligament, right posterior and this is not it. You need to look for signs and symptoms that would lead Dr. Cipher to make the decision to perform those tests.

Take a look at Maria's complaint of "neck pain." This would certainly lead the doctor to want to check her cervical spine to investigate what damage might have occurred as a result of the car accident. The neck pain is not a component symptom of the strained sacroiliac ligament so it will need to be coded separately.

In the alphabetic index of ICD-9-CM, you will find

Pain
   Neck NEC 723.1
      Psychogenic 307.89

There is no mention that Maria's neck pain is psychogenic, so turn to the tabular list and check out code 723.1.

√4ᵗʰ 723 Other disorders of cervical region. The EXCLUDES note does not refer to any condition for our patient, so read down and review all of the choices for the required fourth digit and determine the correct code:

723.1 Cervicalgia, Pain in neck

Great! This diagnosis code supports the provision of the C Spine x-rays.

Therefore, our claim form for Maria Whitson's visit with Dr. Cipher on September 16 will show:

Diagnosis codes:	**846.1**
	723.1
	E812.0

Procedure codes: **99203**

                                            72040

                                            73550

Good job!

Case 2. Frances Franklin

Okay, let's look at another case. Let's read through the case of Frances Franklin and identify the key words relating to the diagnosis, or *why* Dr. Victors cared for her on October 17.

COMMUNITY HEALTH CENTER
A Complete Health Care Facility
159 CENTRAL AVENUE • SOMEWHERE, FL 32811 • 407-555-4321

PATIENT: FRANKLIN, FRANCES
ACCOUNT/EHR #:   FRANFR001

Date: 10/17/11

Attending Physician: Valerie R. Victors, MD

S: This 57-year-old female came for her *routine annual physical exam.* Pt does not smoke, drinks alcohol occasionally, and exercises three times per week. Pt states she has no specific health concerns at this time. I last saw her 1 year ago.

O: Ht 5'3" Wt. 145 lb. R 20. HEENT: unremarkable; Respiratory: unremarkable; Musculoskeletal: age appropriate. No sign of osteoporosis. Bone density appropriate. Discussed the importance of keeping up her exercise regimen. Comprehensive metabolic panel done, awaiting results.

A: Pt is in good health.

P: 1. Follow-up prn
     2. Schedule screening mammogram

Valerie R. Victors, MD
VRV/mg D: 10/18/11 09:50:16 T: 10/23/11 12:55:01

The key words are *routine annual physical exam.* There do not seem to be any other statements pointing toward why Ms. Franklin came to the doctor's office.

Generally, the word *exam* would be used to identify a procedure or service, but in this case it will actually provide the medical reason that this healthy woman saw the physician. You may remember that the ICD-9-CM includes codes for such occasions—when a person without a current illness or injury needs to meet with a health care provider. These codes are V codes (think preventive).

Go to the alphabetic index in the ICD-9-CM and look up

Examination (general) (routine) (of)(for) V70.9
    Allergy V72.7
    Annual V70.0

The notes state *routine annual physical exam*. The index suggests code V70.9 for routine exam. There is also a listing for annual exam, with suggested code V70.0. Go to the tabular list, and read the descriptions for both codes very carefully.

√4ᵗʰ V70 General medical examination

Read the notation shown here, instructing you to "Use additional code(s) to identify any special screening examination(s) performed V73.0-V82.9)." Make certain to read the physician's notes to identify any special screening exams. For this encounter with Frances, there are none, so this doesn't apply to this case. Read down and review all of the choices for the required fourth digit.

V70.0 Routine general medical examination at a health care facility

V70.9 Unspecified general medical examination

Honestly, the first code, V70.0 is a more specific code and accurately reports what was done for Frances Franklin. This one code tells the whole story as to *why* Ms. Franklin came to see Dr. Victors. Good!

Now, let's review the notes for documentation on *what* Dr. Victors did for Ms. Franklin.

PATIENT:	FRANKLIN, FRANCES
ACCOUNT/EHR #:	FRANFR001
Date:	10/17/11
Attending Physician:	Valerie R. Victors, MD

S: This 57-year-old female came for her *routine annual physical exam.* Pt does not smoke, drinks alcohol occasionally, and exercises three times per week. Pt states she has no specific health concerns at this time. I last saw her 1 year ago.

O: Ht 5′3″ Wt. 145 lb. R 20. HEENT: unremarkable; Respiratory: unremarkable; Musculoskeletal: age appropriate. No sign of osteoporosis. Bone density appropriate. Discussed the importance of keeping up her exercise regimen. *Comprehensive metabolic panel* done, awaiting results.

A: Pt is in good health.

P: 1. Follow-up prn
   2. Schedule screening mammogram

Interestingly, the same key words that identify the *why* also identify the *what:* routine annual physical exam. It is clear from the notes that this is an office visit; however, as you look through the documentation, you see that there is no description of the three key components required for a typical evaluation and management code. There is no documentation of a patient history being taken, nor is there any indication of medical decision-making. Therefore, you must look elsewhere in the E/M section.

You know that the diagnosis code (V70.0) is one for preventive medicine. Again, there is a direct connection to the procedure code for this encounter. Look up *preventive medicine services* in the CPT book's alphabetic index. The index recommends the range 99381–99397. Just as with ICD-9-CM, you *never, never, never* code from the alphabetic index. So let's turn to the numeric listing (in the E/M code section) and look at the code descriptions for all the codes in the suggested range.

The first thing you should note is the long introduction to this subsection. Be certain to read it carefully because it contains important information that you need to know so you will be able to properly assign codes.

Next, you see that the codes are divided into two categories, just like other subsections of this portion of the CPT: new patient and established patient.

Is Frances Franklin a new patient or an established patient? The notes state, "I last saw her one year ago." She is an established patient.

What else do you need to know from the notes to find the correct code? It appears that the codes change based on the age of the patient. How old is Frances Franklin? She's 57 years old.

These details all come together to point us toward the most accurate code:

99396 Periodic comprehensive preventive medicine reevaluation and management of an individual; established, 40–64 years

Good coding!

But, wait, you are not finished yet. Dr. Victors has her own way of writing her notes. She has indicated that a comprehensive metabolic panel was performed. If it were to be performed elsewhere, this would state that the panel needed to be done or needed to be scheduled (as the screening mammogram is written).

You would all like our physicians to write their notes in the clearest, easiest to understand manner for us to interpret into codes. Some will and some won't. It is our responsibility to work with the information given to us, and ask for confirmation or additional details when needed. You are never to assume, guess, or suppose. If it is not documented clearly, you must query. This is in the job description of a professional coding specialist.

So you must code the comprehensive metabolic panel. Looking this up will require you to use your education and knowledge. There are two ways you can find the correct code:

1. You will need to know that the comprehensive metabolic panel is a blood test, and look it up that way in the CPT alphabetic index. You will find:

   Blood Tests

   Panels

   Metabolic Panel, Basic

   Comprehensive..............80053

2. You will need to know that the comprehensive metabolic panel is a lab test, and turn to the Pathology and Laboratory section of the CPT book, the codes that begin with 8.

Either way, you should find the correct code for the test:

80053 Comprehensive metabolic panel

This brings us to the three codes that report the entire story of Frances Franklin and her visit to Dr. Victors on October 17:

Diagnosis code:	V70.0
Procedure codes:	99396
	80053

Good work!

CHAPTER SUMMARY

Abstracting physician's notes is a very important part of a professional coding specialist's responsibilities. It is the only way that you can assure yourself, and those for whom you work, that you are using the codes that most accurately report the diagnoses and procedures relevant to a particular encounter.

As you read through the notes, you must be careful to identify the key words that relate to why the health care provider cared for this patient during the visit. In addition, if the patient is injured or has been poisoned, you must also use codes to notify the third-party payer how and where it happened. The information will also be used so you can send the claim form to the correct insurance carrier.

You need to pull out the key words regarding the procedures and services provided to the patient. Be certain to use modifiers, when appropriate, to report special circumstances.

Remember that ancillary services such as durable medical equipment and professionally administered medications are coded from the HCPCS Level II book and services of all kinds provided to a patient who had been admitted into the hospital (an inpatient) will be coded from the ICD-9-CM volume 3 to reimburse the hospital for what was done.

Following the "Seven Steps of Coding" will help remind you how to determine the most accurate codes and gain optimal reimbursement for your provider.

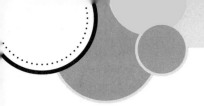

Chapter Review

1. The seven steps of coding include all except

   a. Query the health care provider who wrote the notes.
   b. Abstract the notes to identify key words.
   c. Code from the superbill only.
   d. Link every procedure code to at least one diagnosis code.

2. Key words used to indicate the reason why the provider is caring for the patient during this encounter will lead you to the correct

   a. Diagnosis code.
   b. Procedure code.
   c. Evaluation and management code.
   d. HCPCS Level II code.

3. Medical necessity is the confirmation that the procedures provided were done so within

   a. The physician's office.
   b. Standards of medical care.
   c. Coding guidelines.
   d. With the latest technology.

4. HCPCS Level II codes report the provision of all except

   a. Durable medical equipment.
   b. Transportation services.
   c. Health care supplies.
   d. Prescriptions that are self-administered.

5. ICD-9-CM volume 3 procedure codes are used to report services and procedures provided to

   a. Patients in an ambulatory care center.
   b. Physician's office.
   c. Hospital inpatient.
   d. Clinic.

6. In SOAP notes, you will most likely find the patient's chief complaint in the section marked

   a. Subjective.
   b. Objective.
   c. Assessment.
   d. Plan.

7. The health care provider will document his or her observations and results of the physical examination and any diagnostic tests in the section marked

   a. Subjective.
   b. Objective.
   c. Assessment.
   d. Plan.

8. Narrative or progress notes are most often used by

   a. Radiologists.
   b. Family physicians.
   c. Specialists.
   d. Pathologists.

9. When abstracting notes, the identification of what the provider did for and to the patient will lead you to the correct

   a. Diagnosis codes.
   b. Procedure codes.
   c. E codes.
   d. V codes.

10. When the patient's signs and symptoms, as stated in the S portion of the notes, lead the physician to identify a specific diagnosis, codes should identify

    a. The signs only.
    b. The symptoms only.
    c. The diagnosis only.
    d. All of these.

Identify the key word or main term identifying the diagnostic condition or the procedure, service, or treatment.

1. Epinephrine was injected into the superior aspect of the right orbit of the left eye.

   a. Epinephrine
   b. Injected
   c. Superior aspect
   d. Orbit of the eye

2. A temporal limbal corneal incision was made.

   a. Temporal
   b. Limbal
   c. Corneal
   d. Incision

3. The metal rod was inserted during surgery to keep the spine straight until the vertebrae bonded permanently. This completed the spinal fusion.

   a. Metal rod
   b. Vertebrae
   c. Bonded
   d. Spinal fusion

4. The examination confirms an intracranial contusion.

   a. Examination
   b. Confirms
   c. Intracranial
   d. Contusion

5. Dr. Thomas determined the patient had acute and chronic primary cardiomyopathy.

   a. Acute
   b. Chronic
   c. Primary
   d. Cardiomyopathy

6. An episode of moderate retrosternal chest pressure.

   a. Episode
   b. Moderate
   c. Retrosternal
   d. Pressure

7. Evidence of inferolateral ischemia was present in the left ventricular myocardium.

   a. Inferolateral
   b. Ischemia
   c. Ventricular
   d. Myocardium

8. The radiographic tests confirmed arteriohepatic dysplasia.

   a. Radiographic
   b. Tests
   c. Arteriohepatic
   d. Dysplasia

9. Patient had a thrombosis of the right superior ophthalmic vein.

   a. Thrombosis
   b. Superior
   c. Ophthalmic
   d. Vein

10. An anterior longitudinal cervical sprain was observed.

   a. Anterior
   b. Longitudinal
   c. Cervical
   d. Sprain

Allergy and Immunology Cases and Patient Records

INTRODUCTION

The following case studies are from an allergy/immunology office. In a physician's office of this type, a professional coding specialist is likely to see many different health situations.

Allergists, also known as immunologists, are physicians who specialize in the diagnosis and treatment of conditions and diseases that involve the immune system. These health care professionals treat individuals with such concerns as asthma; allergies to food, medications, animals, or environmental elements such as pollen; and autoimmune diseases including human immunodeficiency virus (HIV) and lupus erythematosus.

Allergy/immunology specialists may focus on treating a specific type of condition, such as rheumatoid arthritis, or they may specialize in patients of certain age groups, such as pediatric allergists, who only treat children.

Allergists can be board-certified by the Board of Allergy and Immunology, which is recognized by the American Board of Medical Specialties.

You can use the following cases to practice coding diagnoses, E/M, procedures, DME, or other HCPCS Level II items, as applicable, code for the physician or the facility:

1. Code for the physician.
2. Code for the anesthesiologist, when applicable.
3. Code for the hospital, when applicable.
4. Code for the pathology and laboratory, when applicable.
5. Code HCPCS Level II codes, when applicable.

MORRIS, SHALLERT & ASSOCIATES
Allergy & Immunology
975 CENTRAL AVENUE • SOMEWHERE, FL 32811 • 407-555-4321

PATIENT: BAPTISMA, CORRINE
ACCOUNT/EHR #:   BAPTCO001
Date: 09/16/11

Attending Physician: Suzanne R. Shallert, MD

This 55-year-old female was admitted for a high fever and obtundation. She had been treated with oral antibiotics for left ear fullness (clogged up) and decreased hearing for one week. Three days ago, I saw the patient in the office and her left ear spontaneously drained.

On PE, the patient appeared confused and febrile. Her left ear continued to drain. Spinal fluid is turbid and showed 6250 WBC, 330 mg% protein, and 21 mg% glucose.

Two blood cultures are positive for arbovirus. She responded to antimicrobial therapy and except for the reduction of hearing on the left, there are no neurologic sequelae. If patient continues to improve, she can be discharged home tomorrow.

DX. Meningitis due to arbovirus, urban; acute suppurative otitis media

Suzanne R. Shallert, MD

SRS/pw   D: 09/16/11 09:50:16   T: 09/18/11 12:55:01

You Code It!

What are the best, most accurate codes?

Diagnosis Codes: _____

Procedure Codes: _____

Anesthesia Codes (when applicable): _____

HCPCS Level II codes (when applicable): _____

MORRIS, SHALLERT & ASSOCIATES
Allergy & Immunology
975 CENTRAL AVENUE • SOMEWHERE, FL 32811 • 407-555-4321

PATIENT: WRIGHT, LEA

ACCOUNT/EHR #:   WRIGLE001

Date: 08/11/11

Consulting Physician: Marcus Morris, MD

Attending Physician: Willard B. Reader, MD

Dr. Reader asked me to consult on this patient, due to PMH of HIV-positive status.

Patient was admitted by Dr. Reader into the cardiology unit with a chief complaint of shortness of breath of approximately 1-week duration. PMH: HIV positive in March 2000; manifestation of AIDS in August 2003.

Patient reports that she has lost approximately 12 pounds within the last 4 weeks.

T 102.58 Wt 115 lb. Ht 5'7" Red and blue skin lesions are noted in her mouth, specifically the upper palate. Lesions biopsied earlier today are positive for Kaposi's. Explained diagnosis and treatment options with patient and family at bedside. They will call me when a decision is made.

DX. Kaposi's sarcoma of the palate, secondary to AIDS

Marcus Morris, MD

MM/pw   D: 08/11/11 09:50:16   T: 08/13/11 12:55:01

You Code It!

What are the best, most accurate codes?

Diagnosis Codes: _____

Procedure Codes: _____

Anesthesia Codes (when applicable): _____

HCPCS Level II codes (when applicable): _____

MORRIS, SHALLERT & ASSOCIATES
Allergy & Immunology
975 CENTRAL AVENUE • SOMEWHERE, FL 32811 • 407-555-4321

PATIENT: BASCINTRASEN, ERNEST
ACCOUNT/EHR #:   BASCER001
Date: 07/23/11

Attending Physician: Suzanne R. Shallert, MD

History: This 47-year-old male has a history of chronic sinusitis with perennial nasal allergy and several attempts at desensitization using allergy injections. He had several sinus surgery procedures for chronic sinusitis and removal of nasal polyps. He is seen today for the first time and volunteered that he has been "sick all his life." He complained of nasal stuffiness, sinus pressure, ear pressure, and constant postnasal drainage. He had episodes of asthma that were particularly bad in May when boating on a lake. He frequently felt short of breath with wheezing and had sinus headaches through the frontal and maxillary areas. He had the diagnosis of celiac disease made through a blood test and avoids wheat and gluten. He had eczema as a child and still has occasional patches on the elbows. His previous allergy treatment was at a local hospital where he was treated with antihistamines and topical nasal steroids as well as Atrovent and albuterol lung inhalers.

EXAM: He had small nasal polyps bilaterally with much lymphoid hyperplasia in the posterior pharynx and postnasal drainage. The exam was otherwise normal.

SKIN TESTING: Performed today in our office, he reacted quite strongly to dust and dust mites and to the molds and formalin but did not react to ragweed mixture, grass mixture, or Midwest tree mixture.

PROGRESS NOTE: The patient will be started on treatment 7/24/11 with sublingual antigens appropriate for the testing results for dust, dust mite, *Alternaria, Cladosporium, Aspergillus, Penicillium*, and four other mold mixtures. (He also reacted to formaldehyde, and this was included in the sublingual antigen.) He was given a prescription for Sporanox capsules to be taken twice weekly for yeast and mold colonization. He should continue the sublingual antigens and will be seen again in 4 to 6 weeks.

Suzanne R. Shallert, MD

SRS/pw   D: 07/23/11 09:50:16 T: 07/27/11 12:55:01

You Code It!

What are the best, most accurate codes?

Diagnosis Codes: _____

Procedure Codes: _____

Anesthesia Codes (when applicable): _____

HCPCS Level II codes (when applicable): _____

MORRIS, SHALLERT & ASSOCIATES
Allergy & Immunology
975 CENTRAL AVENUE • SOMEWHERE, FL 32811 • 407-555-4321

PATIENT: BASCINTRASEN, ERNEST
ACCOUNT/EHR #:   BASCER001
Date: 09/06/11

Attending Physician: Suzanne R. Shallert, MD

Progress notes: Patient shows a very dramatic response. Treatment was effective in just five weeks. Primary allergic treatment using sublingual antigens and Sporanox to decrease mold and yeast growth rapidly has helped him to do better than he has in years. Sublingual treatment will be continued, and he will be seen every six months until testing of the inhalants is negative or near negative. He will be given antibiotics for any acute respiratory infection, followed with antifungals if needed.

Suzanne R. Shallert, MD

SRS/pw   D: 09/06/11 09:50:16   T: 09/18/11 12:55:01

You Code It!

What are the best, most accurate codes?

Diagnosis Codes: _____

Procedure Codes: _____

Anesthesia Codes (when applicable): _____

HCPCS Level II codes (when applicable): _____

MORRIS, SHALLERT & ASSOCIATES
Allergy & Immunology
975 CENTRAL AVENUE • SOMEWHERE, FL 32811 • 407-555-4321

PATIENT: BRANCH, BETHANY
ACCOUNT/EHR #:   BRANBE001
Date: 08/11/011

Attending Physician: Willard B. Reader, MD

This 58-year-old female was admitted with cough of 13 weeks duration. Pt also complained of headache and nasal discharge.

History—She has a history of urticaria and multiple drug allergies, including ampicillin, ibuprofen, and diclofenac.

Previously any drug given to her for pain resulted in skin rashes, pruritus, and facial edema. She was administered oral paracetamol (500 mg) on admission at 0930. At about 1110, the patient developed severe itching and rash all over the body along with facial edema and swelling of lips. This was quickly followed by change in voice and tachypnea.

Examination: Her blood pressure was 124/80 mm Hg on admission. Respiratory system examination was unremarkable except for tenderness over frontal sinuses. After intake of paracetamol, she was found to have hypotension and altered sensorium. Diffuse rhonchi were heard on auscultation.

Diagnosis: Anaphylactic shock

Testing: Her blood counts revealed hemoglobin of 12.7 g/dl and total leukocyte count of 9,100/mm^3 with 3% eosinophils. Radiology department reports chest x-ray and electrocardiogram were normal. X-ray paranasal sinuses were suggestive of frontal sinusitis.

Treatment: Injection adrenaline 0.5 mL (1:1000) was given intramuscularly and rapid infusion of normal saline along with high-flow nasal oxygen was started. Intravenous dopamine in normal saline was also started, as blood pressure was not recordable. Nebulized salbutamol was given every 15 minutes till bronchospasm was controlled. Hydrocortisone (200 mg) was given intravenously and patient was kept under close monitoring. Injection adrenaline was repeated after 20 minutes and infusion of normal saline and dopamine continued till systolic blood pressure had risen to above 90 mm Hg.

Patient recovered fully within 2 hours.

Willard B. Reader, MD

WBR/pw   D: 08/11/11 09:50:16   T: 08/13/11 12:55:01

You Code It!

What are the best, most accurate codes?

Diagnosis Codes: _____

Procedure Codes: _____

Anesthesia Codes (when applicable): _____

HCPCS Level II codes (when applicable): _____

MORRIS, SHALLERT & ASSOCIATES
Allergy & Immunology
975 CENTRAL AVENUE • SOMEWHERE, FL 32811 • 407-555-4321

PATIENT: CARLTON, NELSON
ACCOUNT/EHR #:   CARLNE001
Date: 08/11/11

Attending Physician: Marcus Morris, MD

Patient is a 67-year-old male brought into the emergency department by ambulance with increasing dyspnea, productive cough, and progressive weakness.

His condition deteriorated quickly, and he was sent up immediately to the ICU on the second floor. I was called in on consultation.

The patient was intubated and mechanically ventilated. Broad-spectrum antibiotics were ordered and administered. IV was ordered for septic shock, respiratory failure, and *Hemophilus influenza* pneumonia.

DX: Septic shock with respiratory failure, pneumonia due to H. influenza

_____

Marcus Morris, MD

MM/pw   D: 08/11/11 09:50:16   T: 08/13/11 12:55:01

You Code It!

What are the best, most accurate codes?

Diagnosis Codes: _____

Procedure Codes: _____

Anesthesia Codes (when applicable): _____

HCPCS Level II codes (when applicable): _____

MORRIS, SHALLERT & ASSOCIATES
Allergy & Immunology
975 CENTRAL AVENUE • SOMEWHERE, FL 32811 • 407-555-4321

PATIENT: WRIGHT, PAUL
ACCOUNT/EHR #: WRIGPA001
Date: 09/15/11

Attending Physician: Suzanne R. Shallert, MD

S: This new Pt is a 5-year-old male brought to this office by his father. He has been suffering from fatigue and appears to be experiencing moderate edema. Two weeks ago, the father states that the boy had a sore throat. This was treated with over-the-counter medications.

O: Ht 3'3" Wt. 45 lb. R 23. BP 100/80. UA reveals proteinuria and hematuria. CBC indicates RBC, WBC and mixed cell casts common in urinary sediment. Elevated serum creatinine levels, and low creatinine clearance with impaired glomerular filtration evident. Elevated antistreptolysin-O titers, elevated streptozyme and anti-DNase titers, and low serum complement levels. Throat culture shows group A beta-hemolytic streptococcus. Renal ultrasound is unremarkable.

A: Acute poststreptococcal glomerulonephritis secondary to streptococcal pharyngitis

P: 1. Bed rest, fluids
   2. Diet should be no/low sodium
   3. Rx diuretic; antibiotic 7-10 days
   4. Return in 2 weeks for follow-up

Suzanne R. Shallert, MD

SRS/pw   D: 09/15/11 09:50:16   T: 09/17/11 12:55:01

You Code It!

What are the best, most accurate codes?

Diagnosis Codes: _____

Procedure Codes: _____

Anesthesia Codes (when applicable): _____

HCPCS Level II codes (when applicable): _____

MORRIS, SHALLERT & ASSOCIATES
Allergy & Immunology
975 CENTRAL AVENUE • SOMEWHERE, FL 32811 • 407-555-4321

PATIENT: HAYES, LEONARD
ACCOUNT/EHR #:   HAYELE001
Date: 09/15/11

Attending Physician: Suzanne R. Shallert, MD

This 55-year-old male comes in with a complaint of bilateral hearing loss and allergy symptoms. He states that his hearing loss has been going on for several years, but he feels the right ear is worse than the left. He does admit to using Q-tips. He was seen by his primary care physician back in August and was told he had no wax impactions. He has had no otorrhea or tinnitus. He has no history of ear surgery, recent skull trauma, or noise exposure.

The review of systems, past medical history, family history, and social history are per the new patient history sheet dated September 15th.

PE: BP 100/62. HR: 68 T 98.3. The patient is a well-developed, well-nourished male in no apparent distress. Voice is normal. Face: symmetrical with normal salivary glands, and normal facial strength. Pinnae, external auditory canals, and tympanic membranes are normal with no evidence of middle ear effusion, acute infection, or cerumen impaction. The external nose is normal. Nasal cavity has no polyps or purulent drainage. The septum is essentially straight.

Oral cavity shows no masses or lesions. Normal mucosa. Lips, teeth, and gums are normal. The true vocal cords are mobile bilaterally with no nodules, polyps, or masses in the larynx or hypopharynx. No lymphadenopathy, masses, or thyromegaly.

Audiogram: This revealed essentially normal hearing throughout the frequencies with 100 percent discrimination on the right and 96 percent on the left. Tympanograms were Type A bilaterally.

Impression: Perception of auditory loss; however, no evidence of significant hearing loss by audiogram. Allergic rhinitis that has responded well to allergy shots in the past.

Suzanne R. Shallert, MD

SRS/pw   D: 09/15/11 09:50:16   T: 09/17/11 12:55:01

You Code It!

What are the best, most accurate codes?

Diagnosis Codes: _____

Procedure Codes: _____

Anesthesia Codes (when applicable): _____

HCPCS Level II codes (when applicable): _____

MORRIS, SHALLERT & ASSOCIATES
Allergy & Immunology
975 CENTRAL AVENUE • SOMEWHERE, FL 32811 • 407-555-4321

PATIENT: RAYTHES, DEAN
ACCOUNT/EHR #:   RAYTDE001
Date: 09/15/11

Attending Physician: Marcus Morris, MD

This 15-year-old male came to the emergency room with complaints of fever, headache, malaise, and generalized myalgias. He stated the symptoms have lasted several days. The day of admission, he acutely developed painful swelling of his right wrist.

 On examination of his extremities, a lesion was noted on his left shin just below the knee. He had several other lesions on his right arm near the elbow.

DIAGNOSIS: Disseminated gonorrhea (arthritis dermatitis syndrome)

TREATMENT: Antiinflammatory drug therapy, plus passive range-of-motion exercises including stretching; active range of motion and muscle strengthening should be done at least twice daily.

Marcus Morris, MD

MM/pw D: 09/15/11 09:50:16 T: 09/17/11 12:55:01

You Code It!

What are the best, most accurate codes?

Diagnosis Codes: _____

Procedure Codes: _____

Anesthesia Codes (when applicable): _____

HCPCS Level II codes (when applicable): _____

MORRIS, SHALLERT & ASSOCIATES
Allergy & Immunology
975 CENTRAL AVENUE • SOMEWHERE, FL 32811 • 407-555-4321

PATIENT: CHESDRAKE, SARAH
ACCOUNT/EHR #:   CHESSA001
Date: 08/11/11

Attending Physician: Willard B. Reader, MD

Patient is a 23-month-old female seen in our emergency facility. She was brought in by ambulance, accompanied by her father, Roger. Father states that the patient was complaining of pain in her abdomen. He also noted that she was having a bad case of diarrhea. When her stool turned to bright red bloody, he called 911. In addition, he said he also has been having abdominal cramps and a bit of diarrhea himself. Last weekend, he said, Sarah was watching an old Popeye cartoon when she came into the kitchen. He was eating a fresh spinach salad, and she wanted to try it. She ate several mouthfuls.

  Pt is listless and showing signs of dehydration. T102, BP 80/65 Immunoassay antigen detection for E. coli, multi-step method ordered. Stool culture confirms the presence of E. coli bacteria.

DX: Hemolytic uremic syndrome due to E. coli bacteria

Admit to PCCU.

_____

Willard B. Reader, MD

DRC/pw   D: 08/11/11 09:50:16   T: 08/13/11 12:55:01

You Code It!

What are the best, most accurate codes?

Diagnosis Codes: _____

Procedure Codes: _____

Anesthesia Codes (when applicable): _____

HCPCS Level II codes (when applicable): _____

MORRIS, SHALLERT & ASSOCIATES
Allergy & Immunology
975 CENTRAL AVENUE • SOMEWHERE, FL 32811 • 407-555-4321

PATIENT: GARRISON, JUSTIN
ACCOUNT/EHR #:   GARRJU001
Date: 08/11/11

Attending Physician: Willard B. Reader, MD

This 31-year-old male came in with complaints of clogged sinuses. I have not seen this patient since last year when he was experiencing severe hay fever symptoms. Patient states that he recently started dating a woman who has a pet cat. He noted symptoms the first time he visited her home.

HEENT: His sinuses appear to be congested. Throat and nasal passages are mildly inflamed. Upon visual inspection, the ears appear unremarkable. Because complete allergy testing had not been done previously, we performed full-spectrum, percutaneous (scratch) testing. Tests confirmed some mild food allergies and a severe allergy to cat dander.

DX: Allergy to animal dander (cat)

RX: Allegra

PLAN: Patient states he does not want to be dependent on medication for the rest of his life. After discussions of benefits and concerns, he opts to begin weekly desensitization injections.

Willard B. Reader, MD

DRC/pw   D: 08/11/11 09:50:16 T: 08/13/11 12:55:01

You Code It!

What are the best, most accurate codes?

Diagnosis Codes: _____

Procedure Codes: _____

Anesthesia Codes (when applicable): _____

HCPCS Level II codes (when applicable): _____

MORRIS, SHALLERT & ASSOCIATES
Allergy & Immunology
975 CENTRAL AVENUE • SOMEWHERE, FL 32811 • 407-555-4321

PATIENT: GARRISON, JUSTIN
ACCOUNT/EHR #:   GARRJU001
Date: 08/30/11

Supervising Physician: Willard B. Reader, MD

Preparation and provision of serum for allergen immunotherapy: single allergen, six doses; single injection of allergenic extract

DX: Allergy to animal dander (cat)

_____

Jonelle Harrison, RN

You Code It!

What are the best, most accurate codes?

Diagnosis Codes: _____

Procedure Codes: _____

Anesthesia Codes (when applicable): _____

HCPCS Level II codes (when applicable): _____

MORRIS, SHALLERT & ASSOCIATES
Allergy & Immunology
975 CENTRAL AVENUE • SOMEWHERE, FL 32811 • 407-555-4321

PATIENT:	TRUMAINE, BARRY
ACCOUNT/EHR #:	TRUMBA001
Date:	09/09/11

Attending Physician: Suzanne R. Shallert, MD

S: The patient comes in today for follow-up. He has had allergic rhinitis, along with a rash that was difficult to make go away. After doing significant exploration, he finally determined that it was Entex that was causing him to get the rash repeatedly. He apparently has taken Sudafed since then, without substantial rash. He states he still continues to smoke. He needs a refill on his Zyrtec. He would like to, perhaps, try Zyrtec D, if that is not going to cause him a rash. I warned him against using guaifenesin, as that is likely his allergic component.

O: Blood pressure 102/70, pulse 86, respirations 18, weight 149 pounds. Tympanic membranes clear bilaterally. Nares congested with clear rhinorrhea. Pharynx clear. Neck supple with full range of motion. No adenopathy. No thyromegaly. Lungs clear to auscultation bilaterally. Heart regular rate and rhythm.

A: Allergic rhinitis

P: The patient will be given Zyrtec D, 1 tablet twice a day (#10 samples given). The patient will follow up as necessary. Should he develop a rash or reaction to medication, he is to stop immediately and use Benadryl. The patient will otherwise follow up as directed. Should he experience any problems, he will follow up accordingly.

Suzanne R. Shallert, MD

SRS/pw   D: 09/09/11 09:50:16   T: 09/15/11 12:55:01

You Code It!

What are the best, most accurate codes?

Diagnosis Codes: _____

Procedure Codes: _____

Anesthesia Codes (when applicable): _____

HCPCS Level II codes (when applicable): _____

Cardiology and Cardiovascular Cases and Patient Records

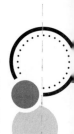

INTRODUCTION

Cardiologists are physicians who specialize in identifying and treating diseases or conditions of the heart and blood vessels, including conditions such as chest pain (angina), irregular heart rhythms, high blood pressure, congenital cardiac problems, and myocardial infarctions (heart attacks).

These health care professionals run diagnostic procedures to identify the functionality of a person's heart. Therapeutic procedures performed by cardiologists include cardiac catheterizations and angioplasties. Cardiac subspecialties include interventional cardiology, which uses mechanical treatments, such as angioplasty and electrophysiology, in which treatments involve the heart's electrical system.

Cardiovascular surgeons are the specialists who perform surgery on the heart and blood vessels. Most often, these operations are done to open a blockage in the blood vessels leading to the heart, such as in coronary artery disease, or problems with heart valves, such as mitral insufficiency or aortic stenosis.

Cardiologists can be board-certified through the Board of Internal Medicine, and cardiovascular surgeons can be board-certified by the Board of Surgery in general surgery or vascular surgery. The American Board of Medical Specialties recognizes both of these certifications.

You can use the following cases to practice coding diagnoses, E/M, procedures, DME, or other HCPCS Level II items, as applicable; code for the physician or the facility; code inpatient and outpatient services, as applicable:

1. Code for the physician.
2. Code for the anesthesiologist, when applicable.
3. Code for the hospital, when applicable.
4. Code for the pathology and laboratory, when applicable.
5. Code HCPCS Level II codes, when applicable.

WINTER HILLS CARDIOLOGY
420 VENTURA BYPASS • CENTRAL, FL 32811 • 407-555-4798

PATIENT: CAPOZZI, VINCENT
ACCOUNT/EHR #:   CAPOVI001
Date: 08/11/11

Attending Physician: Willard B. Reader, MD

Patient is a 62-year-old male previously seen by Dr. David Bush 18 months ago. The patient has a history of coronary artery disease and hyperlipidemia. He underwent coronary bypass surgery in 1973 by Dr. Howard that involved a left internal mammary artery to left anterior descending. In 1989, he underwent a redo operation consisting of a right internal mammary artery to left anterior descending, saphenous vein graft to circumflex, and saphenous vein graft to right coronary artery.

He did well until yesterday afternoon when he developed an episode of moderate retrosternal chest pressure radiating to the right shoulder, which was prolonged and lasted until 3:00 a.m., at which time he presented to the ED. He apparently was given one nitroglycerin sublingual, with resolution of symptoms.

The patient is currently asymptomatic on examination and his review of systems is noncontributory.

PE: He is alert, oriented times three, in no acute distress. HEENT: unremarkable. Lungs: clear. Cardiovascular: Regular rate and rhythm. No murmurs and no gallops. Abdomen: Benign. Extremities: No edema. EKG: Normal sinus rhythm with myocardial changes. Lab tests completed here, today: Lipid panel: all unremarkable except for a cholesterol of 255. CBC: within normal limits. PT and PTT within normal limits. Cardiac enzymes times one: negative. Radiology report states chest x-ray: unremarkable.

Admitting DX: Prolonged chest pain with negative electrocardiogram and negative enzymes times one.

Admit for observation to Telemetry. In view of the atypical nature of prolonged chest pain, we will proceed with a screening Cardiolite stress test later today. Nitroglycerin paste was applied on admission; however, it will be held until the stress test is completed. One aspirin a day was started. Further recommendation and interventions will depend on the results from the stress test.

Discharge DX: Coronary atherosclerosis of native coronary artery

Willard B. Reader, MD

DRC/pw   D: 08/11/11 09:50:16   T: 08/13/11 12:55:01

You Code It!

What are the best, most accurate codes?

Diagnosis Codes: _____

Procedure Codes: _____

Anesthesia Codes (when applicable): _____

HCPCS Level II codes (when applicable): _____

WINTER HILLS CARDIOLOGY
420 VENTURA BYPASS • CENTRAL, FL 32811 • 407-555-4798

PATIENT: KLACKSON, KEVIN
MRN: KLACKE01
Date: 15 September 2011

Diagnosis: Primary cardiomyopathy with chest pain
Procedure: Arterial catheterization

Physician: Frank Vincent, MD
Anesthesia: Local

PROCEDURE: The patient was placed on the table in supine position. Local anesthesia was administered. Once we were assured that the patient had achieved no nervous stimuli, the incision was made and the catheter was introduced percutaneously. The incision was sutured with a simple repair. The patient tolerated the procedure well and was transferred to the recovery room.

Frank Vincent, MD

FV/mg D: 09/15/11 09:50:16   T: 09/15/11 12:55:01

You Code It!

What are the best, most accurate codes?

Diagnosis Codes: _____

Procedure Codes: _____

Anesthesia Codes (when applicable): _____

HCPCS Level II codes (when applicable): _____

WINTER HILLS CARDIOLOGY
420 VENTURA BYPASS • CENTRAL, FL 32811 • 407-555-4798

PATIENT: CRAINE, JACOB
ACCOUNT/EHR #: CRAJA001
Date: 10/15/11

Consulting Physician: Taylor Duggan, MD
Attending Physician: Faron Macavoy, MD

HISTORY OF PRESENT ILLNESS: The patient is a 57-year-old white male with a longstanding history of hypertension, coronary artery disease, and chronic obstructive pulmonary disease who was admitted for chest pain. The patient has recurrent pain episodes and is followed by South City Cardiology. The patient has had a stress test prior to admission, which did not reveal any ischemia. The patient is ruled out for myocardial infarction and was stable over two nights in the hospital. He also had a CT scan negative for dissection. The patient was discharged to home in good condition without any further pain. He is to follow up with his primary care physician, Dr. Lorrenez, in 1-2 weeks after discharge and with Dr. Macavoy, his cardiologist, two weeks after discharge. He is to resume his home medications.

Taylor Duggan, MD

TD/bje   10/13/11 11:47:39

You Code It!

What are the best, most accurate codes?

Diagnosis Codes: _____

Procedure Codes: _____

Anesthesia Codes (when applicable): _____

HCPCS Level II codes (when applicable): _____

WINTER HILLS CARDIOLOGY
420 VENTURA BYPASS • CENTRAL, FL 32811 • 407-555-4798

PATIENT: FELIZ, MARIA
ACCOUNT/EHR #:   FELMA001
Date: 10/15/11

Attending Physician: Taylor Duggan, MD
Chief Complaint: Chest pain

HISTORY OF PRESENT ILLNESS: The patient is a 43-year-old Hispanic female with numerous visits to the emergency room and hospital for chest pain and to rule out MI. The patient also has a longstanding history of drug-seeking behavior. She has a history of coronary artery disease, status post PTCAx5, the last episode per her occurred three months ago. The patient was seen in her cardiologist's office today for a Persantine thallium test and was experiencing chest discomfort. She reported shortness of breath, some nausea, no vomiting, some diaphoresis with the pain; the pain was substernal and not pleuritic in nature. She denied any fever or chills. She denied any cough. She denied any lower extremity swelling. The patient is a nonsmoker and has a longstanding history of asthma and COPD. She is on multiple medications for her asthma and COPD.

PAST MEDICAL HISTORY: Hypertension, elevated cholesterol, coronary artery disease, status post-stenting x5, COPD, anxiety, chronic pain syndrome.

ALLERGIES: Talwin, Keflex

MEDICATIONS: Lasix, Singulair, Zoloft, Theo-Dur, Colace, OxyContin, Baclofen, Levaquin, Norvasc, aspirin, Xanax, Neurontin, Deltasone, Pravachol MDI, Zanaflex, Zantac

SOCIAL HISTORY: The patient does not smoke or drink or use illegal drugs

FAMILY HISTORY: Noncontributory

PHYSICAL EXAMINATION

VITAL SIGNS: T 97.3; P 115, R 28, BP 154/106. Repeat value of 133/86. O2 saturation 96% on two liters.

GENERAL APPEARANCE: In general, the patient is slightly obese, in no acute distress currently.

HEENT: Normocephalic, atraumatic. Pupils are equal, round, and reactive to light and accommodation, extraocular movements are intact.

NECK: Supple; no JVD or lymphadenopathy

HEART: Regular rate and rhythm, without bruits

CHEST: Coarse, with fine bronchial rales throughout

ABDOMEN: Soft, nontender, no distention, positive bowel sounds

PELVIC/RECTAL:

EXTREMITIES: No clubbing, cyanosis, or edema. 2 distal pulses.

LABORATORY VALUES: Chest x-ray shows bilateral pulmonary scarring and an elevated right hemidiaphragm; otherwise, no acute pulmonary process. Electrocardiogram shows sinus tachycardia at 111 beats per minute with no acute ST-T wave changes. BMP is normal except for a sodium of 130. CBC reveals a white blood cell count of 14,800; hemoglobin of 14.4 and platelet count of 501,000. D-dimer is greater than 0.5, less than 1. Troponin is pending.

Continued

IMPRESSION:
1. Acute chest pain syndrome in a patient with known coronary heart disease
2. History of coronary artery disease, status post-PTCA (percutaneous transluminal coronary angioplasty) x5; the last was 3 months ago
3. History of COPD and asthma
4. Hypertension
5. History of drug-seeking behavior and chronic pain syndrome
6. Anxiety
7. Elevated cholesterol
8. Leukemoid reaction probably secondary to steroids

RECOMMENDATIONS:
1. This patient has a long-standing history of multiple admissions and visits to the emergency room for chest pain. She has a long-standing history of drug-seeking behavior and noncompliance; however, the patient does not have known coronary disease and had a stress test performed at the office of Grosspoint Cardiology on the morning of admission. For this reason, we will admit her for 23-hour observation and rule her out for a myocardial infarction.
2. Will consult Grosspoint Cardiology. The patient is known to them and they may review the results of the stress test from today with her.
3. Will continue her home medications including aspirin and MDI. The patient is not on a beta-blocker secondary to her COPD and asthma. Nitroglycerin will be used p.r.n.
4. CT scan of the chest is pending, as performed by the emergency room staff to rule out PE and dissection.

Taylor Duggan, MD

TD/bje   10/13/11 11:47:39

You Code It!

What are the best, most accurate codes?

Diagnosis Codes: _____

Procedure Codes: _____

Anesthesia Codes (when applicable): _____

HCPCS Level II codes (when applicable): _____

PATIENT: WALLACE, LEO
ACCOUNT/EHR #:   WALLE001
Date: 10/15/11

Primary Care Physician: Quentin David, MD

Attending Physician: Faron Macavoy, MD
Presenting Complaint/Chief Complaint: Right Leg DVT

HISTORY OF PRESENT ILLNESS: The patient is a 59-year-old male patient, presenting to my office today with a 4-day history of right leg discomfort and swelling. Patient also complaining of hematuria and smelly urine with no fever or chills nor dysuria. Patient was sent to have an urgent venous Doppler as he was found on clinical exam to have varicose veins with right calf tenderness and right leg edema. The urgent venous Doppler results were called to me, which is positive for acute right leg DVT. Patient's urinalysis is also positive for blood and urinary tract infection.

PAST MEDICAL HISTORY: Parkinson's disease. Patient stated he had DVT ten years ago in the left leg for which he was treated only with aspirin. He denies any past medical history of urinary tract infection or renal stones.

ALLERGIES: None.

MEDICATIONS: Sinemet, dose unknown, which he is taking three times a day. He is also on Eldepryl 5 mg p.o. daily.

SOCIAL HISTORY: Lives alone. He is a widower for 6 years. Does not smoke.

FAMILY HISTORY:

REVIEW OF SYSTEMS: Denies any fever. No flank pain, no suprapubic pain, no vomiting, no headache, no shortness of breath, no palpitations.

PHYSICAL EXAMINATION

GENERAL APPEARANCE: He is comfortable

VITAL SIGNS: His vitals are stable. He is afebrile. Pulse is 80 beats per minute, BP 122/90

HEENT: Unremarkable

NECK: Supple. No goiter. No carotid bruits

LUNGS: Clear bilaterally

ABDOMEN: Soft. No suprapubic or costovertebral angle tenderness

EXTREMITIES: Examination of his lower extremities reveals bilateral varicose veins. Right calf tenderness is present, as well as right leg edema.

NEUROLOGIC: Neurologic exam reveals Parkinsonian tremors with increased rigidity.

PELVIC/RECTAL:

LABORATORY DATA: Urinalysis, which was done in the office, is positive for blood, nitrate, and also leukocytes. Venous Doppler, as I mentioned above, is positive for acute DVT, right leg.

Continued

ASSESSMENT:
1. Acute DVT, right leg
2. Urinary tract infection
3. Parkinson's disease

PLAN: Patient is admitted to the Mason Hospital for anticoagulation therapy. We will also get routine blood tests, including CBC, chest x-ray, ECG, INR/prothrombin time. Patient will be started on Coumadin. He is also started on Levaquin. We will get sonogram of his kidneys and bladder to rule out any underlying renal pathology for current urinary tract infection. Patient will be managed by Winter Hills Cardiology.

Faron Macavoy, MD

FM/bje   10/13/11 11:47:39

You Code It!

What are the best, most accurate codes?

Diagnosis Codes: _____

Procedure Codes: _____

Anesthesia Codes (when applicable): _____

HCPCS Level II codes (when applicable): _____

WINTER HILLS CARDIOLOGY
420 VENTURA BYPASS • CENTRAL, FL 32811 • 407-555-4798

PATIENT: FINNEGAN, IAN
ACCOUNT/EHR #: FINIA001
Date: 10/15/11

Consulting Physician: Taylor Duggan, MD
Attending Physician: Faron Macavoy, MD

REASON FOR VISIT: Patient is here for preoperative clearance. Dr. Macavoy is the surgeon to repair an aneurysm behind his left knee. He denies any cardiac discomfort or SOB at present.

HISTORY OF PRESENT ILLNESS: This 61-year-old male is scheduled for popliteal aneurysm surgery per Dr. Macavoy. The patient has a history of thoracoabdominal aneurysm operated on by Dr. Macavoy approximately 1 year ago. Catheterization at that time revealed the right coronary artery to be a dominant vessel diffuse plaquing with two areas of eccentric stenosis of approximately 60-70% in the midportion. The circumflex was a small and nondominant vessel. Ejection fraction was approximately 6%. Medical management was recommended.

At the present time, there are no symptoms of angina, heart failure or arrhythmias. The patient remains compliant with his diet and medication.

MEDICATIONS: Dynabac 250 mg qd; Rhinocort 4 sp qhs, Darvocet p.r.n.

ALLERGIES: ASA

PHYSICAL EXAMINATION

VITAL SIGNS: BP 148/78; P 80; R 18; Ht 5'5"; Wt 199

NECK: Neck veins are flat. Carotid upstrokes are symmetrical and without bruits

CHEST: Clear to auscultation and percussion

HEART: Regular rate and rhythm

ABDOMEN: Benign

EXTR: Palpable aneurysms in both popliteal areas. There is no edema.

CLINICAL IMPRESSION/PLAN:
This information reviewed at length with the patient. Clinically, he remains asymptomatic. In view of his upcoming surgery, I have recommended that he undergo a Persantine Cardiolite stress test. Coronary intervention would be recommended only if a significant amount of reversible ischemia is demonstrated.

Taylor Duggan, MD

TD/bje   10/13/11 11:47:39

You Code It!

What are the best, most accurate codes?

Diagnosis Codes: _____

Procedure Codes: _____

Anesthesia Codes (when applicable): _____

HCPCS Level II codes (when applicable): _____

WINTER HILLS CARDIOLOGY
420 VENTURA BYPASS • CENTRAL, FL 32811 • 407-555-4798

PATIENT:	HAYMAN, ALANA
ACCOUNT/EHR #:	HAYAL001
Date:	10/15/11
Attending Physician:	Taylor Duggan, MD
Chief Complaint:	Uncontrolled palpitations with dyspnea

HISTORY OF PRESENT ILLNESS: The patient is a pleasant and elderly 78-year-old Caucasian female with atherosclerotic peripheral vascular disease. She is admitted to the hospital today with new onset uncontrolled atrial fibrillation. She presents with symptomatic palpitations, shortness of breath, and generalized weakness with exertional dizziness. She denies exertional angina pectoris, although her exertional dyspnea is now quite limiting with her palpitations. No dependent edema.

She reports a several-month history of worsening left-leg claudication. A previous arterial ultrasound has documented a stenosis in her proximal left-leg arterial system.

PAST MEDICAL HISTORY: The patient is allergic to PENICILLIN and PREVACID. Environmental allergies to feathers and trees. Gastric intolerance to Mevacor. Historic hypercholesterolemia and peptic ulcer disease. Recorded illnesses are hiatal hernia, gastroesophageal reflux disorder, osteopenia with lumbar compression fracture, and controlled but recurrent supraventricular tachycardia (SVT). Status posthysterectomy and bilateral oophorectomy, and right segmental mastectomy.

FAMILY HISTORY: Both the patient's mother and brother are deceased secondary to colon carcinoma.

SOCIAL HISTORY: Patient is a widow, currently living alone. She is a retired biostatistician. No recent tobacco usage.

REVIEW OF SYSTEMS: This is significant, with reported left-leg sciatica, recurrent esophageal pyrosis, anxiety, right knee osteoarthritis, and recurrent sinus posterior drainage due to perennial rhinitis.

PHYSICAL EXAMINATION

GENERAL: This reveals a 78-year-old white female complaining of dyspnea and unrestrained palpitations.

VITAL SIGNS: Respiratory rate increased at 20 per minute, BP 100/64 with an irregular pulse

HEENT/NECK: Normocephalic with some erythema of her nasal turbinates. No jugular venous distention or carotid bruits. Cervical kyphosis.

LUNGS: The lungs are clear to auscultation.

HEART: A soft and systolic murmur present. Heart tones are irregular without a gallop.

ABDOMEN: Soft and nontender to palpitations

EXTREMITIES: No dependent edema. The distal left pedal pulses are reduced.

NEUROLOGIC: Neurologic reflexes symmetric bilaterally.

ADMITTING LAB DATA BASE: The admitting EKG confirms atrial fibrillation.

Continued

IMPRESSION:
1. Paroxysmal and uncontrolled atrial fibrillation
2. Atherosclerotic peripheral vascular disease with left leg claudication
3. Lumbar compression fracture with osteopenia
4. Treated hypercholesterolemia
5. Treated and controlled supraventricular tachycardia
6. Gastroesophageal reflux disorder with hiatal hernia
7. Historical peptic ulcer disease
8. Status posthysterectomy with bilateral oophorectomy
9. Status post–right segmental mastectomy
10. Allergic perennial rhinitis
11. Aortic valvular murmur
12. Gastric intolerance to oral Mevacor
13. Environmental allergies to feathers and trees
14. Drug allergies to PENICILLIN and PREVACID

PLAN: Patient has been admitted to GASTRON MEDICAL CENTER today for control and treatment of her rapid atrial fibrillation. Also, her atherosclerotic peripheral vascular disease and progressive claudication will have to be addressed clinically.

Taylor Duggan, MD

TD/bje   10/16/11 11:47:39

You Code It!

What are the best, most accurate codes?

Diagnosis Codes: _____

Procedure Codes: _____

Anesthesia Codes (when applicable): _____

HCPCS Level II codes (when applicable): _____

WINTER HILLS CARDIOLOGY
420 VENTURA BYPASS • CENTRAL, FL 32811 • 407-555-4798

PATIENT:	LONDON, JOSEPH
ACCOUNT/EHR #:	LONJO001
Date:	10/15/11
Surgeon:	Taylor Duggan, MD
Asst. Surgeon:	Maureen O'Connell, MD
Preop DX:	Severe coronary artery disease with unstable angina
Postop DX:	Same
Operative Procedure:	Cardiac bypass grafting
Anesthesiologist:	Randolph Sullivan, MD
Anesthesia:	General

INDICATIONS: This is a 55-year-old male who underwent evaluation for severe coronary disease. Catheterization demonstrated severe triple vessel coronary disease with a subtotal right coronary artery and significant disease involving the left anterior descending, diagonal, and circumflex. We thought the patient could have four bypasses. The left anterior descending disease appeared diffused. Ventricular function was preserved.

PROCEDURE: With the patient in the supine position under general anesthesia, the chest, abdomen, groin, and legs were prepped and draped in standard fashion. Saphenous vein was taken from the right leg and this wound was closed in routine fashion. Simultaneously, the chest was opened through a median sternotomy and the left internal mammary was prepared. The mammary was densely adherent to the back of the sternum at the top and we ended up dividing it at this point. The proximal end was oversewn with 3-0 Prolene and then with #2 silk and the mammary was prepared as a free graft.

We then opened the pericardium and heparinized and cannulated the aorta and right atrium. We went on bypass and cooled down. The aorta was cross-clamped and cardioplegia was infused in the root. We then bypassed the right coronary artery just beyond the acute angle of the heart. It was about 2.0 mm. We then bypassed a marginal, which was in about midposition; this was about a 2.5-mm vessel.

We then bypassed a diagonal, which was also 2.5 mm. The left internal mammary, used as a free graft, was then used to bypass a 2.0-mm left anterior descending. The aortic cross-clamp was removed and three vein anastomoses were made to the ascending aorta. We then sutured the left internal mammary to the hood of the diagonal vein graft. With flow established in all four grafts, we weaned from bypass with good hemodynamics. The heart was decannulated, protamine was administered, and Hemostasis was obtained. Atrial and ventricular pacing wires were attached, and chest tubes were inserted. The mediastinum was copiously irrigated out, and we closed in layers. The patient tolerated this well and left the operating room for intensive care in stable condition.

Taylor Duggan, MD

TD/bje   10/16/11 09:15:39

You Code It!

What are the best, most accurate codes?

Diagnosis Codes: _____

Procedure Codes: _____

Anesthesia Codes (when applicable): _____

HCPCS Level II codes (when applicable): _____

WINTER HILLS CARDIOLOGY
420 VENTURA BYPASS • CENTRAL, FL 32811 • 407-555-4798

PATIENT:	DEL FINNIO, MARTA
ACCOUNT/EHR #:	DELMA001
Date:	10/15/11
Surgeon:	Taylor Duggan, MD
Asst. Surgeon:	Maureen O'Connell, MD
Preop DX:	1. Coronary artery disease
	2. Unstable angina pectoris
	3. Left carotid artery disease
Postop DX:	Same
Operative Procedure:	Cardiac bypass grafting
Anesthesiologist:	Randolph Sullivan, MD
Anesthesia:	General

INDICATIONS: This is a 61-year-old female who was admitted at another hospital with unstable angina. At that time, the patient underwent cardiac catheterization. There was some anterior apical hypokinesis. The left anterior descending had an 85 percent proximal narrowing. The right coronary artery had proximal 75 percent narrowing. Carotid ultrasound, arteriogram revealed very significant, severe disease in the carotids.

INTRAOPERATIVE FINDINGS: Cardiac-wise, there were no intrapericardial adhesions. They were normal without palpable plaque. The ventricular function was quite preserved. The left anterior descending measured 2.2 mm in diameter and had excellent brisk flow through the left internal mammary artery. The right coronary artery measured 2.4 mm in diameter and the right internal mammary artery had excellent brisk flow.

OPERATION: With satisfactory insertion of monitoring line, induction of anesthesia, standard prepping and draping, for the chest operation, a median sternotomy was performed. We dissected both internal mammary arteries and their pedicles, opened the pericardium, and heparinized and cannulated routinely. Cardiopulmonary bypass was initiated. Temperature dropped to 32 degrees. Myocardium was immediately arrested with aortic cross-clamping and infusion of aortic root blood cardioplegia initially, supplemented by retrograde cardioplegia through the coronary sinus. We performed two end-to-side distal anastomoses, using the mammary artery. The left internal mammary artery was passed toward the left anterior descending through a vent made on the left side of the pericardium. As we did with the right internal mammary artery passing through a vent on the right side of the pericardium. Both distal anastomoses were done with continuous running suture of 7-0 Prolene. Rewarming was in progress. Cross-clamp released. Myocardial activity resumed spontaneously. Temporary atrial and ventricular wires were placed and pleural and mediastinal cavities drained appropriately with chest tubes. There was satisfactory hemostasis. Decannulation followed. Heparinization reversed with protamine sulfate. Sternotomy approximated with interrupted #6 wires. The linea alba, fascia, subcutaneous tissue and skin were closed in the usual manner with continuous and interrupted sutures. The patient was transported to the ICU in satisfactory condition.

Taylor Duggan, MD

TD/bje   10/15/11 05:05:39

You Code It!

What are the best, most accurate codes?

Diagnosis Codes: _____

Procedure Codes: _____

Anesthesia Codes (when applicable): _____

HCPCS Level II codes (when applicable): _____

WINTER HILLS CARDIOLOGY
420 VENTURA BYPASS • CENTRAL, FL 32811 • 407-555-4798

PATIENT: SUSNOW, FRANK
ACCOUNT/EHR #:   SUSFR001
Date: 10/16/11

Surgeon: Taylor Duggan, MD

Asst. Surgeon: Ethan Harrison, MD
Preop DX: Status post–coronary artery bypass grafting, remote, with closed bypasses.
Postop DX: Same
Operative Procedure: 1. Redo median sternotomy and open-heart 2. Cardiac bypass grafting

Anesthesiologist: Randolph Sullivan, MD
Anesthesia: General

INDICATIONS: This is a 49-year-old male patient who underwent previous coronary artery bypass at the VA Hospital with closure of all the grafts and, most recently, very unstable angina pectoris. At the time of surgery, which was approached through a redo median sternotomy due to poor peripheral pulses, we elected to cannulate again the ascending aorta. The left internal mammary artery was a good vessel, which was anastomosed to the junction of the diagonal and the upper left anterior descending. This was a good vessel. We elected to do distal anastomosis to the distal left anterior descending, as well as bypass the circumflex on the right. The operation was accomplished through a redo median sternotomy.

OPERATION: Following placement of Swan-Ganz catheter and induction of anesthesia, the chest was carefully re-entered. Adhesions were lysed. The patient was heparinized, and we cannulated the ascending aorta. It is worth mentioning the fact that the patient was markedly ischemic with PA pressures in the mid-50s. We instituted cardiopulmonary bypass and hypothermia. The aorta was cross-clamped. Cardioplegia solution was given through the aortic root. Following dissection of the mammary, individual segments of saphenous vein were anastomosed to the circumflex, distal left anterior descending and anastomosed to the circumflex, distal left anterior descending and right coronary artery, which were good vessels. The left internal mammary artery was anastomosed to the upper left anterior descending diagonal junction. The two proximal anastomoses for the right coronary artery and the left anterior descending were performed with aortic cross-clamp in the anterior portion of the ascending aorta. Cross-clamp time was 40 minutes. We released the aortic cross-clamp, following which we performed the proximal anastomoses of the graft to the circumflex to the side of the graft to the left anterior descending. We rewarmed and experienced no difficulty in weaning the patient from cardiopulmonary bypass. Routine decannulation and closure was performed. The patient was taken to the cardiac surgical intensive care unit in satisfactory condition.

Taylor Duggan, MD

TD/bje   10/17/11 10:41:20

You Code It!

What are the best, most accurate codes?

Diagnosis Codes: _____

Procedure Codes: _____

Anesthesia Codes (when applicable): _____

HCPCS Level II codes (when applicable): _____

PATIENT: CALLMAN, DELMAR
ACCOUNT/EHR #:   CALDE001
Date: 10/18/11

Referring Cardiologist: Simon R. Blackman, MD

Primary Physician: Curtis Le Fran, MD
Office Consultation

CHIEF COMPLAINT: Referral from Dr. Blackman for evaluation for aortic valve replacement due to aortic insufficiency.

HISTORY OF PRESENT ILLNESS: Patient is a 39-year-old black male who relates a history of increasing fatigue as well as occasional palpitations. He denies chest pain, orthopnea, PND, pedal edema, syncope, or presyncope. The patient has a three-month history of a known cardiac murmur. This has been evaluated through Dr. Blackman's office. Transesophageal echocardiogram was performed on June 8 at Gaston Medical Center by Dr. Blackman, which showed PA 36/25, mean wedge 19. There is no significant gradient across the aortic value. The left main coronary artery is free of stenosis. The LAD is free of stenosis. The circumflex is free of stenosis. The right coronary artery is free of stenosis. There are no anomalous coronaries noted. Ejection fraction was noted to be 40%. The LV was markedly dilated. The aortic root injection demonstrated severe aortic regurgitation. Because of these findings, the patient is referred for evaluation for aortic valve replacement.

PAST HISTORY

PAST MEDICAL HISTORY: History of fractured ankles, secondary

ALLERGIES: No known drug allergies

MEDICATIONS: Zestril 20 mg p.o. qd; Alprazolam p.r.n. dose unknown

FAMILY HISTORY: Father has an unknown heart problem. Older brother has had a stroke. Mother has a history of high blood pressure.

SOCIAL HISTORY: The patient has a 30-pack/year history of cigarette smoking. He continues to smoke. He relates daily vodka intake of 2-3 oz. He also relates marijuana use. He works as a delivery driver.

REVIEW OF SYSTEMS: Hematopoietic: The patient denies chronic anemia, easy bruising, or previous blood transfusion reaction. HEET: He denies chronic headaches or sinus problems or dental problems. RESPIRATORY: The patient denies chronic cough, wheeze, sputum production, hemoptysis, TB or pneumonia. CARDIAC: See HPI. He denies varicose veins or claudication. GASTROINTESTINAL: He denies nausea, vomiting, hematemesis, or melena. GENITOURINARY: He denies dysuria, urgency, frequency, hematuria. MUSCULOSKELETAL: The patient denies acutely swollen, painful, or warm joints or history of DVT. ENDOCRINE: The patient denies diabetes mellitus or thyroid disease. NEUROLOGIC: The patient denies stoke, TIA, amaurosis fugax, and syncope.

PHYSICAL EXAMINATION: Well-developed, well-nourished male in no apparent distress. Ht 5'7", wt 157 lb., BP 150/60, P 60 and regular, R 18 and unlabored, T 98.3.

HEENT: Normocephalic, atraumatic. Pupils equal, round, and reactive to light and accommodation bilaterally. sclerae nonicteric, conjunctivae pink. Oral mucosa is well hydrated, and pink.

NECK: The trachea is midline. There is no jugular venous distension. Carotid pulses are bilateral without bruit. There is no thyromegaly noted.

CHEST: The lungs are clear to auscultation and percussion. Excursion is satisfactory. Chest wall is nontender.

Continued

HEART: Regular rate and rhythm. Grade III/VI systolic murmur heard at the base. Grade III/VI diastolic murmur heard at the apex and at the base.

ABDOMEN: Positive bowel sounds, nontender, no organomegaly detected. Abdominal aorta is nonenlarged. There is no abdominal bruit heard.

EXTREMITIES: Radial pulses are bilateral. Femoral pulses are with water hammer pulse. Pedal pulses are intact. There is no peripheral edema, clubbing, or cyanosis noted.

NEUROLOGIC: The patient is alert and oriented x3. The affect is appropriate. No motor deficits are seen.

IMPRESSION: Severe aortic insufficiency

DISCUSSION AND PLAN: The patient was seen and evaluated by me. Records were reviewed. However, the echocardiogram did not accompany the patient nor did the cardiac catheterization. This will be reviewed at a later date. Aortic valve replacement, device options, autologous blood donation, alternatives, risks, and imponderables were discussed in detail with the patient and his wife. They seem to understand and wish us to proceed. We will consult Dr. Blackman perioperatively for medical evaluation and treatment of medical management problems.

Taylor Duggan, MD

TD/bje   10/18/11 07:20:39

You Code It!

What are the best, most accurate codes?

Diagnosis Codes: _____

Procedure Codes: _____

Anesthesia Codes (when applicable): _____

HCPCS Level II codes (when applicable): _____

PATIENT: HASSAN, SUNIL
ACCOUNT/EHR #:   HASSU001
Date: 10/19/11

Surgeon: Taylor Duggan, MD
Asst. Surgeon: Carole Franks, PA and Wayne Hanson, RN
Preop DX: Severe aortic valve incompetence with class II congestive heart failure and moderately severe left ventricular dysfunction
Postop DX: Same
Operative Procedure: Aortic valve replacement with St. Jude model #25A-101, serial #88073284; transesophageal echocardiography; temporary cardiopulmonary bypass with moderate hypothermia; sanguinous cardioplegia with topical hypothermia and warm blood cardioplegic reperfusion.

Anesthesiologist: Randolph Sullivan, MD
Anesthesia: General

INDICATIONS: This 43-year-old male was found to have severe aortic valve incompetence with moderately severe left ventricular dysfunction and early onset of symptoms. Operation is undertaken for relief of symptoms, preservation of ventricular function, and prolongation of life.

OPERATIVE FINDINGS: The left ventricle was enlarged grade 4/6, and hypertrophied grade 3/6, with reduced LV function diffusely. The ascending aorta was normal. The aortic valve was a tricuspid structure with myxomatous degeneration and prolapse, particularly of the noncoronary cusp.

OPERATION: After induction of general endotracheal anesthesia and placement of appropriate monitoring devices, the patient's chest and legs were sterilely prepped and draped. Primary median sternotomy was performed. The pericardium was opened and pericardial stays placed. Pursestrings were placed in the distal ascending aorta and right atrium. The patient was systemically heparinized and adequate anticoagulation was confirmed. He was cannulated and temporary cardiopulmonary bypass instituted at 2.4 l/min/m^2 at 32 degrees throughout most of the 58-minute bypass time. The patient was core cooled and topically cooled until ventricular fibrillation ensured. The aortic cross-clamp was placed. The left ventricular vent was placed through the right superior pulmonary vein. Right cardioplegia followed by subsequent direct ostial antegrade cardioplegia was administered and repeated at 20-minute intervals throughout the 39-minute cross-clamp time. An oblique aortotomy was performed. The valve was precisely excised after achieving effective cardiac arrest. The annulus comfortably accepted the 25-mm prosthesis. Interrupted nonpledgeted 2-0 Tycron sutures were placed circumferentially around the annulus, then passed through the sewing ring of the valve. The valve was seated and the sutures tied and cut. The valve seated nicely. The mechanism worked well. The root was irrigated and as we allowed the left heart to fill with blood, the aortotomy was closed with a double row

Continued

of running 4-0 Prolene suture. With strong suction on the aortic needle vent and the patient in Trendelenburg position after a dose of warm blood cardioplegia followed by warm blood, the aortic cross-clamp was removed with a 34-minute ischemic time. The heart regained spontaneous rhythm but subsequently required DC cardioversion after some air entered the coronary arteries. The rhythm thereafter remained stable. We completed de-airing by TE guidance, rewarmed the patient. Temporary pacing wires were left on the surface of the right atrium and right ventricle. Two mediastinal tubes were placed at separate water-seal suction and to the autotransfusion device. He was weaned from cardiopulmonary bypass without difficulty. Protamine sulfate was administered, the patient decannulated. Hemostasis was achieved with electrocautery and the wounds closed in layers in the usual fashion. Sterile dressings were applied. The sponge, needle, lap, and instrument counts were noted as correct. The patient was transported directly to the CVRR in satisfactory condition.

Taylor Duggan, MD

TD/bje   10/19/11 11:17:39

You Code It!

What are the best, most accurate codes?

Diagnosis Codes: _____

Procedure Codes: _____

Anesthesia Codes (when applicable): _____

HCPCS Level II codes (when applicable): _____

WINTER HILLS CARDIOLOGY
420 VENTURA BYPASS • CENTRAL, FL 32811 • 407-555-4798

PATIENT: GASDEN, ADELE
ACCOUNT/EHR #: GASAD001
Date: 10/21/11

Physician: Taylor Duggan, MD
Consulting: Garrett Kildare, MD

PROCEDURE: Intraoperative transesophageal echocardiogram. Intraoperative transesophageal echocardiography was performed and the procedure note is reported separately. This is an echocardiographic interpretation.

FINDINGS: Transesophageal and some transgastric views were obtained. The left ventricle is well visualized. There is mild-to-moderate global left ventricular systolic dysfunction with left ventricular dilation and an ejection fraction estimated at 45%. The left ventricle is moderately dilated with end-diastolic dimension approximately 6.5 cm by transesophageal. The aortic valve is well visualized, and it is clearly tricuspid. The aortic root is moderately dilated. The mitral valve appears to have normal structure and motion with no evidence of prolapse or stenosis. The aortic valve does not appear to have prolapse. There is no stenosis. The tricuspid valve has normal structure and motion. The pulmonic valve is not visualized. There is no pericardial effusion or abnormal calcifications seen.

DOPPLER: The aortic valve shows moderate-to-severe aortic insufficiency by color Doppler. Measurements of the aortic valve annulus appear to be 23-24 mm. The right-sided structures appear to be normal. A PA catheter is identified.

IMPRESSION:
1. Significant left ventricular dilation with moderately depressed left ventricular systolic function. Ejection fraction estimated at 40%.
2. Structurally normal aortic valve, which is tricuspid with a dilated aortic root, with associated aortic insufficiency. Taken together, these are findings of left ventricular volume overload due to significant aortic insufficiency.
3. Postoperative St. Jude's valve has been placed in the aortic position. There is central trace insufficiency, which is within the designed parameters of the valve. There is no perivalvular leak or rocking seen. There is no pericardial effusion or other pericardial abnormalities identified. The left ventricular systolic function is moderately reduced and estimated at 35-40%.
4. Hemodynamically significant aortic insufficiency with dilated cardiomyopathy secondary to volume overload on the left ventricle.
5. Status postaortic valve replacement with a St. Jude's prosthesis appears to be stable and functioning normally postoperatively.

Taylor Duggan, MD

TD/bje 10/21/11 11:47:39

You Code It!

What are the best, most accurate codes?

Diagnosis Codes: _____

Procedure Codes: _____

Anesthesia Codes (when applicable): _____

HCPCS Level II codes (when applicable): _____

WINTER HILLS CARDIOLOGY
420 VENTURA BYPASS • CENTRAL, FL 32811 • 407-555-4798

PATIENT:	ROLANE, JACK
MRN:	ROLAJA01
Date:	19 September 2011
Diagnosis:	Atrial fibrillation
Procedure:	Internal cardiac defibrillator
Physician:	Frank Vincent, MD
Anesthesia:	Moderate sedation

CLINICAL INFORMATION: A 71-year-old male with a history of paroxysmal atrial fibrillation, on antibiotic therapy, continued paroxysms of atrial fibrillation, now for an atrial defibrillator. We discussed the risks and benefits of this procedure, including 1% less risk of bleeding, infection; injury to the cephalic vein, subclavian vein, and right atrium and right ventricular structures; cardiac perforation; clot formation and lead resistance and distal embolization to arms, legs, kidneys; stroke; death; and lead dislodgement. He understood and agreed to proceed.

The patient was then taken to the EP laboratory and given Versed and fentanyl for sedation. After receiving 1 gram of Vancomycin for antibiotic prophylaxis, the whole anterior thorax was prepped and draped in the sterile fashion. Pre-gelled electrodes were placed in the posterior thorax with access to the anesthesia-monitoring machine. Pre-gelled electrode pads were placed in the anterior and posterior and care taken to verify that the heart had been adequately interfaced between the two pads. After this, patient was prepped and draped in a sterile fashion. 1% lidocaine was then used to anesthetize the left prepectoral area. A 7-cm incision was made in the medial to lateral direction with care taken to verify that the deltopectoral groove was within the incision line. Blunt dissection electrocautery was then used to make the ICD pocket, and venotomy technique was then used to cut down to the cephalic vein and introduce the leads. Using venotomy technique, a 0.3 G-tipped guide wire was passed to the level of the left cephalic vein to the subclavian vein. This was then used to pass a 9 French safe sheath to the level of the left subclavian vein. Guide wire remained in place, and then the guide wire was removed and the second guide wire was put in place and the sheath was then removed. An 11 French safe sheath was then passed over one of the guide wires. The guide wire dilator was removed, and the ventricular lead, a Medtronic lead 6942, 65, serial #TCB115488V, was then passed to the level of the inferior vena cava. Under fluoroscopic visualization, leads were then placed in the right ventricular apex. The lead was then sutured in the prepectoral muscle using 2-0 Vicryl suture. Over the second guide wire, a 9 French safe sheath was then passed, guide wire and dilator were removed, and an atrial lead Medtronic 6940, 65, serial #TCB023468V, was then passed to the level of the right atrium. This is an activation lead and was actively fixed. The following pacing thresholds were noted upon implant. A sense P wave of 4.4 mV, sensory R wave of 10.5 mV, with a capture threshold in the atrium and 1.2 volts at 0.5 msec, the ventricle 0.3 volts at 0.5 msec, lead impedance in the atrium is 819 and the ventricle 518. Each lead was sutured in the prepectoral muscle using 2-0 nylon absorbable suture. The lead in the ICD was then

Continued

placed in the pocket. The ICD was a Medtronic 7258H, dual AF, serial number of PID, 102351R. Under fluoroscopic visualization, the leads were verified to be in stable position and the ICD was sutured to the prepectoral muscle using 2-0 nonabsorbable suture. A total of two inductions of ventricular fibrillation were then induced; each time it was quickly detected, and terminated with an 18-joule biphasic shock, designating the RV electrode and cathode. Defibrillation pressure was established at less or equal to 18 joules. Atrial fibrillation was then induced two times, each time was quickly detected and terminated with a 4-joule biphasic shock. The atrial defibrillation threshold established was less than or equal to 4 joules. The patient tolerated the procedure well. The wound was then copiously irrigated with a G-U irrigant and closed in layers, using 2-0 Vicryl suture for the first fascial layer, 3-0 Vicryl suture for the second fascial layer, and 4-0 Vicryl suture for subcuticular layer. Steri-strips and sterile occlusive dressing were then placed for final wound approximation. The patient was then taken to the recovery room for further monitoring.

Frank Vincent, MD

FV/mg   D: 09/19/11 09:50:16   T: 09/15/1108 12:55:01

You Code It!

What are the best, most accurate codes?

Diagnosis Codes: _____

Procedure Codes: _____

Anesthesia Codes (when applicable): _____

HCPCS Level II codes (when applicable): _____

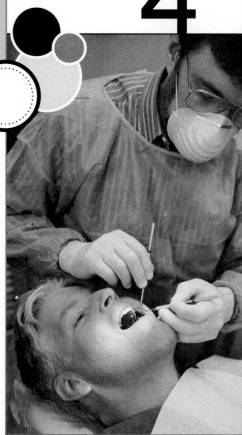

Dentistry Cases and Patient Records

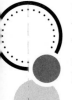

INTRODUCTION

The following case studies are from a dental practice. In a dentist's office, a professional coding specialist is likely to see many different types of health situations, especially preventive health care services.

Dentists are health professionals who specialize in the prevention, diagnosis, and treatment of health problems in the mouth and of the teeth. They will clean out and fill cavities, remove diseased teeth, embed dental implants, and provide cosmetic procedures, such as whitening teeth.

Dentists may specialize, such as:

- Periodontist, who specializes in treating diseases of the gum
- Orthodontist, who straightens crooked teeth
- Endodontist, who specializes in treating nerves of the teeth
- Oral surgeon, who performs surgical procedures on the mouth and gums
- Prosthodontist, who specializes in tooth restoration

Some dentists may specialize in treating particular age groups, such as pediatric dentists, who treat only children, or those who might only work with those needing dentures.

You can use these cases to practice coding diagnoses, E/M, procedures, DME, or other HCPCS Level II items, as applicable; code for the physician or the facility; code inpatient and outpatient services, as applicable:

1. Code for the physician.
2. Code for the anesthesiologist, when applicable.
3. Code for the hospital, when applicable.
4. Code for the pathology and laboratory, when applicable.
5. Code HCPCS Level II codes, when applicable.

DENTAL ASSOCIATES OF ARRINGTON
9550 ENAMEL BLVD. • MOLAR, FL 32811 • 407-555-4703

PATIENT: PRIESTLY, ERIK
ACCOUNT/EHR #:   PRIER001
Date: 10/15/11

This patient is a 2-year-old boy, brought to the offce by his mother, with concerns that he has not been eating normally and has many dark spots on his teeth. He might be having dental pain, but she is not sure. Acetaminophen has been given, and this might be helping to some degree. His mother reports trying to wean him off the bottle. She typically feeds him at night, and he refuses to go to sleep without a bottle of milk or apple juice. She doesn't brush his teeth because he doesn't like it. She has never taken him to a dentist before due to financial reasons. His past medical history and family history are unremarkable.

EXAM: VS T 37.50C. He appears alert and active in no apparent distress. Intraorally, there are opaque brown and grey specks on the enamel surface of several upper primary teeth. The upper central and lateral incisors show extensive decay and are slightly loose. The gingival tissues above the upper right central incisor are slightly swollen. Moderate lesions are visible in the upper canines, upper first molars, and lower first molars. The upper and lower second molars are just emerging through the gingiva. The lower canines and incisors are all intact, with no signs of dental decay.

DIAGNOSIS: Early childhood caries (ECC)

PLAN: His mother is told to wean him off the bottle and to brush his teeth at least twice a day. An appointment is made for her to bring him back for treatment of the ECC.

10/15/11 11:47:39

You Code It!

What are the best, most accurate codes?

Diagnosis Codes: _____

Procedure Codes: _____

Anesthesia Codes (when applicable): _____

HCPCS Level II codes (when applicable): _____

DENTAL ASSOCIATES OF ARRINGTON
9550 ENAMEL BLVD. • MOLAR, FL 32811 • 407-555-4703

PATIENT: WOZNIAK, LEONARD
ACCOUNT/EHR #:   WOZLE001
Date: 10/15/11

Leonard is a 41-year-old male with limited finances who is concerned about the appearance of his teeth. He is seeking the best treatment plan for the least amount of money.

MEDICAL HISTORY: The patient is alert, normally developed, and is in no distress. Patient takes no medications and denies all organ system disease and allergies.

DENTAL HISTORY: He has received intermittent treatment, and the following teeth were extracted due to caries: #14, 15, 19, 20, 21, 30, 31.

CLINICAL FINDINGS: Generalized plaque and calculus with staining are evident. There are focal white rough lesions on the mandibular left and right alveolar ridges. These white lesions are asymptomatic and do not rub off.

TREATMENT: A complete series, including bitewings, are taken. Prophylaxis is completed.

PLAN: Patient to return in 1 week to discuss treatment options for cosmetic measures.

10/15/11 12:15:05

You Code It!

What are the best, most accurate codes?

Diagnosis Codes: _____

Procedure Codes: _____

Anesthesia Codes (when applicable): _____

HCPCS Level II codes (when applicable): _____

DENTAL ASSOCIATES OF ARRINGTON
9550 ENAMEL BLVD. • MOLAR, FL 32811 • 407-555-4703

PATIENT: OPPENHEIM, CALLIE
ACCOUNT/EHR #:   OPPCA001
Date: 10/17/11

Patient is a 19-year-old female who has requested a routine examination.

MEDICAL HISTORY: No abnormalities are identified.

DENTAL HISTORY: Patient had a congenitally missing permanent tooth and a retained deciduous tooth. The patient's last dental visit was 2 years ago. The patient has good oral hygiene. She uses a stiff toothbrush and brushes with the left hand.

CLINICAL FINDINGS: A localized white plaque is present on the attached gingiva buccal to the mandibular right second premolar. The lesion is nontender, slightly thickened, firm, rough, and fixed to the surface mucosa and underlying structures. The lesion does not rub off. The patient was unaware of the lesion.

TREATMENT: Complete x-ray series including bitewings. Adjunctive prediagnostic exam for mucosal abnormality identification. Patient to return to discuss lab results.

10/17/11 08:55:39

You Code It!

What are the best, most accurate codes?

Diagnosis Codes: _____

Procedure Codes: _____

Anesthesia Codes (when applicable): _____

HCPCS Level II codes (when applicable): _____

DENTAL ASSOCIATES OF ARRINGTON
9550 ENAMEL BLVD. • MOLAR, FL 32811 • 407-555-4703

PATIENT: MITCHELL, BRENT
ACCOUNT/EHR #:   MITBR001
Date: 10/19/11

Patient is a 15-year-old male who comes to this office requesting a routine examination.

MEDICAL HISTORY: Patient reports acne. No other abnormalities are identified.

DENTAL HISTORY: The patient has had intermittent dental care. The last dental visit was 4 years ago.

CLINICAL FINDINGS: White patches are present diffusely and bilaterally on the hard and soft palate, buccal mucosa, dorsum of the tongue, and some areas of the gingiva. The lesions are nontender, thickened, firm, rough, and will not rub off. All the white patches are fixed to the surface mucosa, but they are fixed to underlying structures only on the hard palate and gingiva. The patient reports that the lesions are asymptomatic, have been present as long as the patient can remember, have always been in the same location, and have not changed. Other members of the patient's family have had white patches in their mouths.

TREATMENT: Comprehensive oral evaluation, complete x-ray series including bitewings, and accession of tissue samples, both gross and microscopic, including the assessment of surgical margins for presence of disease, of lesions.

DIAGNOSIS: Vitiligo

10/19/11 11:10:25

You Code It!

What are the best, most accurate codes?

Diagnosis Codes: _____

Procedure Codes: _____

Anesthesia Codes (when applicable): _____

HCPCS Level II codes (when applicable): _____

DENTAL ASSOCIATES OF ARRINGTON
9550 ENAMEL BLVD. • MOLAR, FL 32811 • 407-555-4703

PATIENT: ULSTER, AARON
ACCOUNT/EHR #:   ULSAA001
Date: 10/23/11

Patient is a 69-year-old male, new to the area. He was referred by Miriam Sanderson.

CHIEF COMPLAINT: The patient complains of a persistent, progressive, erythematous area of 3 months duration involving the mandibular left retromolar pad. The area is slightly sore. Topical therapy with Nystatin and Triamcinolone acetonide have had no effect on the lesion.

MEDICAL HISTORY: No abnormalities are identified.

DENTAL HISTORY: The patient has worn complete maxillary and mandibular dentures for seven years. The current dentures are 6 years old. The patient does not wear the dentures at night.

CLINICAL FINDINGS: The lesion is a localized erythematous area involving the crest and lingual aspect of the mandibular left retromolar pad. The lesion is nonpalpable, mildly tender, and fixed to surface mucosa but not to underlying structures.

TREATMENT: Comprehensive periodontal evaluation, new patient; adjustment to complete denture, maxillary, and mandibular.

PLAN: Patient to return if this adjustment does not solve the problem.

10/23/11 11:47:39

You Code It!

What are the best, most accurate codes?

Diagnosis Codes: _____

Procedure Codes: _____

Anesthesia Codes (when applicable): _____

HCPCS Level II codes (when applicable): _____

DENTAL ASSOCIATES OF ARRINGTON
9550 ENAMEL BLVD. • MOLAR, FL 32811 • 407-555-4703

PATIENT: DAVIDS, SARAH
ACCOUNT/EHR #: DAVSA001
Date: 10/05/11

Patient is a sixteen-year-old female whom I have not seen in 6 months.

CHIEF COMPLAINT: The patient has had a sore mouth associated with a white lesion for 3 weeks. Drinking orange juice makes the discomfort worse. The lesion has been in the same location during the 3 weeks. The patient has not recently burned the roof of her mouth.

MEDICAL HISTORY: The patient is taking Erythromycin, 250 mg, twice a day for acne.

DENTAL HISTORY: No abnormalities are identified.

CLINICAL FINDINGS: Soft, white plaques, which rub off, are diffusely present on the hard palate. The mucosa underlying the plaques is tender and erythematous.

TREATMENT: Limited oral evaluation—problem-focused; microorganisms collected for culture and sensitivity tests.

DX: Leukoplakia of oral mucosa

10/05/11 11:21:39

You Code It!

What are the best, most accurate codes?

Diagnosis Codes: _____

Procedure Codes: _____

Anesthesia Codes (when applicable): _____

HCPCS Level II codes (when applicable): _____

DENTAL ASSOCIATES OF ARRINGTON
9550 ENAMEL BLVD. • MOLAR, FL 32811 • 407-555-4703

PATIENT: GLOUSTINE, MONICA
ACCOUNT/EHR #:   GLOMO001
Date: 11/15/11

Patient is a thirteen-year-old female who requests a routine examination.

MEDICAL HISTORY: The patient recently completed a regimen of penicillin for strep throat.

DENTAL HISTORY: The patient's last dental appointment was 8 months ago.

CLINICAL FINDINGS: A sharply delineated erythematous area is located at the midline of the posterior dorsum of the tongue. The erythematous area is nonthickened, nontender, and does not bleed. Several compressible, tender submandibular lymph nodes are palpable bilaterally. The patient was unaware of the lesion.

TREATMENT: Periodic oral examination; bitewings (2); adjunctive prediagnostic tests to determine status of lesion.

DX: Plicated tongue

PLAN: No caries identified. Unremarkable dental examination. Patient to return in 2 weeks, once results of tests have returned from lab.

11/15/11 11:47:39

You Code It!

What are the best, most accurate codes?

Diagnosis Codes: _____

Procedure Codes: _____

Anesthesia Codes (when applicable): _____

HCPCS Level II codes (when applicable): _____

DENTAL ASSOCIATES OF ARRINGTON
9550 ENAMEL BLVD. • MOLAR, FL 32811 • 407-555-4703

PATIENT: VAN HOUSEN, PAUL
ACCOUNT/EHR #:   VANPA001
Date: 12/03/11

Patient is a 48-year-old male.

CHIEF COMPLAINT: The patient is concerned about mucosal lesions of the palate and gingiva covering the mandibular third molars. The palatal lesion is nonpainful. The patient has been aware of it for 3 weeks, during which time it has increased in size. It has not been treated. The gingival lesions cover the mandibular third molars. Purple patches are present on the skin of the temples bilaterally.

MEDICAL HISTORY: The patient reports hypotension. He states that he was hospitalized for hepatitis-B 6 years ago. He reports purple skin lesions on the temples and anterior neck of 2 weeks duration.

DENTAL HISTORY: The patient seeks routine dental treatment every 2 to 3 years. He had a dental evaluation of the gingival swelling covering the mandibular third molars approximately 2 months ago.

CLINICAL FINDINGS: A 3 x 2 cm, purple, surface lesion is present on the hard palate. Purple surface lesions are present around the mandibular third molars, on the temples bilaterally, and on the neck. The skin lesions and the oral mucosal lesions are thickened but flat. All the thickened lesions are compressible, nontender, fixed to surface mucosa and underlying structures, and blanch upon pressure. Ecchymotic areas present at the junction of the hard and soft palate are not thickened. Anterior and posterior cervical lymph nodes and posterior auricular lymph nodes are enlarged, firm, and nontender. The posterior auricular nodes are fixed to surrounding structures.

DIAGNOSIS: Spontaneous ecchymoses

PLAN: Referral to dermatologist

12/03/11 11:47:39

You Code It!

What are the best, most accurate codes?

Diagnosis Codes: _____

Procedure Codes: _____

Anesthesia Codes (when applicable): _____

HCPCS Level II codes (when applicable): _____

DENTAL ASSOCIATES OF ARRINGTON
9550 ENAMEL BLVD. • MOLAR, FL 32811 • 407-555-4703

PATIENT: MAC KAY, TRENT
ACCOUNT/EHR #:   MACTR001
Date: 12/13/11

Patient is a four-year-old male.

CHIEF COMPLAINT: The patient's parents are concerned about a pigmented area on the lower lip. The pigmentation has been present for 6 weeks and is asymptomatic but is becoming progressively darker. The parents state that the child spends a lot of time in the sun.

MEDICAL HISTORY: No abnormalities are identified.

DENTAL HISTORY: No abnormalities are identified.

CLINICAL FINDINGS: A localized area of pigmentation about 3 mm in diameter is present on the midline of the lower lip. The lesion is nonthickened, is nontender, and does not blanch.

DX: Purpura annularis telangiectodes

12/13/11 11:47:39

You Code It!

What are the best, most accurate codes?

Diagnosis Codes: _____

Procedure Codes: _____

Anesthesia Codes (when applicable): _____

HCPCS Level II codes (when applicable): _____

DENTAL ASSOCIATES OF ARRINGTON
9550 ENAMEL BLVD. • MOLAR, FL 32811 • 407-555-4703

PATIENT: ASSRHAM, RANDIWAH
ACCOUNT/EHR #:   ASSRA001
Date: 10/17/11

Patient is a 41-year-old female.

CHIEF COMPLAINT: Patient requests a routine examination.

MEDICAL HISTORY: No abnormalities identified.

DENTAL HISTORY: No abnormalities identified. The patient does not wear dentures.

CLINICAL FINDINGS: Multiple blue-to-black areas with irregular borders are located on the right maxillary tuberosity, hard palate, and soft palate. The pigmented lesions are nontender and smooth to palpation. They do not blanch and do not rub off. Some of the lesions are flat and nonthickened, while other areas are thickened and firm to palpation. All the pigmented areas are fixed to the surface mucosa, but only the thickened areas are fixed to the underlying structures. No radiographic abnormalities are identified. The patient was unaware of the lesions. There are no palpable lymph nodes or other palpable masses. No skin lesions are identified.

TREATMENT: Complete series x-rays, including bitewings; periodic oral examination

DX: Dyschromia

10/17/11 11:47:39

You Code It!

What are the best, most accurate codes?

Diagnosis Codes: _____

Procedure Codes: _____

Anesthesia Codes (when applicable): _____

HCPCS Level II codes (when applicable): _____

DENTAL ASSOCIATES OF ARRINGTON
9550 ENAMEL BLVD. • MOLAR, FL 32811 • 407-555-4703

PATIENT: CARR, ROSEMARY
ACCOUNT/EHR #:   CARRO001
Date: 11/21/11

Patient is a 27-year-old female.

CHIEF COMPLAINT: Patient complains of painful oral ulcers of 5 days duration. The patient has not noticed blisters. The lesions have occurred five times previously, always in the same location. The lesions resolved in 2 weeks for each episode.

MEDICAL HISTORY: No abnormalities identified.

DENTAL HISTORY: An amalgam restoration was placed in a maxillary right tooth 1 week ago.

CLINICAL FINDINGS: Multiple ulcers are present on the right hard palate in the first molar region. The lesions are tender when palpated and are not thickened.

DX: Ulcerative stomatitis

RX: Steroidal cream

11/21/11 12:33:51

You Code It!

What are the best, most accurate codes?

Diagnosis Codes: _____

Procedure Codes: _____

Anesthesia Codes (when applicable): _____

HCPCS Level II codes (when applicable): _____

DENTAL ASSOCIATES OF ARRINGTON
9550 ENAMEL BLVD. • MOLAR, FL 32811 • 407-555-4703

PATIENT: DIAZ, LANCE
ACCOUNT/EHR #: DIALA001
Date: 12/04/11

Patient is a 25-year-old male.

CHIEF COMPLAINT: Patient requests a routine examination.

MEDICAL HISTORY: No abnormalities are identified.

DENTAL HISTORY: No abnormalities are identified.

CLINICAL FINDINGS: Tooth #32 is unerupted and displaced by a well-circumscribed radiolucent lesion associated with the crown of the tooth.

TREATMENT: Comprehensive periodontal evaluation, new patient; complete series x-rays w/bitewings

DX: Displaced tooth #32; radicular cyst.

12/04/11 11:47:39

You Code It!

What are the best, most accurate codes?

Diagnosis Codes: _____

Procedure Codes: _____

Anesthesia Codes (when applicable): _____

HCPCS Level II codes (when applicable): _____

DENTAL ASSOCIATES OF ARRINGTON
9550 ENAMEL BLVD. • MOLAR, FL 32811 • 407-555-4703

PATIENT: MILTON, SILVESTER
ACCOUNT/EHR #: MILSI001
Date: 11/30/11

Patient is a 58-year-old male.

CHIEF COMPLAINT: The patient reports swelling in the left mandible of 3 months duration. The swelling is not painful.

MEDICAL HISTORY: No abnormalities are identified.

DENTAL HISTORY: No abnormalities are identified.

CLINICAL FINDINGS: Nontender bony expansion is palpated in the left body of the mandible. Radiographic examination reveals a radiolucent lesion with well-defined, corticated borders. No other abnormalities are identified.

DX: Torus mandibularis

11/30/11 14:10:39

You Code It!

What are the best, most accurate codes?

Diagnosis Codes: _____

Procedure Codes: _____

Anesthesia Codes (when applicable): _____

HCPCS Level II codes (when applicable): _____

DENTAL ASSOCIATES OF ARRINGTON
9550 ENAMEL BLVD. • MOLAR, FL 32811 • 407-555-4703

PATIENT: INGRAM, MARK
ACCOUNT/EHR #: INGMA001
Date: 12/21/11

Patient is a 37-year-old male.

CHIEF COMPLAINT: Patient requests a routine examination.

MEDICAL HISTORY: No abnormalities are identified.

DENTAL HISTORY: No abnormalities are identified.

CLINICAL FINDINGS: During routine radiographic examination (complete series), a radiolucent lesion with sharply defined, corticated borders is noted in the mandibular right body of the mandible. The lesion demonstrates radiopaque areas within the radiolucent region.

DX: Latent bone cyst of the jaw

12/21/11 11:47:39

You Code It!

What are the best, most accurate codes?

Diagnosis Codes: _____

Procedure Codes: _____

Anesthesia Codes (when applicable): _____

HCPCS Level II codes (when applicable): _____

DENTAL ASSOCIATES OF ARRINGTON
9550 ENAMEL BLVD. • MOLAR, FL 32811 • 407-555-4703

PATIENT: MC PHERSON, SALLY
ACCOUNT/EHR #: MCPSA001
Date: 12/23/11

Patient is a 1-year-old female.

CHIEF COMPLAINT: Patient referred for evaluation of mobile teeth and gingival swelling.

MEDICAL HISTORY: Alert, ill-appearing girl. The patient has a history of intermittent malaise, fever, and irritability during the past 2 months. The patient has recently been evaluated by the University Hospital. Examination there revealed axillary lymphadenopathy and marked hepatosplenomegaly. Radiographic examination of the skull revealed numerous, well-demarcated radiolucent lesions of the cranium. Bone marrow biopsy did not reveal abnormal cellular infiltrates. No other abnormalities are identified.

DENTAL HISTORY: No abnormalities are identified.

CLINICAL FINDINGS: The gingival surrounding the erupting deciduous first molars is enlarged, erythematous, nontender and spongy to palpation. The erupting teeth exhibit marked mobility. Panoramic radiograph reveals diffuse horizontal alveolar bone loss.

DX: Alveolar mandibular hypoplasia

12/23/11 15:53:39

You Code It!

What are the best, most accurate codes?

Diagnosis Codes: _____

Procedure Codes: _____

Anesthesia Codes (when applicable): _____

HCPCS Level II codes (when applicable): _____

DENTAL ASSOCIATES OF ARRINGTON
9550 ENAMEL BLVD. • MOLAR, FL 32811 • 407-555-4703

PATIENT: ALLINGTON, CHAD
ACCOUNT/EHR #:   ALLCH001
Date: 12/15/11

Patient is a 68-year-old male.

CHIEF COMPLAINT: Patient requests routine dental care.

MEDICAL HISTORY: Alert, normally developed, in no distress. Carcinoma of prostate treated by surgical excision 2 years ago. Previous history of cystitis and urinary incontinence subsequent to prostate surgery. No symptoms or abnormalities in past year. Denies cardiovascular, pulmonary, gastrointestinal, allergic disease or abnormality.

DENTAL HISTORY: Multiple tooth extractions secondary to dental caries. No extractions in past 6 years. Maxillary partial denture constructed 10 years ago. Patient does not wear partial at night. Has never had mandibular prosthetic appliance.

CLINICAL FINDINGS: Periodontitis type II, missing teeth, calculus. Complete x-ray series w/bitewings show circumscribed radiolucent area in the left mandibular edentulous second and third molar region. No other abnormalities identified.

12/15/11 11:47:39

You Code It!

What are the best, most accurate codes?

Diagnosis Codes: _____

Procedure Codes: _____

Anesthesia Codes (when applicable): _____

HCPCS Level II codes (when applicable): _____

DENTAL ASSOCIATES OF ARRINGTON
9550 ENAMEL BLVD. • MOLAR, FL 32811 • 407-555-4703

PATIENT: CAUFIELD, MEGAN
ACCOUNT/EHR #:   CAUME001
Date: 12/18/11

Patient is a 15-year-old female.

CHIEF COMPLAINT: The patient complains of a sore mouth of 4 days duration. The lesions are painful and bleed when the patient eats. The patient has had difficulty eating or drinking for the past 2 days because of the discomfort.

MEDICAL HISTORY: No abnormalities are identified.

DENTAL HISTORY: No abnormalities are identified.

CLINICAL FINDINGS: The gingival mucosa and soft tissue distal to the mandibular second molars are swollen, erythematous, compressible, and blanch upon pressure. Ulcerations are present on the dorsum of the tongue, soft palate, and soft tissue distal to the mandibular second molars. The ulcerated areas bleed during examination and are tender to palpation. Submandibular and anterior cervical lymph nodes are enlarged bilaterally, tender to palpation, and slightly compressible.

DX: Ulcerative stomatitis

Accession of tissue, gross and microscopic performed. Report completed and sent to patient's PCP.

12/18/11 11:47:39

You Code It!

What are the best, most accurate codes?

Diagnosis Codes: _____

Procedure Codes: _____

Anesthesia Codes (when applicable): _____

HCPCS Level II codes (when applicable): _____

DENTAL ASSOCIATES OF ARRINGTON
9550 ENAMEL BLVD. • MOLAR, FL 32811 • 407-555-4703

PATIENT: SINGER, ABIGAIL
ACCOUNT/EHR #:   SINAB001
Date: 10/15/11

Patient is a 45-year-old female.

SUMMARY OF VISUALS: Examination of the visuals reveals ulcerations of the buccal mucosa bilaterally, gingival erythema and ulceration, plaque, calculus, and periodontitis.

CHIEF COMPLAINT: The patient reports a sore mouth of 8 to 9 months duration. The discomfort consistently involves the gingiva and buccal mucosa. The discomfort has varied in intensity but has never resolved. Blisters have been observed on the buccal mucosa. The discomfort is worse when the patient drinks fruit juice, when she rinses with peroxide and Listerine, and when her mouth is dry. The patient's physician prescribed Decadron and Kenalog in Orabase. Both of these medications resulted in some improvement but not total resolution of the discomfort. The patient reports soreness of the left eye 5 months ago. This was treated with an unknown ointment, resulting in improvement.

MEDICAL HISTORY: The patient reports hypertension treated with Ser-Ap-Es and occasional arthritis in the left shoulder treated with aspirin. The patient previously used Minipress for hypertension, but this medication caused xerostomia and a sore throat. The patient has had a cholecystectomy (gallbladder removed) because of gallstones, and varicose veins stripped.

DENTAL HISTORY: The patient has had numerous teeth extracted due to caries. Her last dental visit was approximately 1 year ago for adjustment of partial dentures. The patient has used maxillary and mandibular partial dentures for 10 years. She does not wear her partial dentures at night. She has difficulty wearing her partial dentures because they irritate her gingiva. She has difficulty brushing her teeth because of her gingival discomfort.

CLINICAL FINDINGS: Ulcerations are present on the buccal mucosa, attached gingiva, and attached alveolar mucosa. The ulcerations are mildly compressible, tender, and fixed to surface mucosa and underlying structures. A Nikolsky's sign is present. Cervical lymphadenopathy and skin lesions are not present.

DX: Periadenitis mucosa

10/15/11 11:47:39

You Code It!

What are the best, most accurate codes?

Diagnosis Codes: _____

Procedure Codes: _____

Anesthesia Codes (when applicable): _____

HCPCS Level II codes (when applicable): _____

DENTAL ASSOCIATES OF ARRINGTON
9550 ENAMEL BLVD. • MOLAR, FL 32811 • 407-555-4703

PATIENT: ATTARIAN, DIANE
ACCOUNT/EHR #:   ATTDI001
Date: 11/25/11

This is a healthy 14-year-old female who first presented for an initial orthodontic examination.

HISTORY OF THE PRESENT ILLNESS: Radiographs revealed a large radiopaque and radiolucent lesion associated with an impacted tooth 32. It was approximately 3 x 3 x 4 cm in size. The lesion displaced the third molar posteriorly and up the ramus. Clinical examination of the area showed a normal range of the mandibular motion with no evidence of bony expansion. The overlying and surrounding oral mucosa was unremarkable.

PAST MEDICAL HISTORY: The patient's medical history is unremarkable. She has no known allergies and is not on any medications.

CLINICAL FINDINGS: This lesion was discovered on the initial orthodontic panoramic radiograph. There was a normal range of mandibular motion with no evidence of bony expansion. The oropharyngeal examination was unremarkable and oral mucosa was healthy. The panoramic and periapical radiographs demonstrate a large radiopaque mass associated with an impacted third molar (tooth #32). There was no evidence of cortical expansion or pain.

The panoramic view of the primary tumor taken at the initial presentation for orthodontic treatment shows an impacted tooth #32 with a large radiopaque mass associated with the crown of the tooth.

INCISIONAL AND EXCISIONAL BIOPSY: The decalcified specimen revealed multiple tooth-like structures surrounded by a dental follicle with epithelial lining. The tooth-like structures were for the most part coalesced and are made up of dentin, enamel matrix, cementum, and dental pulp.

DX: Odontoma

11/25/11 11:47:39

You Code It!

What are the best, most accurate codes?

Diagnosis Codes: _____

Procedure Codes: _____

Anesthesia Codes (when applicable): _____

HCPCS Level II codes (when applicable): _____

DENTAL ASSOCIATES OF ARRINGTON
9550 ENAMEL BLVD. • MOLAR, FL 32811 • 407-555-4703

PATIENT: SENACRUZ, VICTOR
ACCOUNT/EHR #:   SENVI001
Date: 4/09/11

This is a 16-year-old male who presented with a history of increasing swelling without pain in the left mandible.

HISTORY OF THE PRESENT ILLNESS: His mother noted the swelling and took him to the family dentist, Dr. Kahn, for a clinical evaluation where a periapical radiograph was taken. Dr. Kahn then referred this patient to me. A panoramic radiograph, taken upon the patient's arrival today, revealed a large scalloped radiolucency in the left posterior mandible extending into the ramus. There is a hint of multilocular appearance of the radiograph. Also identified were multiple missing teeth. There was no impacted third molar in the site. He had no soft tissue swelling or pain at the site and no paresthesia.

PAST MEDICAL HISTORY: The patient is otherwise healthy with no significant medical or family history.

CLINICAL FINDINGS: At presentation, a swelling in the left mandible was identified. The swelling was not painful. Panoramic view at first presentation demonstrating large radiolucency with scalloped border and a hint of multilocular appearance extending high into the ramus. Absence of teeth #17 and #18 is noted. The swelling started at the left posterior mandible and extended into the ramus. The radiograph revealed multiple missing teeth with no impacted third molar tooth in the site. There was no evidence of soft tissue swelling or paresthesia. The CT scan revealed a radiolucent lesion with no mass or evidence of tumor.

INCISIONAL AND EXCISIONAL BIOPSY: Histologic examination revealed multiple pieces of hard and soft tissue made up of ribbons of loose and vascular connective tissue and early bone formation. In one area, a piece of loose connective tissue with cholesterol clefts and multinucleated foreign body type giant cells were present. The specimen also contained small aggregates of extravasated erythrocytes which were interpreted to be surgically induced.

DX: Traumatic bone cavity/cyst

04/09/11 11:47:39

You Code It!

What are the best, most accurate codes?

Diagnosis Codes: _____

Procedure Codes: _____

Anesthesia Codes (when applicable): _____

HCPCS Level II codes (when applicable): _____

Dermatology and Burns Cases and Patient Records

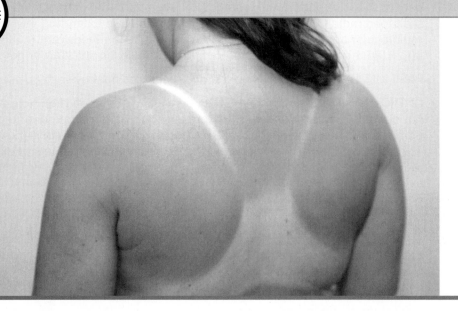

INTRODUCTION

The following case studies are from a dermatology practice. In a physician's office of this type, a professional coding specialist is likely to see many different kinds of health situations.

Dermatologists are physicians specializing in the diagnosis and treatment of diseases and conditions of the integumentary system—skin, hair, and nails. These health care professionals care for patients with such conditions as impetigo, acne, alopecia, rosacea, and melanoma.

Dermatologists can be board-certified by the Board of Dermatology, which is recognized by the American Board of Medical Specialties.

You can use these cases to practice coding diagnoses, E/M, procedures, DME, or other HCPCS Level II items, as applicable; code for the physician or the facility; code inpatient and outpatient services, as applicable:

1. Code for the physician.
2. Code for the anesthesiologist, when applicable.
3. Code for the hospital, when applicable.
4. Code for the pathology and laboratory, when applicable.
5. Code HCPCS Level II codes, when applicable.

DERMATOLOGY ASSOCIATES OF CAULDWELL
469 EPIDURAL LANE • SUBQUE, FL 32711 • 407-555-7539

PATIENT: JABELONE, JAMAL
MRN: JABJA01
Admission Date: 09 October 2011
Discharge Date: 09 October 2011
Date: 09 October 2011

Preoperative DX: Lacerations of arm, hand, and leg
Postoperative DX: Same
Procedure: Layered repair of leg laceration; simple repair of arm and hand lacerations

Surgeon: Geoff Conner, MD
Assistant: None
Anesthesia: General

INDICATIONS: The patient is a 4-year-old male brought to the emergency room by his father. He was helping his father install a new window when the window fell and shattered. The boy suffered lacerations on his left hand, left arm, and left leg.

PROCEDURE: The patient was placed on the table in supine position. Satisfactory anesthesia was obtained. The area was prepped, and attention to the deeper laceration of the left thigh, right above the patella, was first. A layered repair was performed and the 5.1 cm laceration was closed successfully with sutures. The lacerations on the upper extremity, 2-cm laceration on the left hand at the base of the fifth metacarpal and 3-cm laceration on the left arm, just below the joint capsule in the posterior position, were successful closed with 4-0 Vicryl, as well. The patient tolerated the procedures well and was transported to the recovery room.

10/09/11 01:19:47

You Code It!

What are the best, most accurate codes?

Diagnosis Codes: _____

Procedure Codes: _____

Anesthesia Codes (when applicable): _____

HCPCS Level II codes (when applicable): _____

DERMATOLOGY ASSOCIATES OF CAULDWELL
469 EPIDURAL LANE • SUBQUE, FL 32711 • 407-555-7539

PATIENT: BERN, BEBE
MRN: BERBE01
Date: 19 October 2011

Physician: Collin L. Jonston, MD

This new patient is a 19-year-old female who comes in with a complaint of blisters all over her hands. She works in the mailroom of a large international corporation and is very concerned that this may be a reaction to anthrax exposure.

VITALS: T 98.8, R 16, P regular.

EXAM: Visual inspection of skin disruption reveals no inflammation. Skin scraping is negative for anthrax or other poisons under microscopic investigation.

DX: Pimples

10/19/11 11:47:39

You Code It!

What are the best, most accurate codes?

Diagnosis Codes: _____

Procedure Codes: _____

Anesthesia Codes (when applicable): _____

HCPCS Level II codes (when applicable): _____

DERMATOLOGY ASSOCIATES OF CAULDWELL
469 EPIDURAL LANE • SUBQUE, FL 32711 • 407-555-7539

PATIENT: HEINZ, HARRISON
MRN: HEIHA01
Date: 11 October 2011

Physician: Collin L. Jonston, MD

This 27-year-old male was brought to the emergency room via ambulance after sustaining severe chemical burns to his face, neck, arms, and both hands while working at the chemical plant.

Examination reveals third degree burns on his face and both hands, and second degree burns on his neck and arms. Patient is wrapped in sterile gauze and transferred to the Burn Unit.

10/11/11 13:25:55

You Code It!

What are the best, most accurate codes?

Diagnosis Codes: _____

Procedure Codes: _____

Anesthesia Codes (when applicable): _____

HCPCS Level II codes (when applicable): _____

DERMATOLOGY ASSOCIATES OF CAULDWELL
469 EPIDURAL LANE • SUBQUE, FL 32711 • 407-555-7539

PATIENT: VAN DYKE, ROBERTA

MRN: VANRO01

Date: 29 October 2011

HISTORY & PHYSICAL EXAM: A 20-year-old African-American female presented to the emergency room with complaints of malaise, myalgia, chills, sore throat, fever, photophobia, diarrhea, neck stiffness, headache, chest pain, and "bruise on leg." The patient was in her usual state of health until the day prior to presentation.

On exam, the patient was lethargic, complaining of chest pain, with a blood pressure of 89/36. She had a faint, purpuric rash and scattered petechiae on the lower extremities.

LABS: WBC: 27K PLT: 223 PT: 31 INR: 1.23 PTT: 31

Skin biopsy was performed.

DX: Meningococcemia

_____

Suzanna A. Maconi, MD

SAM/ghh 10/29/11 11:47:39

You Code It!

What are the best, most accurate codes?

Diagnosis Codes: _____

Procedure Codes: _____

Anesthesia Codes (when applicable): _____

HCPCS Level II codes (when applicable): _____

DERMATOLOGY ASSOCIATES OF CAULDWELL
469 EPIDURAL LANE • SUBQUE, FL 32711 • 407-555-7539

PATIENT: FORRESTER, MATHIAS
MRN: FORMA01
Date: 21 October 2011

HISTORY OF PRESENT ILLNESS: This is a 57-year-old African-American male with history of acute lymphocytic lymphoma (ALL) status post–bone marrow transplant. He has a history of graft versus host disease. He was recently hospitalized for sepsis. This consult by dermatology was ordered to evaluate a scaly rash of his scalp and feet that has been present for one year. Patient denies pain or pruritus of this eruption. He had been treated with topical triamcinolone with no improvement.

PMH: ALL, GVHD, CMV, bacterial sepsis, DVT

MEDS: Prograf, prednisone, acyclovir, bactrim, MS Contin, vancomycin, Cipro, Lexapro

PHYSICAL EXAMINATION: Diffuse, hyperkeratotic, crusted plaques of the face, scalp, chest, arms, legs and feet. Thickened dystrophic nails.

DX: Crusted (Norwegian) Scabies

PLAN: RX Permethrin 5% cream
        Follow-up in office one week.

Suzanna A. Maconi, MD

SAM/ghh 10/21/11 11:47:39

You Code It!

What are the best, most accurate codes?

Diagnosis Codes: _____

Procedure Codes: _____

Anesthesia Codes (when applicable): _____

HCPCS Level II codes (when applicable): _____

DERMATOLOGY ASSOCIATES OF CAULDWELL
469 EPIDURAL LANE • SUBQUE, FL 32711 • 407-555-7539

PATIENT: DUFFY, DENNIS
MRN: DUFDE01
Date: 29 October 2011

HISTORY OF PRESENT ILLNESS: Patient is a 58-year-old white male with a history of colon cancer diagnosed in 1999 that was treated with resection and chemotherapy. Three months after surgery, he began to notice the growth of abnormal facial hair. This hair growth progressively worsened, and he presented to the VA Dermatology Clinic in March 2004. At the time of presentation, there was no evidence of recurrence of the primary malignancy; however, the patient was being followed for a one-and-a-half year history of hoarseness and unexplained mediastinal lymphadenopathy.

PHYSICAL EXAM: Excess growth of fine, lightly pigmented hairs on cheeks, eyelids, nose, and ears.

DX: Hypertrichosis lanuginosa acquisita (malignant down)

PLAN: Topical therapy with Epi-Stop and Vaniqa

Suzanna A. Maconi, MD

SAM/ghh 10/29/11 11:47:39

You Code It!

What are the best, most accurate codes?

Diagnosis Codes: _____

Procedure Codes: _____

Anesthesia Codes (when applicable): _____

HCPCS Level II codes (when applicable): _____

DERMATOLOGY ASSOCIATES OF CAULDWELL
469 EPIDURAL LANE • SUBQUE, FL 32711 • 407-555-7539

PATIENT: REINGOLD, MELISSA
MRN: REIME01
Date: 21 October 2011

HISTORY OF PRESENT ILLNESS: This 51-year-old Caucasian woman presented to the dermatology outpatient clinic for a skin examination and was noted to have a red papule on her left breast. The lesion had been present for one year and was asymptomatic. The patient has a past medical history notable for papillary carcinoma of the same breast two years prior, which was treated with breast conservation surgery and radiation.

PHYSICAL EXAMINATION: The lesion appeared as a firm and nontender erythematous papule, 4 mm. There was no clinical evidence of ulceration. A punch excision of the lesion was performed in clinic.

DX: Atypical Vascular Proliferation

PROCEDURE: Simple excision is performed.

_____

Suzanna A. Maconi, MD

SAM/ghh 10/21/11 11:47:39

You Code It!

What are the best, most accurate codes?

Diagnosis Codes: _____

Procedure Codes: _____

Anesthesia Codes (when applicable): _____

HCPCS Level II codes (when applicable): _____

DERMATOLOGY ASSOCIATES OF CAULDWELL
469 EPIDURAL LANE • SUBQUE, FL 32711 • 407-555-7539

PATIENT: PARKS, CLIFTON
MRN: PARCL01
Date: 11 November 2011

HISTORY OF PRESENT ILLNESS: Patient is a 70-year-old African-American male who presented to the dermatology clinic complaining of a painless, slowly enlarging growth on the left side of his nose. The patient noted that the lesion has been present for at least 15 years.

PHYSICAL EXAMINATION: A 2 cm x 1 cm soft skin-colored pedunculated nodule was present on the inferior edge of the left nasal ala.

DX: Polypoid Sebaceous Hamartoma with connective tissue and organoid features

PROCEDURE: Simple excision is performed, with 0.5 margins.

Suzanna A. Maconi, MD

SAM/ghh 11/11/11 11:47:39

You Code It!

What are the best, most accurate codes?

Diagnosis Codes: _____

Procedure Codes: _____

Anesthesia Codes (when applicable): _____

HCPCS Level II codes (when applicable): _____

DERMATOLOGY ASSOCIATES OF CAULDWELL
469 EPIDURAL LANE • SUBQUE, FL 32711 • 407-555-7539

PATIENT: EVERSON, REGINA
MRN: EVERE01
Date: 23 October 2011

HISTORY OF PRESENT ILLNESS: This 24-year-old black female developed fevers one week after Cesarean section for twins. She presented to her primary gynecologist who prescribed Keflex for a postoperative wound infection. The patient's fever persisted, and she presented to her local hospital. During the patient's hospitalization, she developed an episode of transient visual loss and confusion that was diagnosed as hysterical blindness. She also developed generalized pustules and worsening mental status. She was transferred to the Hospital Medical ICU. I was then called in for this dermatologic consultation.

PHYSICAL EXAM: The patient had fever (41C), confusion, and a faint systolic ejection murmur heard best at the apex. Her initial dermatologic exam was significant for diffuse pustules on the face, trunk, and extremities. Her recent surgical scar was erythematous with purulent discharge.

TESTING: The patient developed splinter hemorrhages, Roth spots, Janeway lesions, and Osler's nodes over the next few days. The patient's pustules, blood, and CSF were sent for gram stain and culture. She was empirically started on Vancomycin for extended gram-positive coverage. All body fluids sent grew oxacillin-resistant Staphylococcus aureus.

DX: ORSA (oxacillin-resistant Staphylococcus aureus) endocarditis with septic emboli to skin.

PLAN: IV antibiotics

_____

Suzanna A. Maconi, MD

SAM/ghh 10/23/11 17:17:45

You Code It!

What are the best, most accurate codes?

Diagnosis Codes: _____

Procedure Codes: _____

Anesthesia Codes (when applicable): _____

HCPCS Level II codes (when applicable): _____

DERMATOLOGY ASSOCIATES OF CAULDWELL
469 EPIDURAL LANE • SUBQUE, FL 32711 • 407-555-7539

PATIENT: DONNELLSON, CARLA
MRN: DONCA01
Date: 19 October 2011

HISTORY OF PRESENT ILLNESS: A 51-year-old Caucasian female presented to our dermatology clinic with a painful, itchy rash present for one year. Her past medical history is significant for an extensive hot water burn 13 years prior requiring skin grafting. Her review of systems was significant for dull muscle aches, primarily affecting her back and lower legs.

PHYSICAL EXAMINATION: Cutaneous examination revealed multiple violaceous papules and plaques along the edges of graft sites. The upper extremities, lower extremities, and torso were primarily affected, with sparing of the head and neck.

A skin biopsy was performed.

DX: Cutaneous Sarcoidosis

PLAN: Multiple short-term courses of prednisone for temporary relief of her rash and myalgias.

_____

Suzanna A. Maconi, MD

SAM/ghh 10/19/11 11:47:39

You Code It!

What are the best, most accurate codes?

Diagnosis Codes: _____

Procedure Codes: _____

Anesthesia Codes (when applicable): _____

HCPCS Level II codes (when applicable): _____

DERMATOLOGY ASSOCIATES OF CAULDWELL
469 EPIDURAL LANE • SUBQUE, FL 32711 • 407-555-7539

PATIENT: CRAWFORD, VELMA

MRN: CRAVE01

Date: 07 October 2011

HISTORY OF PRESENT ILLNESS: The patient is a 43-year-old woman with a history of acute myelogenous leukemia, in remission six weeks after allogeneic bone marrow transplantation, who presented with an eruption of asymptomatic pink papules on her trunk that has appeared over the previous two weeks.

PHYSICAL EXAM: On her lower back and abdomen were scores of firm, pink papules, 4–10 mm in size.

DX: Leukemia cutis

PLAN: Referral for chemotherapy

Suzanna A. Maconi, MD

SAM/ghh 10/07/11 08:53:39

You Code It!

What are the best, most accurate codes?

Diagnosis Codes: _____

Procedure Codes: _____

Anesthesia Codes (when applicable): _____

HCPCS Level II codes (when applicable): _____

DERMATOLOGY ASSOCIATES OF CAULDWELL
469 EPIDURAL LANE • SUBQUE, FL 32711 • 407-555-7539

PATIENT: WORTHINGTON, WILMA
MRN: WORWI01
Date: 27 October 2011

HISTORY OF PRESENT ILLNESS: This is a 59-year-old white female who over the past five months noticed a progressive thickening and darkening of the skin of her palms, dorsal hands, and ventral wrists. She has also noticed a texture change involving the roof of her mouth.

PHYSICAL EXAM: On full-body skin exam she had rugose thickening of the palms with dermatoglyphic accentuation and a velvety appearance. On the soft palate was a velvety-appearing plaque. There were fine vellus hair growth on the forehead, nose, and cheeks. She has otherwise been feeling well without weight loss, fatigue, or other systemic complaints. She is on no medications.

CBC, comprehensive metabolic panel, and liver function tests, chest x-ray, mammogram, and colonoscopy all report negative.

DX: Tripe Palms and Florid Mucosal Acanthosis

PLAN: With the high association of her skin findings with internal cancer, further work-up is indicated.

Suzanna A. Maconi, MD

SAM/ghh 10/27/11 11:47:39

You Code It!

What are the best, most accurate codes?

Diagnosis Codes: _____

Procedure Codes: _____

Anesthesia Codes (when applicable): _____

HCPCS Level II codes (when applicable): _____

DERMATOLOGY ASSOCIATES OF CAULDWELL
469 EPIDURAL LANE • SUBQUE, FL 32711 • 407-555-7539

PATIENT: KOLOZVARY, ADAM
MRN: KOLAD01
Date: 04 October 2011

HISTORY OF PRESENT ILLNESS: The patient is a 30-year-old graduate student who presented after vacationing for the summer in Ecuador. He had developed an itchy rash on both feet and right thigh that started prior to his return to the United States. The lesions continue to spread.

PHYSICAL EXAMINATION: The dorsum of his feet showed several erythematous, papular and vesicular, serpiginous lesions. Minimal crusting was present over several toes.

DX: Cutaneous Larva Migrans (creeping eruption)

RX: Thiabendazole, 500 mg tabs x3, p.o. bid for two successive days

___

Suzanna A. Maconi, MD

SAM/ghh 10/04/11 11:47:39

You Code It!

What are the best, most accurate codes?

Diagnosis Codes: _____

Procedure Codes: _____

Anesthesia Codes (when applicable): _____

HCPCS Level II codes (when applicable): _____

DERMATOLOGY ASSOCIATES OF CAULDWELL
469 EPIDURAL LANE • SUBQUE, FL 32711 • 407-555-7539

PATIENT: BECK, JOSEPH
MRN: BECJO01
Date: 23 October 2011

HISTORY OF PRESENT ILLNESS: This patient is an 80-year-old white male with no significant past medical history who was referred to the dermatology clinic because of several pink "bumps" on his face and trunk. The patient reports that these lesions developed over a period of several months prior to presentation. They are asymptomatic, and are not rapidly growing in size. The patient denies a history of skin cancer or other skin disease.

PHYSICAL EXAMINATION: The patient has several 0.4- to 0.6-cm pink, pearly, telangiectatic papules scattered on the face, chest, and upper arms.

LABORATORY EVALUATION: A complete blood count showed mild thrombocytopenia with platelet count of 60,000. Peripheral blood smear showed mild monocytosis and rare immature myeloid cells.

DX: Multiple xanthogranulomas, associated with chronic myelomonocytic leukemia.

PLAN: Due to the unusual diagnosis of adult xanthogranuloma, as well as the abnormal CBC, a full work-up was initiated to evaluate the possibility of an underlying systemic malignancy.

REFERRAL to oncology for bone marrow biopsy

RX: Intralesional corticosteroids

Suzanna A. Maconi, MD

SAM/ghh 10/23/11 11:47:39

You Code It!

What are the best, most accurate codes?

Diagnosis Codes: _____

Procedure Codes: _____

Anesthesia Codes (when applicable): _____

HCPCS Level II codes (when applicable): _____

DERMATOLOGY ASSOCIATES OF CAULDWELL
469 EPIDURAL LANE • SUBQUE, FL 32711 • 407-555-7539

PATIENT: SCHUMMER, ANISHA
MRN: SCHAN01
Date: 19 October 2011

HISTORY OF PRESENT ILLNESS: This patient is a 24-year-old woman G2P1 at 34 weeks gestation who presented with a "rash" on her hands evident since the first trimester. She denied pain or pruritus and had a similar eruption during her first pregnancy, which resolved after delivery. Her past medical history was significant only for gestational diabetes.

PHYSICAL EXAM: The patient had well-demarcated erythematous patches symmetrically over her distal phalanges as well as her thenar and hypothenar eminences. The areas completely blanched with pressure.

DX: Pregnancy-associated palmar erythema

PLAN: No treatment. Condition is expected to spontaneously resolve after delivery.

Suzanna A. Maconi, MD

SAM/ghh 10/19/11 11:47:39

You Code It!

What are the best, most accurate codes?

Diagnosis Codes: _____

Procedure Codes: _____

Anesthesia Codes (when applicable): _____

HCPCS Level II codes (when applicable): _____

DERMATOLOGY ASSOCIATES OF CAULDWELL
469 EPIDURAL LANE • SUBQUE, FL 32711 • 407-555-7539

PATIENT: LIGHTFOOT, YAMIDRA
MRN: LIGYA01
Date: 15 November 2011

HISTORY OF PRESENT ILLNESS: This is a 21-year-old Caucasian female who was referred to this dermatology clinic for a history of a pruritic eruption secondary to either natural light or tanning beds. The patient states she discontinued tanning and limited her exposure to sunlight over the past six months because of an increasing sensitivity to light. She stated that she would react within a few minutes to light exposure.

PE: The patient was placed in a UVA light box for 40 seconds. As a result of an absence of response, she was immediately placed in a UVB light box for 50 seconds. No reaction to the light occurred, and the patient went to the neighboring SunKiss tanning beds. She returned to our clinic with erythematous plaques after less than one minute in the tanning bed. This rash resolved within 30 minutes. Skin biopsy was performed.

DX: Solar urticaria

PLAN: RX: Antihistamines and light treatment for hardening

_____

Suzanna A. Maconi, MD

SAM/ghh 11/15/11 11:47:39

You Code It!

What are the best, most accurate codes?

Diagnosis Codes: _____

Procedure Codes: _____

Anesthesia Codes (when applicable): _____

HCPCS Level II codes (when applicable): _____

DERMATOLOGY ASSOCIATES OF CAULDWELL
469 EPIDURAL LANE • SUBQUE, FL 32711 • 407-555-7539

PATIENT: MC KENZIE, DANIEL
MRN: MCKDA01
Date: 17 October 2011

HISTORY OF PRESENT ILLNESS: This 20-year-old white man presented to the dermatology clinic for evaluation of draining facial nodules. The patient is a member of the military and is anticipating imminent deployment to the Middle East. His history is notable for being stationed in southern California several months previously, while in basic training. In addition, his family recently adopted a stray kitten that has been sleeping in the same bed with the patient.

The patient reported that when the eruption first appeared, 4-6 weeks prior to his presentation in our office, the lesions looked like "ringworm," with circular pink scaly patches. His primary care physician, Dr. Alendar, treated him at that time with Lotrisone (clotrimazole/betamethasone dipropionate) twice daily. Because the lesions worsened, becoming more painful and swollen, with purulent drainage, his physician then treated him with a course of cephalexin, followed by a course of azithromycin, and finally a course of Augmentin, all the while continuing his Lotrisone. The patient also reported that two large "boils" on his face were drained by Dr. Alendar. The patient reported moderate clinical improvement on Augmentin.

The patient presents today for a second opinion. He was concerned this eruption would interfere with his deployment.

PE: Upon presentation, the patient appears as a healthy male in no distress. He is afebrile and vitals are stable. On examination, he is noted to have erythema and inflammation of his lower face and neck, with draining red nodules along his jawline. In addition, he has two pink scaly plaques on his abdomen, each with central pustules.

Four punch biopsies are performed: two for tissue culture and two for histopathologic examination. In addition, wound cultures from the pustules on his abdomen are obtained. A PPD is placed to rule out tuberculosis and is found to be nonreactive. A chest x-ray is within normal limits.

LAB RESULTS: Tissue and wound cultures taken from the abdomen and the left face revealed the diagnosis.

DX: Tinea barbae secondary to Trichophytin mentagrophytes

RX: Sporanox, 150 mg, daily for three weeks; topical antifungal cream and a low-potency topical steroid

---

Suzanna A. Maconi, MD

SAM/ghh 10/17/11 11:47:39

You Code It!

What are the best, most accurate codes?

Diagnosis Codes: _____

Procedure Codes: _____

Anesthesia Codes (when applicable): _____

HCPCS Level II codes (when applicable): _____

DERMATOLOGY ASSOCIATES OF CAULDWELL
469 EPIDURAL LANE • SUBQUE, FL 32711 • 407-555-7539

PATIENT: TROTTIER, MARSHALL
MRN: TROMA01
Date: 09 December 2011

HISTORY OF PRESENT ILLNESS: This premature male was born via C-section at 29 weeks of gestation to a 29-year-old G4P2Ab1 female with a monochorionic triplet pregnancy. Marshall was born with extensive skin defects involving the trunk, scalp, and extremities. Triplet B died in utero at 14 weeks of gestation. Triplet C died of hydrops fetalis at delivery.

PHYSICAL EXAMINATION: The flanks, abdomen, and scalp showed sharply demarcated lesions covered with a glistening membrane and an absence of the epidermis and dermis with prominent vasculature. No syndactyly, limb reduction, or cleft palate was present. Corneal opacities and glaucoma were present.

LABORATORY FINDINGS: An MRI of the head revealed cerebral dysmorphism posteriorly with absence of the corpus callosum. Colpocephaly, schizocephaly, & lissencephaly were also found. Abdominal film revealed mild left hydronephrosis.

DX: Aplasia Cutis Congenita

PLAN: A skin flap is performed to repair the defect on the vertex of the scalp with good results. The other areas were covered with AlloDerm, and skin grafting will be carried out in the future.

Suzanna A. Maconi, MD

SAM/ghh 12/09/11 11:47:39

You Code It!

What are the best, most accurate codes?

Diagnosis Codes: _____

Procedure Codes: _____

Anesthesia Codes (when applicable): _____

HCPCS Level II codes (when applicable): _____

DERMATOLOGY ASSOCIATES OF CAULDWELL
469 EPIDURAL LANE • SUBQUE, FL 32711 • 407-555-7539

PATIENT: STRICKLAND, JADE
MRN: STRJA01
Date: 13 November 2011

HISTORY OF PRESENT ILLNESS: This patient is a 49-year-old African-American female presenting with a 1-month history of a diffuse-skin eruption. She reported that the eruption was at first mild and became severe one week prior to presentation. The eruption was pruritic and not painful. She denied eye pain, abdominal pain, dysuria, chest pain, dyspnea, myalgia, or arthralgias. She reported an intermittent fever for three weeks and facial edema. Past medical history was significant for a subarachnoid hemorrhage six weeks prior to presentation from a ruptured aneurysm which was treated with cerebral aneurysm clipping. She started Dilantin at this time (six weeks prior to presentation) as seizure prophylaxis. Other medications included atenolol, lisinopril, and aspirin.

PHYSICAL EXAMINATION: Vital signs at presentation were: T 39.4C, BP 140/90, heart rate 118, and respiratory rate 18. She has significant facial edema with numerous pustules and yellow crust. Her skin reveals an erythroderma with red papules on her arms and legs, some of which were vesiculated. Her lips had yellow crust, but she did not have mucosal involvement of the oropharynx, conjunctiva, or vagina. She has an enlarged right anterior cervical lymph node.

LAB FINDINGS: Electrocardiogram revealed sinus tachycardia. Laboratory analysis revealed a WBC of 4.6 x 103/ mcL, hemoglobin of 11.6 g/dL, and platelet count of 33 x 103/mcl. The platelet count normalized without transfusion of platelets, suggesting that the initial value was a laboratory error. Her eosinophil count was 1.1 x 103/mcL (24% of the WBC). A complete metabolic panel was significant for a slightly elevated AST and ALT of 63 and 58, respectively.

DX: Drug reaction with eosinophilia and systemic symptoms (DRESS), formerly referred to as drug hypersensitivity syndrome.

PLAN: RX: Systemic corticosteroids

Suzanna A. Maconi, MD

SAM/ghh 11/13/11 11:47:39

You Code It!

What are the best, most accurate codes?

Diagnosis Codes: _____

Procedure Codes: _____

Anesthesia Codes (when applicable): _____

HCPCS Level II codes (when applicable): _____

DERMATOLOGY ASSOCIATES OF CAULDWELL
469 EPIDURAL LANE • SUBQUE, FL 32711 • 407-555-7539

PATIENT: SAFKEN, ANTONIA
MRN: SAFAN01
Date: 30 October 2011

HISTORY OF PRESENT ILLNESS: Patient is a previously healthy 7-year-old girl presenting from an outside hospital for evaluation and treatment of swelling of the head and neck. The patient's mother reports that the patient was sleeping on a rarely used hide-a-bed when she awoke in middle of the night crying and complaining of lip pain. Within hours, the patient's mother noted significant swelling of the left lip and face. The patient was taken to a small local hospital. Despite treatment with antihistamines, epinephrine, and IV steroids at the outside hospital, the patient experienced rapidly progressing facial and neck swelling requiring transfer to Children's Hospital. Shortly after admission, the patient was intubated due to a compromised airway. The patient remained intubated in the pediatric intensive care unit for five days. As the swelling slowly resolved, a necrotic papule became apparent on the left lower lip. A dusky depressed linear plaque in a gravitational pattern also developed along the left chin and mandible.

TEST RESULTS: All laboratory results were within normal limits. Imaging of the head and neck revealed extensive soft tissue swelling. As the edema improved and the area of necrosis became visible, a brown recluse bite was suspected. Upon further interview, the patient's father reported seeing a brown spider in the area of the hide-a-bed. On the basis of the patient's history, the presence of a brown spider, and a clinically compatible lesion, a diagnosis of probable brown recluse bite was made.

DX: Life-threatening head and neck edema secondary to probable brown recluse spider bite of the lip

PLAN: Thorough cleansing followed by rest, ice, compression, and elevation (RICE) is indicated for mild localized lesions without systemic involvement. RX: Antibiotics, to prevent secondary infection. Aspirin can be used to counteract platelet aggregation. Parents are warned that heat should be avoided as it potentiates the venom's enzymatic activity.

Suzanna A. Maconi, MD

SAM/ghh 10/30/11 11:47:39

You Code It!

What are the best, most accurate codes?

Diagnosis Codes: _____

Procedure Codes: _____

Anesthesia Codes (when applicable): _____

HCPCS Level II codes (when applicable): _____

DERMATOLOGY ASSOCIATES OF CAULDWELL
469 EPIDURAL LANE • SUBQUE, FL 32711 • 407-555-7539

PATIENT: VALENTIN, KERI
MRN: VALKE01
Date: 17 November 2011

HISTORY OF PRESENT ILLNESS: This patient is a 43-year-old Caucasian male who was admitted to the hospital with a two year history of petechial lesions on the bilateral lower extremities and a two week history of swelling and pain of the right ankle. He denies any history of trauma, bites, tick exposure, or new medications. Additional findings are significant for submucosal hemorrhage of the oral mucosa and gingival hypertrophy with bleeding gums.

PAST MEDICAL HISTORY: Noncontributory.

SOCIAL HISTORY: Significant for heavy alcohol consumption of approximately 12 beers/day.

MEDICATIONS: Patient denies any medications at time of admission and denies using recreational drugs.

LABORATORY DATA: Significant for anemia (hemoglobin – 11.6, hematocrit – 34.1) and leucopenia (WBC 2.1). CMP panel was within normal limits.

DX: Scurvy

PLAN: Supplementation with Vitamin C, 100 mg 3-5x/day until a total of 4g is reached then 100mg qd. Patient is counseled to have a diet rich in fruits and vegetables such as grapefruit, lemons, broccoli, green peppers, tomatoes, and cabbage.

Suzanna A. Maconi, MD

SAM/ghh 11/17/11 11:47:39

You Code It!

What are the best, most accurate codes?

Diagnosis Codes: _____

Procedure Codes: _____

Anesthesia Codes (when applicable): _____

HCPCS Level II codes (when applicable): _____

DERMATOLOGY ASSOCIATES OF CAULDWELL
469 EPIDURAL LANE • SUBQUE, FL 32711 • 407-555-7539

PATIENT: CROWE, CASSANDRA
MRN: CROCA01
Date: 03 October 2011

HISTORY OF PRESENT ILLNESS: This is a 54-year-old woman complaining of a painless, nonpruritic, nonhealing ulcer on her left nipple that has been evident for six months. The patient denies any discharge.

PAST MEDICAL HISTORY: Hypertension

FAMILY HISTORY: Positive for breast cancer of unknown type in her sister and aunt. Mammogram and ultrasound showed a hypervascular nipple mass.

PHYSICAL EXAM: On physical exam she has a 1.3 x 1.5-cm palpable mass covering 90% of her nipple. There was no peripheral infiltration, no discharge, and no axillary lymphadenopathy. The left nipple is 2 cm higher than the right nipple. Nipple to midline distance is 12 cm on the left and 11 cm on the right. She has moderate fibrocystic changes throughout both breasts.

DX: Erosive adenomatosis of the nipple

PLAN: Make appointment to perform successful local excision, tumorectomy, liquid nitrogen and Mohs.

Suzanna A. Maconi, MD

SAM/ghh 10/03/11 11:47:39

You Code It!

What are the best, most accurate codes?

Diagnosis Codes: _____

Procedure Codes: _____

Anesthesia Codes (when applicable): _____

HCPCS Level II codes (when applicable): _____

DERMATOLOGY ASSOCIATES OF CAULDWELL
469 EPIDURAL LANE • SUBQUE, FL 32711 • 407-555-7539

PATIENT: BEGAMMO, SHENIKA
MRN: BEGSH01
Date: 17 December 2011

HISTORY OF PRESENT ILLNESS: This 64-year-old Caucasian female presents to the emergency room with a 10-year history of a progressively enlarging ulcer on the right arm. The lesion has never been biopsied or treated. She has not seen a physician for any complaint for 20 years. The patient has hidden the lesion from her family until it was noticed two days prior to her presentation by her son, who brought her to the hospital. She denies pain or decreased range of motion of the right arm. She denies systemic symptoms.

PAST MEDICAL HISTORY: Patient denied any medical conditions.

MEDICATIONS: None.

PHYSICAL EXAMINATION: A large ulcer is present on the right arm, ulcerated to muscle, with rolled, infiltrated borders. There is a palpable 2-cm right axillary lymphadenopathy. A 2.5 x 1-cm slightly brown, telangiectatic, irregularly shaped plaque is present on the right back.

LABORATORY DATA: CBC: WBC: 6.0 (3.8-9.8); Hgb: 2.9 (12.1-15.1); Hct: 10.6 (36.1-44.3); Plt: 445K (140-440K); MCV 52.7 (74-115) CMP: Sodium: 137 (135-145); Potassium: 3.9 (3.3-4.9); Chloride: 106 (97-110); Bicarbonate: 21 (20-28); Creatinine: 0.8 (0.6-1.4); BUN: 10 (8-25); Glucose: 124 (65-199);

Plasma protein: 7.8 (6.5-8.5); Albumin: 3.1 (3.6-5.0); Bili: 0.4 (0.3-1.1); Alk Phos: 82 (38-126); AST: 13 (11-47); ALT: 25 (7-53); INR: 1.31 (0.8-1.2): PTT: 32.8 (23-35)

RADIOGRAPHY: Chest and right humerus radiographs revealed multiple poorly defined nodules over the right lung field, slightly enlarged right hilar shadow, with normal left lung field and cardiac silhouette and no effusion. A large soft tissue defect was present over the proximal humerus.

DX: Basal cell carcinomas, metastatic

PROCEDURE: Surgery to remove carcinoma on humerus to be followed by chemotherapy [Cis-platinum]

Suzanna A. Maconi, MD

SAM/ghh 12/17/11 11:47:39

You Code It!

What are the best, most accurate codes?

Diagnosis Codes: _____

Procedure Codes: _____

Anesthesia Codes (when applicable): _____

HCPCS Level II codes (when applicable): _____

DERMATOLOGY ASSOCIATES OF CAULDWELL
469 EPIDURAL LANE • SUBQUE, FL 32711 • 407-555-7539

PATIENT: SLATE, ASHTON
MRN: SLAAS01
Date: 17 November 2011

HISTORY OF PRESENT ILLNESS: This patient is a 39-year-old African-American male who works as a roofer with significant occupational exposure to pigeon droppings and who presented last week to the emergency department with a two week history of fever, chills, nausea, fatigue, and a 20-pound weight loss. A chest x-ray revealed hilar lymphadenopathy, and presumptive treatment for pneumonia was begun with oral levofloxacin.

He returned today with an additional onset of diffuse lymphadenopathy, decreased visual acuity, a tender effusion of the left wrist, and new skin lesions. It is at this time that he was referred to me.

PHYSICAL EXAMINATION: Skin exam reveals multiple skin-color papules and nodules over the face, ranging in size from 3-15 mm. Some of the lesions have central crusting and ulceration. He additionally has a 5-cm firm left submental mass and diffuse lymphadenopathy over his entire body.

LABORATORY STUDIES: HIV: Negative. Three 4-mm punch biopsies are performed for culture and H&E.

DX: Disseminated Cryptococcus in an apparently immunocompetent patient

RX: Fluconazole, p.o.

PLAN: Long-term follow-up to discover whether he has an occult disease causing immunosuppression

___

Suzanna A. Maconi, MD

SAM/ghh 11/17/11 11:47:39

You Code It!

What are the best, most accurate codes?

Diagnosis Codes: _____

Procedure Codes: _____

Anesthesia Codes (when applicable): _____

HCPCS Level II codes (when applicable): _____

DERMATOLOGY ASSOCIATES OF CAULDWELL
469 EPIDURAL LANE • SUBQUE, FL 32711 • 407-555-7539

PATIENT: MARTINEZ-ORTIZ, ALIZA
MRN: MARAL01
Date: 30 September 2011

HISTORY OF PRESENT ILLNESS: This is a 45-year-old Hispanic female, with a past medical history significant only for rectal fissures in the 1980's, presenting for an evaluation of a plaque present for 5-6 years on her right temple. The lesion began as a small pink papule. However, throughout the years, it has noticeably been increasing in size. She denies any pruritus, pain, or other symptoms associated with the lesion. Moreover, she has no personal or family history of diabetes mellitus. She had two biopsies performed on the lesion in the past. She states the first biopsy was consistent with a keratinous cyst and the second biopsy demonstrated a nonspecific dermatitis.

PERTINENT MEDICATIONS: Prempro

PHYSICAL EXAM: Physical exam demonstrates a thin, Hispanic female. On the right temple, there is a 5.3 cm by 6.3 cm plaque, which has a pearly, yellow atrophic center that contains prominent telangiectasias. Surrounding the atrophic center, there is a palpable, red-brown border. There are no other similar plaques located anywhere else on her body.

DX: Necrobiosis Lipoidica located on the face

RX: Thalidomide was initiated at 50 mg each night. In order to reduce the potential risk of thrombosis associated with the usage of Thalidomide, especially given the concurrent use of Prempro and her history of tobacco use, aspirin 81 mg daily was also prescribed. Smoking cessation was encouraged.

Suzanna A. Maconi, MD

SAM/ghh 09/30/11 11:47:39

You Code It!

What are the best, most accurate codes?

Diagnosis Codes: _____

Procedure Codes: _____

Anesthesia Codes (when applicable): _____

HCPCS Level II codes (when applicable): _____

DERMATOLOGY ASSOCIATES OF CAULDWELL
469 EPIDURAL LANE • SUBQUE, FL 32711 • 407-555-7539

PATIENT: PICARD, TERRELL
MRN: PICTE01
Date: 9 October 2011

HISTORY OF PRESENT ILLNESS: This is a 55-year-old white male with a one year history of worsening rash on his face, back, elbows, hips, knees, and palms. He was referred here for evaluation of pruritus and possible tinea versicolor.

PAST MEDICAL HISTORY: Remarkable for primary biliary cirrhosis (PBC), and he is awaiting a liver transplant. In the meantime, he is being treated with ursodiol (Actigall) for his PBC.

PHYSICAL EXAM: Cachectic WM with diffuse jaundice. Periorbital yellow papules and plaques and facial telangiectasias. A large V-shaped yellow plaque on his chest, back, and upper extremities with a distinct line of demarcation. Red-yellow papules and nodules on bilateral elbows and knees. A well-demarcated yellow plaque on his right hip and yellow discoloration of his palmar surfaces were also noted.

LABORATORY VALUES: Total Cholesterol 678, HDL 14, LDL 607, Triglycerides 190. Alkaline phosphatase 721, Bilirubin 6.7, AST 89, ALT 36

DX: Xanthomatosis secondary to PBC-related hyperlipidemia

IMPRESSION: The hypercholesterolemia in PBC is due to reduction in cholesterol secretion, and the treatment mainstay is liver transplantation. Although responses to systemic medications have been poor, ursodiol (Actigall) has been shown in some studies to increase survival and time to transplant and to reduce cholesterol levels. Other agents that may be helpful include azathioprine and cyclosporine. Unfortunately, none of these treatments have been shown to reliably improve xanthomatosis, and this patient will eventually require liver transplantation for survival.

Suzanna A. Maconi, MD

SAM/ghh 10/9/11 11:47:39

You Code It!

What are the best, most accurate codes?

Diagnosis Codes: _____

Procedure Codes: _____

Anesthesia Codes (when applicable): _____

HCPCS Level II codes (when applicable): _____

DERMATOLOGY ASSOCIATES OF CAULDWELL
469 EPIDURAL LANE • SUBQUE, FL 32711 • 407-555-7539

PATIENT: MADERA, RUSSEL
MRN: MADRU01
Date: 29 October 2011

HISTORY OF PRESENT ILLNESS: This patient is a 42-year-old firefighter who suffered a flame burn injury to the skin on the left inner thigh 11 months before presentation. He was treated as an outpatient at one of the burn centers where he received topical antimicrobials and dressing changes. The wound healed by epithelialization and hypertrophic scarring.

    The patient was referred to our clinic because the burn scar had become quite hypertrophic and was unresponsive to compression stocking therapy.

PE: Using a visual analog scale of scar pruritus, the patient scored itch intensity at 6/10 (where 10 is equal to unbearable itching) and itch frequency at 6/10 (where 10 is equal to itching at all times). With time, the scar has continued to progressively increase in thickness.

IMPRESSION: Therapy is initiated with Avogel hydrogel with 3% salicylic acid in a cream base applied to the scar each night and left for 8 to 10 hours.

___

Suzanna A. Maconi, MD

SAM/ghh 10/29/11 11:47:39

You Code It!

What are the best, most accurate codes?

Diagnosis Codes: _____

Procedure Codes: _____

Anesthesia Codes (when applicable): _____

HCPCS Level II codes (when applicable): _____

PATIENT: LUDWIG, HENRIETTA
MRN: LUDHE01
Date: 01 October 2011

HISTORY OF PRESENT ILLNESS: This patient is a 65-year-old woman who underwent open-heart surgery two years ago. She had applied vitamin E topically to the scar for a short period of time without effect. She complained of pain and tenderness, and the scar was very elevated and erythematous.

PE: The patient's scar is 14 cm long, varying from 4 to 6 mm in width, and is elevated by 3 mm to 4 mm. Symptomatic relief from pruritus and tenderness occurred within 48 hours of applying 2% salicylic acid and hydrogel.

   At this follow-up, the patient reports that after one week of the new regimen, she noted a marked decrease in symptoms and decreased erythema in this area. Regression in the size of the scar was less impressive, but symptomatic relief was significant.

PLAN: Patient to return for another appointment in 60 days.

Suzanna A. Maconi, MD

SAM/ghh 10/01/11 11:47:39

You Code It!

What are the best, most accurate codes?

Diagnosis Codes: _____

Procedure Codes: _____

Anesthesia Codes (when applicable): _____

HCPCS Level II codes (when applicable): _____

DERMATOLOGY ASSOCIATES OF CAULDWELL
469 EPIDURAL LANE • SUBQUE, FL 32711 • 407-555-7539

PATIENT: LUDWAX, HENRY
MRN: LUDHE02
Date: 25 October 2011

HISTORY OF PRESENT ILLNESS: This is a 31-year-old white male who was trapped in a burning apartment building when he decided to jump from a window. Pre-assessment by emergency personnel revealed burns to his extremities, scalp, face, thorax, and back (an estimated 90% total body surface area burn). It also appeared he sustained a tibia/fibula fracture of the left leg and a crush injury of the right ankle. He was brought into the emergency room on a 100% oxygen nonrebreathing mask. In the emergency room he was promptly intubated with an oral 7.5 ETT because of suspected inhalation burns. Appropriate analgesics and IV fluids were administered and the patient was placed on mechanical ventilation. He was immediately taken to the burn unit and tanked. He then went to surgery to repair and stabilize his fractures. The following day his total body surface area burns were reassessed from 90% to 60%.

PATIENT COURSE: He developed pleural effusion on the right and right upper lobe pneumonia. Pseudomonas was cultured from his sputum. Escharotomy was required on all ten fingers. Debridement and skin grafting proceeded without complications. The patient had a tracheotomy during the fourth week and is now on 4-hour trachshield trials throughout the day with mechanical ventilatory support at night.

PHYSICAL EXAM IN ER: HR 110, BP 154/110, RR 24, Chest: coarse, CV: RRR
    Pt is alert. IV Fluids started. Burns: 2nd and 3rd degree.

LABS: WBC 16.1 mm3, Gluc 122 mg/dl, Na 141 mEq/L, K 4.0 mEq/L, Cl 105 mEq/L, Ca 9.5 mEq/L, PO4 3.6 mEq/L, Mg 1.9 mEq/L, Bun 22 mg/dl, Cr 0.9 mg/d

IMPRESSION: A restrictive defect may occur anywhere on the body, but from a respiratory standpoint, chest and abdomen burns are the most life-threatening. The burned skin will restrict chest or abdomen movement, decrease chest wall compliance, and make it very difficult to ventilate the patient.

Suzanna A. Maconi, MD

SAM/ghh 10/25/11 11:47:39

You Code It!

What are the best, most accurate codes?

Diagnosis Codes: _____

Procedure Codes: _____

Anesthesia Codes (when applicable): _____

HCPCS Level II codes (when applicable): _____

Emergency Services Cases and Patient Records

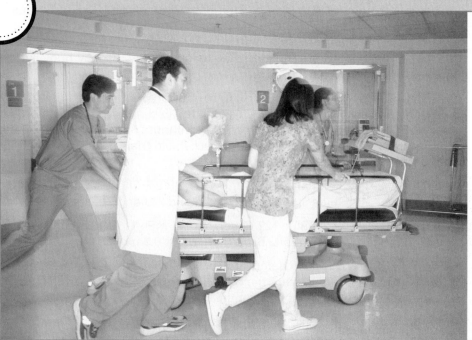

INTRODUCTION

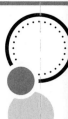

These case studies are from a health care facility providing emergency services. Physicians who specialize in emergency, or urgent, care are called emergency medicine specialists, also known as ER doctors. These health care professionals diagnose and treat multiple health care concerns, often in life-threatening situations where decisions must be made quickly. Unlike many other medical specialists, emergency medical specialists must maintain diagnostic and treatment standards for conditions that affect almost all body and organ systems.

Frequently, emergency medical specialists will diagnose and treat patients to stabilize them and then call in a physician who specializes in the body or organ system involved for a consultation and continued care. Some emergency medicine specialists may choose to have a subspecialty, such as infectious disease medicine or orthopedics.

Emergency medicine doctors are board-certified by the Board of Emergency Medicine, which is recognized by the American Board of Medical Specialties.

You can use these cases to practice coding diagnoses, E/M, procedures, DME, or other HCPCS Level II items, as applicable; code for the physician or the facility; code inpatient and outpatient services, as applicable:

1. Code for the physician.
2. Code for the anesthesiologist, when applicable.
3. Code for the hospital, when applicable.
4. Code for the pathology and laboratory, when applicable.
5. Code HCPCS Level II codes, when applicable.

Note: Despite the fact that most EDs are located in a hospital, these services are considered outpatient services for coding.

TYLER EMERGENCY CLINIC
911 QUICK LANE • ANYTOWN, FL 32711 • 407-555-6248

PATIENT: PARKMAN, SHEILA
ACCOUNT/EHR #   PARKSH001
Date: 10/01/11

Attending Physician: Valerie R. Victors, MD

S: This 29-year-old female was brought to the ED by ambulance after she was found unconscious on her garage floor this afternoon. She regained consciousness within several minutes, complaining of a severe headache with pain in the occipital lobe and nausea. Pt states that the last thing she remembers was climbing on a box to reach a vase on the top of a storage shelf. She lost her footing when the box she was standing on collapsed, and she fell onto the cement floor.

O: Ht 5'7" Wt. 175 lb. R 16. Head: Scalp laceration on the right posterior parietal bone. Bruise indicates trauma to this area. Eyes: PERL. Neck: Neck muscles are tense; there is minor pain upon rotation of the head. Musculoskeletal: All other aspects of the shoulders, arms, and legs are unremarkable. X-rays of skull, two views, and soft tissue of the neck are all benign.

A: Concussion

P: 1. MRI brain to rule out subdural hematoma is negative
      2. Repair laceration and bandage

Valerie R. Victors, MD

VRV/mg   D: 10/01/11 09:50:16 T: 10/05/11 12:55:01

You Code It!

What are the best, most accurate codes?

Diagnosis Codes: _____

Procedure Codes: _____

Anesthesia Codes (when applicable): _____

HCPCS Level II codes (when applicable): _____

TYLER EMERGENCY CLINIC
911 QUICK LANE • ANYTOWN, FL 32711 • 407-555-6248

PATIENT: BLACK, YVONDA
ACCOUNT/EHR #:   BLACYV001
Date: 08/11/11

Attending Physician: Willard B. Reader, MD

Patient is a 35-year-old female seen in our emergency facility. She was brought in by ambulance, accompanied by her daughter. Daughter states that the patient was found unconscious in her bedroom, a bottle of Nytol found empty on the nightstand. Pt exhibited signs of severe depression over the course of the last 3–4 days after being served with divorce papers.

　　　Pt is listless and unresponsive. Respiration labored, BP 80/65, P slow and erratic. Skin pale and moist. Stomach pumped. Pt responding to treatment.

DX: Poisoning by Nytol due to attempted suicide
　　Admit to observation unit.
　　Call for psychiatric evaluation.

Willard B. Reader, MD

DRC/pw   D: 08/11/11 09:50:16   T: 08/13/11 12:55:01

You Code It!

What are the best, most accurate codes?

Diagnosis Codes: _____

Procedure Codes: _____

Anesthesia Codes (when applicable): _____

HCPCS Level II codes (when applicable): _____

TYLER EMERGENCY CLINIC
911 QUICK LANE • ANYTOWN, FL 32711 • 407-555-6248

PATIENT: GARLAN, BENJAMIN
ACCOUNT/EHR #:   GARLBE001
Date: 12/01/11

Attending Physician: Willard B. Reader, MD

S: Pt is a 44-year-old male who comes in with severe pain in the lower right quadrant of his abdomen. He states that the pain is sharp and shoots across his belly from right to left. Patient also states that he has been somewhat nauseated over the last two days.

O: Ht 5'9" Wt. 177 lb. R 21. T 101.6. BP 130/95. Abdomen appears to be tender upon manual examination. Comprehensive metabolic blood test, general health panel blood work-up, and an MRA, abdomen, angiography are taken. Results of all tests confirm diagnosis of appendicitis.

A: Acute appendicitis, w/o peritonitis

P: Pt to go to hospital immediately to be admitted for appendectomy

_____

Willard B. Reader, MD

WBR/pw   D: 12/01/11 09:50:16 T: 12/01/11 12:55:01

You Code It!

What are the best, most accurate codes?

Diagnosis Codes: _____

Procedure Codes: _____

Anesthesia Codes (when applicable): _____

HCPCS Level II codes (when applicable): _____

TYLER EMERGENCY CLINIC
911 QUICK LANE • ANYTOWN, FL 32711 • 407-555-6248

PATIENT: FAWZI, BENITA
ACCOUNT/EHR #:   FAWZBE001
Date: 12/17/11

Attending Physician: Willard B. Reader, MD

S: Pt is a 31-year-old female who comes in with a sharp pain in the center of her torso. She states that the pain, which began approximately one week ago, comes and goes, is more severe at night, and shoots through to her back. The pain is lessened when she drinks a lot of water and worse after meals.

O: Ht 5'4" Wt. 125 lb. R 20. T 98.6. BP 110/80. HEENT: unremarkable. Chest sounds normal. Abdominal, B-scan, ultrasound indicates impacted gallstone without obstruction. Surgery is recommended.

A: Gallstone, impacted, no obstruction

P: Pt to call for appointment for surgery

_____

Willard B. Reader, MD

WBR/pw   D: 12/17/11 09:50:16   T: 12/17/11 12:55:01

You Code It!

What are the best, most accurate codes?

Diagnosis Codes: _____

Procedure Codes: _____

Anesthesia Codes (when applicable): _____

HCPCS Level II codes (when applicable): _____

TYLER EMERGENCY CLINIC
911 QUICK LANE • ANYTOWN, FL 32711 • 407-555-6248

PATIENT: GEORGES, EDWARD
ACCOUNT/EHR #:   GEORED001
Date: 08/11/11

Attending Physician: Willard B. Reader, MD

S: Pt is a 33-year-old male, who was helping his girlfriend move two days ago. He was lifting a box of books when he felt a sharp pain, "like something ripped," in his lower right abdomen. He states that he has had a sharp, steady pain in his groin. He has vomited several times since the incident.

O: Ht 6′1″ Wt. 199 lb. R 18. T 98.6F. BP 110/85. Examination reveals an obvious swelling in the inguinal area, just above the right groin. Palpation of the area, while the patient is doing the Valsalva's maneuver confirms inguinal hernia. Digital exam confirms hernia is indirect. Automated differential WBC count is elevated. X-ray of abdomen confirms partial bowel obstruction.

A: Indirect inguinal hernia, unilateral, with partial bowel obstruction

P: 1. Rx Truss
  2. Referral to surgeon

Willard B. Reader, MD

WBR/pw D: 08/11/11 09:50:16 T: 08/13/11 12:55:01

You Code It!

What are the best, most accurate codes?

Diagnosis Codes: _____

Procedure Codes: _____

Anesthesia Codes (when applicable): _____

HCPCS Level II codes (when applicable): _____

TYLER EMERGENCY CLINIC
911 QUICK LANE • ANYTOWN, FL 32711 • 407-555-6248

PATIENT: BENJAMIN, DAVIDA
ACCOUNT/EHR #:   BENJDA001
DATE: 09/16/11

Attending Physician: Suzanne R. Taylor, MD

S: Pt is a 49-year-old female complaining of abdominal pain. She states that the pain has been consistent since noon and she has been vomiting since 2 P.M. She has been experiencing chills and weakness, as well. No diarrhea. Last BM was a small one at 7 A.M. and again at 2 P.M. She was in good health prior to the symptoms at noon. She also has GERD.

      Patient had a total hysterectomy three years ago and a laparoscopic cholecystectomy 10 years ago. She quit smoking 10 years ago. Current meds: Evista, Prevacid prn.

O: Wt. 140 Ht 5′2″ T99F P 90 R 18 BP 128/73. Abdomen distended, tympanic, tender. CT Scan abd/pelvis: Dilated small bowel loop appears to contain semisolid material in RLQ, compatible with early small bowel obstruction.

EKG: Sinus tachycardia, otherwise normal. Bowel sounds are normal and hypoactive. Breathing pattern is nonlabored, breath sounds clear. Heart rhythm: regular. Neck veins: nondistended. Skin: warm, dry, intact.

Peripheral pulses: Normal CBC w/differential: WBC, RBC, HGB, and HCT are high; MCHC is low; all other results unremarkable. Glucose and BUN/Creat are high; anion gap is low; all other chemistry unremarkable. UA: UR is cloudy, glucose high.

A: Small bowel obstruction; diaphragmatic hernia; esophageal reflux

P: Admit to hospital for surgery

_____

Suzanne R. Taylor, MD

SRT/pw   D: 09/16/11 09:50:16   T: 09/18/11 12:55:01

You Code It!

What are the best, most accurate codes?

Diagnosis Codes: _____

Procedure Codes: _____

Anesthesia Codes (when applicable): _____

HCPCS Level II codes (when applicable): _____

TYLER EMERGENCY CLINIC
911 QUICK LANE • ANYTOWN, FL 32711 • 407-555-6248

PATIENT: KAHN, ARLENE
ACCOUNT/EHR #:   KAHNAR001
Date: 09/16/11

Attending Physician: Suzanne R. Taylor, MD

The patient is a 7-month-old female infant brought in by paramedics with respiratory distress. During transport, EMT Arthur reports that the patient stopped breathing. Bag mask ventilation with CPR was immediately administered and continued until arrival at the ED. On arrival in the ED, the patient is apneic, asystolic, and pulseless. The infant has no IV access. After brief bag mask ventilation, the patient is intubated with a tracheal tube. A colorimetric carbon dioxide capnometer detector device confirms proper tracheal tube placement.

Findings now include:

1) Airway/breathing: Breath sounds are equal bilaterally, and there is good chest movement with ventilation.
2) Circulation: No pulse is palpable without chest compressions, and no heart sounds are heard. ECG shows asystole. Oxygen saturation is not obtainable.
3) Vital signs: Heart rate 0, respiratory rate 0, blood pressure unobtainable.
4) Attempts at IV access are unsuccessful.

Ventilations and chest compressions are continued. Epinephrine 0.5 mg of the 1:1,000 solution is given down the tracheal tube, and an intraosseous line (IO) is inserted into the proximal left tibia. Blood is obtained from the IO needle and is sent for a number of studies including a rapid glucose check. The airway is reassessed, ventilation and chest compressions are continued, and a second dose of epinephrine is given. The patient converts to a sinus bradycardia with a fair blood pressure. After several more minutes of further stabilization, the infant's heart rate is 120 and she is beginning to move and cough against the tracheal tube. The resuscitation is a success.

DX: PCA (pulmocardiac arrest)
        Admit to NICU

_____

Suzanne R. Taylor, MD

SRT/pw   D: 09/16/11 09:50:16   T: 09/18/11 12:55:01

You Code It!

What are the best, most accurate codes?

Diagnosis Codes: _____

Procedure Codes: _____

Anesthesia Codes (when applicable): _____

HCPCS Level II codes (when applicable): _____

TYLER EMERGENCY CLINIC
911 QUICK LANE • ANYTOWN, FL 32711 • 407-555-6248

PATIENT: HADDOX, TYLER
ACCOUNT/EHR #:   HADDTY001
Date: 09/16/11

Attending Physician: Suzanne R. Taylor, MD

This patient is a 3-month-old male infant is brought to the ED by his father due to continued vomiting and diarrhea. Father states that these symptoms have been ongoing for the last four days. Initial findings in the ED include:

AIRWAY: Breath sounds are normal. Airway is patent.

BREATHING: Breathing is regular at 45 breaths per minute, unlabored.

CIRCULATION: Proximal pulses are poor, distal pulses are absent, and extremities are cool. Feeling from the fifth toe upwards, the legs are cool up to the knee. Capillary refill is 8 seconds. Heart rate is 209 beats per minute, and blood pressure is 70mm Hg systolic.

ECG: There are narrow QRS complexes with sinus tachycardia on the monitor.

The infant does not recognize his parents, is extremely lethargic, and responds to pain only, with a minimal grimace.

Due to the size of his veins, we are unable to start an IV line. 100% oxygen is started. The mucous membranes of the mouth are pink. An intraosseous (IO) is placed in the left tibia and 20 cc/kg of normal saline is infused as rapidly as possible. The infant is then reassessed. Airway and breathing remain stable. The heart rate is now 195. A repeat bolus of 20 cc/kg is given and the patient is reassessed. After the third fluid bolus is given, the patient becomes more alert, distal pulses return, and the patient improves throughout resuscitation. The heart rate has come down to 160. However, a rapid bedside glucose analysis reveals a blood sugar of only 32, which is quickly treated.

DX: Compensated hypovolemic shock (and hypoglycemia) secondary to vomiting and diarrhea

---

Suzanne R. Taylor, MD

SRT/pw   D: 09/16/11 09:50:16   T: 09/18/11 12:55:01

You Code It!

What are the best, most accurate codes?

Diagnosis Codes: _____

Procedure Codes: _____

Anesthesia Codes (when applicable): _____

HCPCS Level II codes (when applicable): _____

TYLER EMERGENCY CLINIC
911 QUICK LANE • ANYTOWN, FL 32711 • 407-555-6248

PATIENT: MODAR, SUZANNE
ACCOUNT/EHR #: MODASU001
Date: 09/16/11

Attending Physician: Suzanne R. Taylor, MD

This patient is a 5-year-old female who was hit by a car when she ran out into the street after her baseball. Paramedics report that, when they arrived at the scene, the child was unconscious. Multiple abrasions were on her face, chest, abdomen, and extremities. Her left thigh was noticeably deformed and swollen. Because she demonstrated very shallow respirations, she was immediately intubated with in-line cervical spine immobilization. Two large bore IV lines where placed and she was then rushed to the trauma center.

EXAM: VS T 37.0C, P160, RR ventilated via the tracheal tube at 20, BP 100/80, oxygen saturation 97%. She is still unresponsive and being ventilated via the tracheal tube. Her pupils are briskly reactive to light. There is excellent chest wall rise and fall via ventilation through the tracheal tube. There are numerous abrasions over her face, chest, abdomen and lower extremities. The abdomen is distended with decreased bowel sounds. Her pelvis is stable, but her left thigh is obviously swollen and tense. Distal perfusion to all four extremities seems adequate. The remainder of the physical examination is unremarkable.

A CT scan of her head reveals a small occipital lobe contusion but no cerebral edema or hemorrhage. The CT scan of her abdomen reveals a small splenic laceration and a mild contusion of the right kidney. Chest and extremity x-rays reveal a displaced midshaft left femur fracture and a small right pulmonary contusion. Her cervical spine and pelvic x-rays are normal. After appropriate stabilization interventions, she is admitted to the pediatric intensive care unit. Her intracranial, pulmonary and splenic injuries are managed with supportive care, and her femur fracture is reduced with open reduction and internal fixation.

DX: Displaced midshaft femur fracture, pulmonary contusion, splenic laceration, contusion to the kidney, multiple lacerations

Admit to pediatric unit for observation.

Suzanne R. Taylor, MD

SRT/pw   D: 09/16/11 09:50:16   T: 09/18/11 12:55:01

You Code It!

What are the best, most accurate codes?

Diagnosis Codes: _____

Procedure Codes: _____

Anesthesia Codes (when applicable): _____

HCPCS Level II codes (when applicable): _____

TYLER EMERGENCY CLINIC
911 QUICK LANE • ANYTOWN, FL 32711 • 407-555-6248

PATIENT:	WERNER, JEFFREY
ACCOUNT/EHR #:	WERNJE001
Date:	09/16/11

Attending Physician: Suzanne R. Taylor, MD

This 7-year-old male is brought into the ED by his father due to his inability "to catch his breath." He states that his son has just recently recovered from a cold but has continued to cough. The father reports that the child often coughs in fits with posttussive emesis, will sometimes turn blue in the face, and makes a "gasping-like" noise when he tries to inhale after a coughing episode. Currently, he is complaining about a pain in his chest and shortness of breath. According to the father, the onset of these symptoms began "after one of those coughing fits this morning." There is an ill contact in the house (a grandmother who has been coughing for the last 3 months).

EXAM: VS T 37.1C, HR 94, RR 28, BP 115/77, Oxygen saturation 93-95% in RA, height is 50-75th %ile, and his weight and head circumference are both in the 10-25th %ile. He is sitting on the exam table, leaning forward, taking quick breaths with some nasal flaring. He has slightly asymmetrical chest movements (the right chest wall moves less than the left), and he has decreased breath sounds with hyperresonance and decreased tactile fremitus on the right as well. His PMI and trachea are normally positioned, his sensorium is normal, and he has regular and symmetrical radial and femoral pulses. The nurse, Robin Spinner, places the patient on 2 liters/minute of oxygen via nasal cannula.

   After 45 minutes, the patient's vitals are relatively unchanged except that his oxygen saturation is now 100% on the 2 liters/minute of oxygen. He is switched to a nonrebreather mask with a FiO2 of 100% and sent for a PA and lateral CXR. Radiologist confirms diagnosis.

DX: Right, simple, primary spontaneous pneumothorax, about 12% in size

TX: Admitted to the hospital for observation and continued oxygen therapy.

Suzanne R. Taylor, MD

SRT/pw   D: 09/16/11 09:50:16   T: 09/18/11 12:55:01

You Code It!

What are the best, most accurate codes?

Diagnosis Codes: _____

Procedure Codes: _____

Anesthesia Codes (when applicable): _____

HCPCS Level II codes (when applicable): _____

TYLER EMERGENCY CLINIC
911 QUICK LANE • ANYTOWN, FL 32711 • 407-555-6248

PATIENT: CAPPELLI, JILL
ACCOUNT/EHR #:   CAPPJI001
Date: 12/16/11

Attending Physician: Suzanne R. Taylor, MD

This patient is a 25-year-old female brought to the ED by her roommate with vomiting and nausea. The roommate states that the patient had an argument with her boyfriend last night. She woke up early this morning saying that she feels sick. The patient admits that last night she took some pills at 2100. She has vomited three or four times at home. The roommate brought in the bottle of pills, which she states was just purchased the day prior. The bottle is marked as having acetaminophen 500mg tablets in a quantity of 30 tablets. There are 8 tablets remaining in the bottle (maximum 11 grams of acetaminophen ingested).

EXAM: VS T 37.2, P 88, R 18, BP 110/70, weight 50 kg. She is alert, quiet, shaking her head yes/no to questions, with poor eye contact. Her skin is pink with good perfusion. Her oral mucosa is moist. Heart is regular with a normal rhythm and rate. Lungs are clear with good aeration. Her abdomen is soft, with normoactive bowel sounds, minimal epigastric tenderness, no rebound, and no guarding. She is alert, oriented, and walks about the room without difficulty.

    50 grams of activated charcoal with sorbitol is administered PO. She is also given 10 grams of N-acetylcysteine orally. An acetaminophen level, aspirin level, blood and urine toxicology screen and beta-HCG are drawn. The acetaminophen level drawn at 8.5 hours postingestion is 150 mcg/mL.

DX: Vomiting and nausea caused by poisoning by acetaminophen, attempted suicide

TX: She is hospitalized for further treatment as well as a psychiatric evaluation.

Suzanne R. Taylor, MD

SRT/pw   D: 12/16/11 09:50:16   T: 12/18/11 12:55:01

You Code It!

What are the best, most accurate codes?

Diagnosis Codes: _____

Procedure Codes: _____

Anesthesia Codes (when applicable): _____

HCPCS Level II codes (when applicable): _____

TYLER EMERGENCY CLINIC
911 QUICK LANE • ANYTOWN, FL 32711 • 407-555-6248

PATIENT: ORTNER, LOUISA
ACCOUNT/EHR #:   ORTNLO001
Date: 11/16/11

Attending Physician: Suzanne R. Taylor, MD

This patient is a 27-year-old female who presents to the clinic in obvious pain. She states that she just returned yesterday from a weekend camping trip and is experiencing pain and redness in the antecubital fossa of her right arm. She does not report any known history of trauma or insect bites. Upon further history, it is learned that she had applied an insect repellent containing 50% DEET to exposed areas of the skin including the neck, arms, and lower extremities. She had used lower concentrations of DEET repellents in the past, with no reported history of adverse skin reactions. On this occasion, the insect repellent was applied approximately 18 hours prior to the onset of symptoms. She reports that she did not wash the treated skin at the end of the day. She does not report applying sunscreen or taking any medications prior to the onset of the rash. No other unusual exposures are reported.

EXAM: There is a well-demarcated area of erythema apparent in the right antecubital fossa. It is warm and tender to palpation. There are no other abnormal findings on physical examination.

DX: Erythematous rash, an adverse skin reaction associated with DEET

PLAN: Patient is told to expect that in about 2 days hemorrhagic blisters will form in the erythematous area, and that about two days after that the bullae should spontaneously rupture, leaving a shallow ulceration which will resolve over the course of the following 10 days.

Suzanne R. Taylor, MD

SRT/pw   D: 11/16/11 09:50:16 T: 11/18/11 12:55:01

You Code It!

What are the best, most accurate codes?

Diagnosis Codes: _____

Procedure Codes: _____

Anesthesia Codes (when applicable): _____

HCPCS Level II codes (when applicable): _____

TYLER EMERGENCY CLINIC
911 QUICK LANE • ANYTOWN, FL 32711 • 407-555-6248

PATIENT: FRANCO, ILIANA
ACCOUNT/EHR #: FRANIL001
Date: 12/05/11

Attending Physician: Suzanne R. Taylor, MD

This patient is a 59-year-old female brought in by her daughter. She states she is feeling anxious, hyperventilating, and suffering paresthesia in both hands and feet. She complains of shortness of breath, which she states is worse since taking meds for anxiety. She denies any pain. Pt is currently under the care of a psychiatrist, Dr. Kennedy, for two weeks.

PMH: Pt has history of asthma, depression, and hypertension. Pt states that she lost her husband 2 years ago and has been having trouble since. She was prescribed Zoloft and felt that she has been more anxious since taking it.

Current Meds: 50 mg bid Zoloft, one tab qd lisinopril; 20 mEq qd potassium; 0.5 mg bid lorazepam

EXAM: BP: 155/83; P 95; R 26 ECG: normal sinus rhythm, left ventricular hypertrophy with repolarization abnormality; CBC: all within normal levels; Cardiac enzyme: 65; PT: normal; PTT: slightly low; CXR – PA and Lat: Lungs clear. Pt. calmed down with reassurance and emotional support.

DX: Depressive disorder; anxiety disorder

PLAN: Xanax 1.0 mg PO tid; Pt to follow-up with Dr. Kennedy

_____

Suzanne R. Taylor, MD

SRT/pw   D: 12/05/11 09:50:16   T: 12/07/11 12:55:01

You Code It!

What are the best, most accurate codes?

Diagnosis Codes: _____

Procedure Codes: _____

Anesthesia Codes (when applicable): _____

HCPCS Level II codes (when applicable): _____

PATIENT: OSTERMAN, SHEILA
ACCOUNT/EHR #:   OSTESH001
Date: 10/15/11

Attending Physician: Suzanne R. Taylor, MD

History of present illness: A 77-year-old woman was playing Bingo in a large hall when she suddenly slumped forward and hit her head on the table, scattering game pieces in every direction. No seizure activity is noted, but she had some loss of bladder control. When she awoke five minutes later she was confused and tired. Onlookers called 911, and EMTs brought her into the ED.

On arrival to the ED, the patient is alert and oriented to person, place, and time, though somewhat tired. She complains of some dizziness and a mild headache.

Her vital signs on arrival are BP 188/90, P112, R 16, SaO2 98% on room air and an oral temperature of 99 F.

REVIEW OF SYSTEMS PRIOR TO EPISODE: No headache or aura, no chest pain, no palpitations, no nausea or vomiting, no fever, no cough. Bowel movements regular, no melena or rectal bleeding. The ROS is essentially negative.

PAST MEDICAL HISTORY: COPD treated with inhalers. No history of CAD, no neurologic history. She has never had chest pain or angina.

SOCIAL HISTORY: Former smoker (40 pack year history), quit 15 years ago. No significant alcohol history, widowed with four children living in the Providence area.

MEDICATIONS: Vitamin B12, aspirin (which she takes for aching knees).

PHYSICAL EXAM:
GENERAL: Cachectic-appearing elderly female in no acute distress.

HEENT: Mild frontal contusion, no other apparent injury. Pupils equal, round, and reactive to light. No signs of hemotympanum or oropharyngeal erythema.

NECK: Nontender.

CHEST: Breath sounds clear bilaterally.

CARDIAC: Normal S1S2 with a 2/6 high-pitched apical holosystolic murmur radiating to the axilla.

ABDOMEN: Soft, nontender.

RECTAL EXAM: Deferred.

NEURO: Cranial nerve function intact to careful testing, no cerebellar findings, reflexes brisk but symmetric. No sensorimotor deficit.

LABS:
CBC: Hgb 10.7 (MCV 81), WBC 12.7 (80% PMN's), platelets 242 (slight anemia)

Chem 7: Na 140, K 3.7, Cl 104, CO2 26, BUN 13, Cr 0.7 (all within normal limits)

Cardiac Enzymes: CK 63, AST 32, LDH 467; PT: 11.3, INR 1.0, PTT 23

Chest x-ray: No acute infiltrate or cardiopulmonary process, mild cardiomegaly

The dramatic anterior ST elevations are the most striking feature of this patient's presentation. The ECG, coupled with the history of syncope, make it very tempting to initiate thrombolysis to treat an evolving

Continued

anterior wall myocardial infarction. Given the history of syncope and headache, however, it was decided to obtain a head CT.

   The CT clearly demonstrates a massive subarachnoid hemorrhage. In retrospect, heparinization and thrombolysis do not seem as prudent an option. For starters, the patient's hypertension at presentation is a relative contraindication to thrombolysis—this case provides an argument for taking those contraindications seriously.

   As for our concern for a co-existing myocardial infarction, on subsequent review of the ECG one notes that the prominent ST elevations exist in the absence of any reciprocal ST depressions in the inferior leads. Moreover, the ECG remained static over time, further supporting the notion that no acute event was taking place.

   An emergency echocardiogram of this patient's heart demonstrated an aneurysm of the anterior myocardial wall, an anatomical finding that we felt could explain her ST elevations.

Suzanne R. Taylor, MD

SRT/pw   D: 10/15/11 09:50:16   T: 10/19/11 12:55:01

You Code It!

What are the best, most accurate codes?

Diagnosis Codes: _____

Procedure Codes: _____

Anesthesia Codes (when applicable): _____

HCPCS Level II codes (when applicable): _____

TYLER EMERGENCY CLINIC
911 QUICK LANE • ANYTOWN, FL 32711 • 407-555-6248

PATIENT: CHESSER, EVAN
ACCOUNT/EHR #:   CHESEV001
Date: 09/05/11

Attending Physician: Suzanne R. Taylor, MD

A 31-year-old Hispanic male presents with "the worst headache ever." He states that at 1100 he felt the acute onset of bitemporal as well as occipital headache. The patient admits to accompanying nausea, vomiting, and weakness in the upper extremities, and complains, "It hurts to move my neck." He denies fevers, chills, change in vision, difficulty speaking or swallowing, chest or abdominal pain, dysuria, or change in bowel habits.

MEDICATIONS: Phenytoin 300mg daily

ALLERGIES: NKDA

PMH: Seizure d/o for several years, unknown etiology

SH: Denies tobacco, alcohol, drug use; No HIV risks; Immigrant from Dominican Republic

REVIEW OF SYSTEMS: 2-3 day h/o cough with yellow sputum production and fevers, some dyspnea

PHYSICAL EXAMINATION: In general, he was an alert, oriented male who was holding head in moderate discomfort, moaning.

VS: T 98.0 (t) HR 110 RR 24; BP 148/85; Pox 99% RA

HEENT: PERRLA, EOMI, No icterus, No injected conjunctiva, Fundi are clear, No photophobia.

LUNGS: Decreased BS Right base, crackles, LL-CTA.

CARDIAC: Tachy, regular, no murmurs

ABDOMEN: Soft, ND, NT. No guarding or rebound.

RECTAL: brown, ob negative

EXT: Good peripheral pulses; no edema; grimaces with bilateral leg raising.

Skin: no rashes

Continued

NEURO: Moves all extremities to command, reflexes symmetric, CNS grossly symmetric, No deficits noted.

LABS: WBC 13.5; Hgb/Hct16/46.2; Plt 305; Na 142; K 4.5; Cl 100; Bicarb 23; Glucose 130; BUN/Cr 25/1.0; Coags: Normal; U/A Normal; Dilantin 7

CXR – normal; MRI

DX: Neurocystocercosis

PLAN: Praziquantel. Six month follow-up scheduled.

Suzanne R. Taylor, MD

SRT/pw   D: 09/05/11 09:50:16   T: 09/07/11 12:55:01

You Code It!

What are the best, most accurate codes?

Diagnosis Codes: _____

Procedure Codes: _____

Anesthesia Codes (when applicable): _____

HCPCS Level II codes (when applicable): _____

TYLER EMERGENCY CLINIC
911 QUICK LANE • ANYTOWN, FL 32711 • 407-555-6248

PATIENT: GRANNAU, BEN
ACCOUNT/EHR #:   GRANBE001
Date: 09/05/11

Attending Physician: Suzanne R. Taylor, MD

HPI: A 23-year-old male presents to the ED complaining of back pain since the previous night. The back pain is dull and not localized to any particular area. He also complains of nausea (no vomiting), neck pain, and headache. He has had similar back pain intermittently for months, but it is worse today. His ROS is positive for photophobia, subjective fevers and generalized weakness. He denies dysuria, frequency, urgency, hematuria, visual changes or focal weakness or numbness.

PMH is negative except for "neck surgery" for cancer, which he had several months ago. He takes some medicines, but he doesn't remember what they are, and he didn't bring them along. He is allergic to penicillin ("it makes me swell up").

FH is unremarkable.

SH: He lives with his wife. He does not drink or smoke.

ROS: As in the HPI. He has felt fairly tired with intermittent back pain for months.

PHYSICAL EXAMINATION: T 101.8 po HR 109 RR 22 BP 88/49

Generally, he is a flushed uncomfortable male appearing moderately ill.

HEENT: Normal, with a normal funduscopic examination. Neck was supple, with a well-healed thyroidectomy scar.

Lungs were clear to auscultation.

Cardiac examination: Regular tachycardic rhythm, without murmurs or gallops.

Abdominal examination: Normal. There was normal rectal tone.

Extremities: Some back pain with straight leg raise on the left, full pulses and no evidence of arthropathy.

Skin: Flushed but there were no rashes.

Neurologic examination: Normal mental state (although s/w agitated), fluent Spanish, intact cranial nerves, and normal motor examination.

CBC: WBC 5.2, Hgb 12.3, Hct 37.1, Plt 198. Diff: 81% segs, 12% lymphs, 5% monos; Chem7: Na 140 Cl 100 BUN 8 glc 86; The patient's calcium level was 4.9.; K 3.5 C02 24 Cr 0.7; PT 12.6 PTT 29

Continued

U/A negative; UCG negative; CXR, CTLS spine series normal

CSF no wbcs, no rbcs, protein 11, glucose 57

DX: Parathyroid insufficiency; Hypocalcemia, secondary to hypoparathyroidism

Suzanne R. Taylor, MD

SRT/pw   D: 09/05/11 09:50:16   T: 09/07/11 12:55:01

You Code It!

What are the best, most accurate codes?

Diagnosis Codes: _____

Procedure Codes: _____

Anesthesia Codes (when applicable): _____

HCPCS Level II codes (when applicable): _____

TYLER EMERGENCY CLINIC
911 QUICK LANE • ANYTOWN, FL 32711 • 407-555-6248

PATIENT: CLAIBORNE, WALTER
ACCOUNT/EHR #: CLAIWA001
Date: 09/09/11

Attending Physician: Suzanne R. Taylor, MD

28-year-old male with no significant PMH presented to the ED by ambulance complaining of bilateral lower extremity weakness.

He was in stable health until three weeks prior, when he noted progressive cramping, pain and weakness in his legs. A week after, he was treated at another hospital for low back pain with hydrocodone and a muscle relaxant. His back pain resolved gradually, but bilateral thigh pain and weakness persisted. On the morning of admission, the patient tried to rise out of bed but immediately fell to the floor with lower extremity paraparesis.

He denied recent injury, fevers, viral symptoms, headache, diplopia, paresthesias, numbness, arm weakness, arthralgias, incontinence, nausea, vomiting, diarrhea, or previous neurologic deficits.

PMH: Motorcycle accident seven years ago without sequelae.

MED: None

ALLERGIES: None

SOC: Single, employed as a truck driver. Intermittently chews tobacco. Occasional alcohol. Denied intravenous drug use.

FH: No history of paraparesis, paraplegias, or neurological diseases.

ROS: Anxious over the last month with occasional insomnia. Eight- to twelve-pound weight loss over several months without dieting. No history of recent travel. No blood transfusions. No noted tick or insect bites and no insecticide exposure. No recent URIs.

PHYSICAL EXAMINATION:
VITALS: Temp: 96.2 BP: 127/68 P: 107 R: 20

GENERAL: Thin young man who appears anxious.

HEENT: PERRL, sclera anicteric, fundi unremarkable, dentition poor. Neck supple, no lymphadenopathy, palpable thyroid.

CV: Tachy normal S1/S2, soft 2/6 holosystolic murmur over LSB. CHEST: clear to auscultation.

ABD: Normoactive bowel sounds, no organomegaly.

EXT: No clubbing, cyanosis, or edema; hands and feet warm and dry.

NEURO: Alert and oriented; fluent; CN intact; motor nl bulk, decreased tone in lower extremities, power 4/5 in upper extremities B, 2-3/5 in bilat lower extremities, distal weaker than proximal. Reflexes 2 and brisk diffusely; toes go down to plantar stim; No clonus. Sensation intact to light touch, pinprick, temperature, proprioception. Coordination intact in UEs (limited by weakness in lower extremities). Gait not tested.

EKG: SR, 97 bpm. Otherwise normal.

Continued

LABS:

Chem7: Na 143 K 1.8 CL 109 CO2 23 BUN 15 CR 0.6 GLU 110

CBC: WBC 5.5 HB 14.7 HCT 42.8 PLT 246 DIFF 73 poly 16 lymph

CSF: Normal protein, glucose, cell count and diff.

Etc: ESR 6 Ca 9.8 Mg 1.6 Phos 4.7 CPK 398 U/A normal

LFTs normal.

CXR: Normal; LS Spine Series: Normal

DX: Hypokalemic periodic paralysis, associated with hypothyroidism

Suzanne R. Taylor, MD

SRT/pw   D: 09/09/11 09:50:16   T: 09/13/11 12:55:01

You Code It!

What are the best, most accurate codes?

Diagnosis Codes: _____

Procedure Codes: _____

Anesthesia Codes (when applicable): _____

HCPCS Level II codes (when applicable): _____

Endocrinology Cases and Patient Records

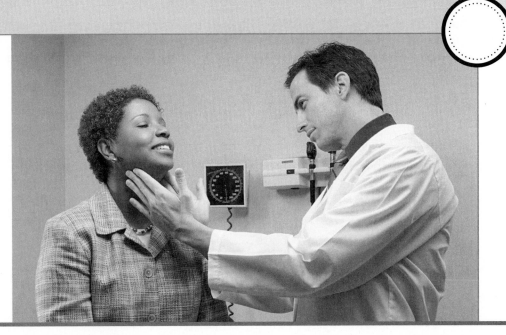

INTRODUCTION

Endocrinologists are physicians whose specialty involves the diagnosis and treatment of abnormalities of the endocrine system. These common health concerns include diabetes insipidus, hypothyroidism, and diabetes mellitus. Such conditions are usually systemic, meaning that they can affect the entire body and are often chronic.

Endocrinologists can be board-certified through the Board of Internal Medicine, which is recognized by the American Board of Medical Specialties.

You can use these cases to practice coding diagnoses, E/M, procedures, DME, or other HCPCS Level II items, as applicable; code for the physician or the facility; code inpatient and outpatient services, as applicable:

1. Code for the physician.
2. Code for the anesthesiologist, when applicable.
3. Code for the hospital, when applicable.
4. Code for the pathology and laboratory, when applicable.
5. Code HCPCS Level II codes, when applicable.

MEDICAL ASSOCIATES OF ENDOCRINOLOGY
6899 LYMPHATIC PATH • NODINE, FL 32811 • 407-555-4661

PATIENT: ROLLINS, KIM
ACCOUNT/EHR #:   ROLLKI001
Date: 09/16/11

Attending Physician: Suzanne R. Taylor, MD

This 53-year-old female came to see me today with complaints of profuse sweating, tremors, and polyuria. I have not seen her for 6 months, when she came for treatment of her carpal tunnel syndrome. She has IDDM.

Glucose test indicated that her diabetes was out of control. I adjusted her dosage. Patient was given Insulin IM. I spent 40 minutes counseling her on the proper manner of giving herself insulin injections and answering other concerns she had related to her disease.

DX: Diabetes mellitus, insulin-dependent, uncontrolled

_____

Suzanne R. Taylor, MD

SRT/pw   D: 09/16/11 09:50:16   T: 09/18/11 12:55:01

You Code It!

What are the best, most accurate codes?

Diagnosis Codes: _____

Procedure Codes: _____

Anesthesia Codes (when applicable): _____

HCPCS Level II codes (when applicable): _____

MEDICAL ASSOCIATES OF ENDOCRINOLOGY
6899 LYMPHATIC PATH • NODINE, FL 32811 • 407-555-4661

PATIENT: STANTON, IMOGENE
ACCOUNT/EHR #: STANIM001
Date: 08/11/11

Attending Physician: Willard B. Reader, MD

S: Pt is a 71-year-old female, visited at home for a regular check of her Type I uncontrolled diabetes mellitus. She exhibited the initial stages of diabetic gangrene on her left lower leg during her last visit, two weeks ago.

O: BP 130/70; She looks well. Her chest is clear and the cardiac examination is unremarkable. Examination of the leg shows no edema, redness, or heat in the lower extremity.

HEENT: unremarkable.

A: Type 1 diabetes uncontrolled; diabetic gangrene

P: 1. Referral to orthopedist, appointment scheduled next week, possible BKA
   2. Continue on meds and treatments prescribed for gangrene
   3. Adjust dosage of insulin to maintain proper glucose levels

_____

Willard B. Reader, MD

WBR/pw   D: 08/11/11 09:50:16   T: 08/13/11 12:55:01

You Code It!

What are the best, most accurate codes?

Diagnosis Codes: _____

Procedure Codes: _____

Anesthesia Codes (when applicable): _____

HCPCS Level II codes (when applicable): _____

PATIENT: PERMANENTE, MORRIS
ACCOUNT/EHR #:   PERMMO001
Date: 09/16/11

Attending Physician: Suzanne R. Taylor, MD

Procedure: Vitrectomy followed by laser panretinal photocoagulation

An ocutome is used to go behind the iris and cut and suction the vitreous mechanically.
     After the vitreous removal, an endolaser is used to treat the remaining retinal disorders in all four retinal quadrants and prevent further retinal hemorrhage.

DX: Juvenile diabetes, insulin-dependent; severe retinal hemorrhage; microaneurysmal diabetic retinopathy

Suzanne R. Taylor, MD

SRT/pw   D: 09/16/11 09:50:16   T: 09/18/11 12:55:01

You Code It!

What are the best, most accurate codes?

Diagnosis Codes: _____

Procedure Codes: _____

Anesthesia Codes (when applicable): _____

HCPCS Level II codes (when applicable): _____

MEDICAL ASSOCIATES OF ENDOCRINOLOGY
6899 LYMPHATIC PATH • NODINE, FL 32811 • 407-555-4661

PATIENT: SHEPARD, CHARLES
ACCOUNT/EHR #: SHEPCH001
Date: 08/11/11

Attending Physician: Willard B. Reader, MD

S: Pt is a 31-year-old male complaining of an unhealed sore on his left foot. He states the sore is of 3 weeks duration with no evidence of healing despite multiple home remedies and over-the-counter treatments. Pt has had type II diabetes for six years.

O: Wt 195, Ht 5'7" T 99F, BP 150/90; HEENT: unremarkable. Left extremity shows a diabetes-related ulcer directly above the third phalange. Ulcer is debrided (skin and subcutaneous tissue), ointment applied, and a bandage placed. Patient is given wound care instructions.

A: Type II diabetes; ulcer of midfoot

P: Pt to return in two weeks for follow-up

Willard B. Reader, MD

WBR/pw   D: 08/11/11 09:50:16   T: 08/13/11 12:55:01

You Code It!

What are the best, most accurate codes?

Diagnosis Codes: _____

Procedure Codes: _____

Anesthesia Codes (when applicable): _____

HCPCS Level II codes (when applicable): _____

MEDICAL ASSOCIATES OF ENDOCRINOLOGY
6899 LYMPHATIC PATH • NODINE, FL 32811 • 407-555-4661

PATIENT: KELLOGG, COLE

ACCOUNT/EHR #:   KELLCO001

Date: 08/11/11

Attending Physician: Willard B. Reader, MD

Surgeon: Colleen Infanti, MD

Patient is a 28-year-old male with insulin-dependent (type I) diabetic nephropathy and chronic renal failure. He presents today for an arteriovenous shunt for dialysis.

    A Cimino-type direct arteriovenous anastomosis is performed by incising the skin of the left antecubital fossa. Vessel clamps are placed on the vein and adjacent artery. The vein is dissected free and the downstream portion of the vein is sutured to an opening in the artery using an end-to-side technique. The skin incision is closed in layers.

Colleen Infanti, MD

CI/pw   D: 08/11/11 09:50:16   T: 08/13/11 12:55:01

You Code It!

What are the best, most accurate codes?

Diagnosis Codes: _____

Procedure Codes: _____

Anesthesia Codes (when applicable): _____

HCPCS Level II codes (when applicable): _____

MEDICAL ASSOCIATES OF ENDOCRINOLOGY
6899 LYMPHATIC PATH • NODINE, FL 32811 • 407-555-4661

PATIENT: JIMENEZ, ANNA
ACCOUNT/EHR #:   JIMEAN001
Date: 07/26/11

Attending Physician: Suzanne R. Taylor, MD

S: This Pt is a 23-year-old female who was diagnosed with juvenile diabetes three years ago. She presents today with complaints of her hands and feet getting numb on occasion. In addition, she has experienced bouts of pain in her extremities.

O: Ht 5'3" Wt. 219 lb. R 23. BP 150/100. Casual plasma glucose values shown to be 220 mg/dL (normal< 199). Feet and hands are cool to the touch indicating poor circulation. Slight edema noticed in left metatarsal and all periphery.

A: Juvenile diabetes mellitus, uncontrolled; Peripheral angiopathy

P: 1. CT of lower extremities
     2. Full blood work up
     3. Adjust insulin dosage
     4. Return in 10 days for follow-up

Suzanne R. Taylor, MD

SRT/pw   D: 07/26/11 09:50:16   T: 07/29/11 12:55:01

You Code It!

What are the best, most accurate codes?

Diagnosis Codes: _____

Procedure Codes: _____

Anesthesia Codes (when applicable): _____

HCPCS Level II codes (when applicable): _____

MEDICAL ASSOCIATES OF ENDOCRINOLOGY
6899 LYMPHATIC PATH • NODINE, FL 32811 • 407-555-4661

PATIENT: DANIELS, GWEN
ACCOUNT/EHR #:   DANIGW001
Date: 11/07/11

Attending Physician: Willard B. Reader, MD

S: Pt is a 41-year-old female who has not been to see a physician in more than five years. She states that she has been experiencing severe headaches, blurry vision, and her skin has become extremely oily. She states that she is suffering from abnormal perspiration (diaphoresis) and abnormal hair growth (hypertrichosis).

O: Ht 5'5" Wt. 133 lb. R 21. T 98.6. BP 125/85. Pt has an enlarged supraorbital ridge and her ears and nose appear thickened. Her lower jaw is projected (prognathism). Her voice sounds deeper and more hollow than I remembered, causing suspicion of laryngeal hypertrophy and paranasal sinus enlargement. Radioimmunoassay testing shows that plasma hGH and somatomedin-C (IL-1) levels are high. Skull x-rays identify a pituitary lesion and a thickening of the occipital and parietal bones.

A: Acromegaly

P: Immediate referral to surgeon for transsphenoidal hypophysectomy

Willard B. Reader, MD

WBR/pw   D: 11/07/11 09:50:16 T: 11/10/11 12:55:01

You Code It!

What are the best, most accurate codes?

Diagnosis Codes: _____

Procedure Codes: _____

Anesthesia Codes (when applicable): _____

HCPCS Level II codes (when applicable): _____

MEDICAL ASSOCIATES OF ENDOCRINOLOGY
6899 LYMPHATIC PATH • NODINE, FL 32811 • 407-555-4661

PATIENT: TESKE, KENDRA
ACCOUNT/EHR #:   TESKKE001
Date: 09/25/11

Attending Physician: Willard B. Reader, MD

S: Pt is a 41-year-old female, who presents today with complaints of malaise and fatigue. She states that she has lost weight without any change in her eating habits and has had a fever recently. Her joints have been achy and sometimes painful, and she has suffered with a rash across her cheeks and nose.

O: Ht 5'7" Wt. 181 lb. R 21. T 99.2. BP 125/85. Pt has butterfly rash over nose and checks. CBC with differential, platelet count, erythrocyte sedimentation rate, and serum electrophoresis. Antinuclear antibody, anti-DNA, and lupus erythematosus cell tests (lupus anticoagulant assay test) are all performed. Anti-DNA test is positive for systemic lupus erythematosus (SLE).

Urine tests show proteinuria in excess of 3.5 g/24h.

A: Systemic lupus erythematosus with nephritic syndrome

P: 1. Rx 325 aspirin prn
      2. Rx flurandrenolide cream for topical treatment of skin lesions
      3. Rx Prednisone, 60 mg, tapering dosage

_____

Willard B. Reader, MD

WBR/pw   D: 09/25/11 09:50:16   T: 09/28/11 12:55:01

You Code It!

What are the best, most accurate codes?

Diagnosis Codes: _____

Procedure Codes: _____

Anesthesia Codes (when applicable): _____

HCPCS Level II codes (when applicable): _____

MEDICAL ASSOCIATES OF ENDOCRINOLOGY
6899 LYMPHATIC PATH • NODINE, FL 32811 • 407-555-4661

PATIENT: WEINGARTEN, LEONORA

ACCOUNT/EHR #:   WEINLE001

Date: 10/26/11

Attending Physician: Valerie R. Victors, MD

S: Pt is a 71-year-old female who I diagnosed with type II diabetes mellitus two years ago. She comes in complaining of cramps and aching in her calves. Pt states that most times she can relieve the symptoms, but lately, the pain has not subsided during rest.

O: Ht. 5'2", Wt 165 lb., comprehensive metabolic panel blood test taken. Each extremity is examined with special attention to lower leg, ankle, and feet. Lab results indicate that glucose levels are abnormal. Gradient compression stockings are applied to each leg, below knee, 18-30 mmHg. Pt is given instructions for proper use of these stockings.

A: Suspected peripheral arterial disease (PAD)
     Uncontrolled diabetes mellitus type II

P: 1. Order for computed tomographic scans of both legs, with contrast
     2. Follow-up after results of CT scans

Valerie R. Victors, MD

VRV/mg   D: 10/26/11 09:50:16 T: 10/27/11 12:55:01

You Code It!

What are the best, most accurate codes?

Diagnosis Codes: _____

Procedure Codes: _____

Anesthesia Codes (when applicable): _____

HCPCS Level II codes (when applicable): _____

MEDICAL ASSOCIATES OF ENDOCRINOLOGY
6899 LYMPHATIC PATH • NODINE, FL 32811 • 407-555-4661

PATIENT: KASSAN, IMAD
ACCOUNT/EHR #: KASIM001
Date: 10/15/11

HISTORY: This is a 50-year-old male, referred by Dr. Simollina for a consultation regarding an enlargement of the left anterior neck. The patient noted increased appetite over past month with no weight gain, and more frequent bowel movements over the same period.

PHYSICAL EXAM: Ht 5'8" Wt 150 lb. Heart rate 82 BP 110/76. There is an ocular stare with a slight lid lag. The thyroid gland is asymmetric to palpation, weighing an estimated 40g (normal = 15-20g). There is a 3 x 2.5 cm firm nodule in left lobe of the thyroid.

A thyroid stimulating hormone (TSH) test is performed here in the office. TSH concentration is markedly decreased. Thyroid scan shows 68% uptake and 54% uptake after treatment with iodine-123 (normal 5-28% uptake at these time points).

A fine needle aspirate (FNA) of the nodule is done and the cytology of the recovered cells identified papillary carcinoma of the thyroid.

DX: Grave's disease with papillary carcinoma

COURSE: The patient will be scheduled for a surgical thyroidectomy followed by thyroid hormone replacement therapy.

Derrick Alexander, MD

10/15/11 11:47:39

You Code It!

What are the best, most accurate codes?

Diagnosis Codes: _____

Procedure Codes: _____

Anesthesia Codes (when applicable): _____

HCPCS Level II codes (when applicable): _____

MEDICAL ASSOCIATES OF ENDOCRINOLOGY
6899 LYMPHATIC PATH • NODINE, FL 32811 • 407-555-4661

PATIENT: MADISON, SALLY ANNE
ACCOUNT/EHR #: MADSA001
Date: 10/15/11

HISTORY: This 28-year-old female came in for a second opinion when her family physician could not resolve her concerns. She states she has had recent tiredness and difficulty concentrating, and has experienced a decline in memory over the last several months. She also noted decreased frequency of bowel movements and an increased tendency to gain weight. She felt chilled without a light sweater, even in warm weather.

FAMILY HISTORY: There was a history of hypothyroidism in her mother and older sister.

PHYSICAL EXAM: Ht 5'5" Wt 125 lb. P 58 beats per min, BP 138/88. She had a slightly puffy face, and her eyebrows were sparse, especially at the lateral margins. The thyroid was firm and bosselated to palpation with an estimated weight of 25 g (normal 15-20 g). The deep tendon reflexes were normally contractive but showed delayed relaxation.

Thyroid stimulating hormone (TSH) test is markedly elevated. Assay of free T4 in serum is also done. Test for anti-thyroid antibodies (anti-thyroglobulin and anti-microsomal) are positive.

DX: Hashimoto's thyroiditis with hypothyroidism

Derrick Alexander, MD

10/15/11 11:47:39

You Code It!

What are the best, most accurate codes?

Diagnosis Codes: _____

Procedure Codes: _____

Anesthesia Codes (when applicable): _____

HCPCS Level II codes (when applicable): _____

MEDICAL ASSOCIATES OF ENDOCRINOLOGY
6899 LYMPHATIC PATH • NODINE, FL 32811 • 407-555-4661

PATIENT: ANDRETTI, JOSHUA
ACCOUNT/EHR #: ANDJO001
Date: 10/15/11

HISTORY: This 6-year-old male presents, accompanied by his mother, with a 6-month history of pubic hair growth. For the past 4 years, he has had a history of rapid somatic growth. Dr. Lukasewski referred his mother to our office.

FAMILY HISTORY: Mother states her obstetric history was unremarkable. He was a full-term infant born to her when she was 34 years old by normal vaginal delivery after an uncomplicated gestation. She is a healthy woman.

PAST MEDICAL HISTORY: His birth weight was normal and there were no neonatal problems. At 9-18 months, his growth was at the 95th percentile for his age; his height at age 2½ was average for 4½ years (his parents were tall). His penis appeared larger than those of his peers at 3 years, he developed some facial acne at 4 years, and pubic hair was seen at 5½ years.

PHYSICAL EXAM: His height is average for 10 years and 3 months, and his weight is average for 9 years and 10 months. BP normal. He is tall, well-proportioned, and muscular with mild facial acne. His penis is large for his age and there is fine pubic hair (Tanner stage II of puberty). The testes are estimated to be 3 mL volume each (small for puberty stage). The neurologic exam is normal.

Test results indicate partial 21-hydroxylase deficiency with simple virilization. Testosterone is markedly elevated, confirming the impression of androgen excess. LH and FSH are not elevated, indicating that a pituitary lesion is not driving the testes to produce androgens. The physical features of the testes (small, without masses) do not suggest a primary testicular lesion.

DX: Congenital adrenal hyperplasia

PLAN: I explained the benefits and adverse effects of hydrocortisone replacement therapy to suppress the pituitary output of ACTH, allowing the adrenal gland to decrease its metabolic output and normalizing the androgen synthesis rate.

Derrick Alexander, MD

10/15/11 11:47:39

You Code It!

What are the best, most accurate codes?

Diagnosis Codes: _____

Procedure Codes: _____

Anesthesia Codes (when applicable): _____

HCPCS Level II codes (when applicable): _____

MEDICAL ASSOCIATES OF ENDOCRINOLOGY
6899 LYMPHATIC PATH • NODINE, FL 32811 • 407-555-4661

PATIENT: MOGDONAVICH, MAGDALENA
ACCOUNT/EHR #:   MOGMA001
Date: 10/15/11

HISTORY: Magdalena is a 27-year-old female referred to me by Dr. Jonas with depression, insomnia, increased facial fullness, and a recent increase in facial hair. She has also had an episode of depression and acute psychosis following uncomplicated delivery of normal baby boy 9 months previously. Her menses have been irregular since their resumption after the birth (she is not breastfeeding).

PHYSICAL EXAM: Heart rate: 90 beats per min, BP 146/110. Her face is puffy with an increase in facial hair and ruddy complexion. There is no truncal obesity, peripheral wasting, or striae.

LABS: Serum electrolytes, white cell count, and hemoglobin and hematocrit are all within normal limits.

DX: Cushing's syndrome

PLAN: Patient to return in one week with her husband to discuss treatment options.

Derrick Alexander, MD

10/15/11 11:47:39

You Code It!

What are the best, most accurate codes?

Diagnosis Codes: _____

Procedure Codes: _____

Anesthesia Codes (when applicable): _____

HCPCS Level II codes (when applicable): _____

MEDICAL ASSOCIATES OF ENDOCRINOLOGY
6899 LYMPHATIC PATH • NODINE, FL 32811 • 407-555-4661

PATIENT: HELGSTROM, INGRID
ACCOUNT/EHR #: HELIN001
Date: 10/15/11

HISTORY: This patient is a 40-year-old female who presents with a 6-month history of increasing fatigue. For the past 3 months she has suffered recurrent upper respiratory infections, poor appetite, abdominal cramps, and diarrhea. During this time, she lost 25 lb. She has also noted joint pains, muscle weakness, and dizzy spells following exercise, and she has not menstruated for the past 3 months. Patient was referred to this office by her family physician, Dr. Farina.

PHYSICAL EXAM: Ht 5' Wt 102 lb. Heart rate 86; BP 120/65 when supine. After one minute of quiet standing, the heart rate is 120, BP 90/58, and she became dizzy. Her thyroid gland was diffusely enlarged, and the bowel sounds were hyperactive.

Initial testing evaluated thyroid, electrolyte, and renal status. Her sodium is significantly low and her potassium is high, consistent with sodium loss and potassium retention by the renal tubules in mineralocorticoid deficiency. TSH is elevated, though not severely so, and is consistent with borderline hypothyroidism. The hemoglobin is also low. The morning cortisol is low, and the ACTH is quite high.

DX: Addison's Disease

PLAN: The patient is instructed to carry an identifying bracelet or card indicating a need for increased steroid dosage during stress or injury. She is informed that thyroid replacement therapy may become necessary in the future.

Derrick Alexander, MD

10/15/11 11:47:39

You Code It!

What are the best, most accurate codes?

Diagnosis Codes: _____

Procedure Codes: _____

Anesthesia Codes (when applicable): _____

HCPCS Level II codes (when applicable): _____

MEDICAL ASSOCIATES OF ENDOCRINOLOGY
6899 LYMPHATIC PATH • NODINE, FL 32811 • 407-555-4661

PATIENT: GRISSOM, MARIETTA
ACCOUNT/EHR #: GRIMA001
Date: 10/15/11

HISTORY: Patient is a 48-year-old female, referred by her psychiatrist, Dr. Knutzon, with a past history of mental illness and a new onset of bizarre psychotic behavior. She has been well for the past two years.

PAST MEDICAL HISTORY: No history of bone pain, recent fractures, or kidney stones. The patient denies use of diuretics (e.g., thiazides, which can raise calcium). Her most recent breast exam, mammography, and chest x-ray, taken two months ago, did not suggest malignancy. Stool analysis for occult blood was negative.

PHYSICAL EXAM: Ht 5'5" tall Wt 138 lb. Heart rate 80; BP 130/75. The physical exam is otherwise normal except that she is confused as to the current location, date, and year.

   Routine hematology and chemistry tests were normal. A blood sample was sent for parathyroid hormone (PTH) analysis. In the meantime, the patient and her family are questioned further.

   Intact parathyroid hormone is mildly elevated in a setting of markedly elevated calcium and depressed phosphate.

DX: Primary hyperparathyroidism

CLINICAL COURSE: Treatment options are discussed with the patient. She agrees to surgery. Exploratory surgery of neck is scheduled for next week.

Derrick Alexander, MD

10/15/11 11:47:39

You Code It!

What are the best, most accurate codes?

Diagnosis Codes: _____

Procedure Codes: _____

Anesthesia Codes (when applicable): _____

HCPCS Level II codes (when applicable): _____

MEDICAL ASSOCIATES OF ENDOCRINOLOGY
6899 LYMPHATIC PATH • NODINE, FL 32811 • 407-555-4661

PATIENT: PETAKKI, WARREN

ACCOUNT/EHR #: PETWA001

Date: 10/15/11

HISTORY: This 35-year-old male has been referred to me by Dr. Waterman with an elevated blood pressure (188/112, seated) at his yearly physical exam. Previous exams noted blood pressures of 160/94 and 158/92. On questioning, patient admits episodes about twice a month of apprehension, severe headache, perspiration, rapid heartbeat, and facial pallor. These episodes had an abrupt onset and lasted 10-15 minutes each.

PHYSICAL EXAM: Thirty minutes after the initial blood pressure measurement, the seated blood pressure is 178/110 with a heart rate of 90. The blood pressure after 3 min of standing is 152/94 with a heart rate of 112. The optic fundi showed moderately narrowed arterioles with no hemorrhages or exudates.

LABS: Routine hematology and chemistry studies are within the reference ranges and a chest film and EKG are essentially normal. A 24-hour urine specimen is collected for analysis of catecholamines and catecholamine metabolites. Plasma catecholamines are also assayed. Urinary catecholamines and catecholamine metabolites are all elevated. Plasma norepinephrine is markedly elevated, but epinephrine is within the normal range. A CT scan of the adrenals revealed an 8-cm mass on the left side.

DX: Pheochromocytoma

CLINICAL COURSE: Treatment options are discussed with the patient. The patient is treated with alpha- and beta-blockers (catecholamine receptor blocking agents) for several weeks. Abdominal surgery for removal of the pheochromocytoma will be scheduled once patient's BP is down.

Derrick Alexander, MD

10/15/11 11:47:39

You Code It!

What are the best, most accurate codes?

Diagnosis Codes: _____

Procedure Codes: _____

Anesthesia Codes (when applicable): _____

HCPCS Level II codes (when applicable): _____

MEDICAL ASSOCIATES OF ENDOCRINOLOGY
6899 LYMPHATIC PATH • NODINE, FL 32811 • 407-555-4661

PATIENT: FEATHERLITE, CARLITA
ACCOUNT/EHR #: FEACA001
Date: 10/15/11

HISTORY OF PRESENT ILLNESS: Referred by her obstetrician, Dr. Laurence, this 26-year-old Caucasian female states that she has been having heart palpitations. She states that the palpitations have been constant over the past 2 weeks but seem worse at nighttime. When asked to describe them, she states that they are regular and it feels as if her heart is going to jump out of her chest. She denies chest pain, shortness of breath, or lightheadedness. She has felt a bit warm of late but denies any frank diaphoresis. It is of note that she recently delivered a normal baby boy during an uncomplicated delivery 5½ weeks before this visit. She says she has loose stools occurring approximately 4 times/day. She complains of feeling tired but is unable to get a good night sleep. She states that she feels as if her mind is racing. She denies any nausea, vomiting, or abdominal pain. She also denies myalgias, arthralgias, fevers, or chills. She denied heat or cold intolerance.

PAST MEDICAL HISTORY: Postpartum status and abnormal thyroid function tests: The patient had a radioactive iodine uptake scan that was normal and subsequently had thyroid auto-antibodies determined positive for antithyroglobulin and antimicrosomal antibodies. A thyroid biopsy was also performed and revealed diffuse, lymphocytic infiltration, a characteristic histologic picture of postpartum thyroiditis.

PHYSICAL EXAMINATION: Patient is a thin, white female in no apparent distress. BP 146/90, pulse 96 and regular, temp 37 C degrees taken orally. Her review of systems revealed clear lungs, normal heart rhythm, normal abdomen, and a normal neurologic response although she showed a fine tremor of the hands. Her neck is supple with no lymphadenopathy and her thyroid is approximately 1.5 times normal in size, symmetrically enlarged, firm, and nontender with carotids palpable bilaterally without bruits.

LAB RESULTS: CBC (WBC 14.2, Hct, 38.6, MCV normal, platelet count normal, differential 56% neutrophiles, 7% bands, 34% lymphocytes and 3% monocytes) and a chemistry screen that included electrolytes (NA 142, K 3.6, Cl 101, CO2 22), glucose 86, BUN 26, creatinine 1. Thyroid panel includes thyroxine 16.2 (NL 4-13), T3 resin uptake 34% (NL 25-35%) and a TSH of 0.05 (NL 0.34 to 5.0).

DX: Postpartum autoimmune thyroid syndrome

PLAN: Rx for beta-blockers to reduce the heart palpitations.

Derrick Alexander, MD

10/15/11 11:47:39

You Code It!

What are the best, most accurate codes?

Diagnosis Codes: _____

Procedure Codes: _____

Anesthesia Codes (when applicable): _____

HCPCS Level II codes (when applicable): _____

MEDICAL ASSOCIATES OF ENDOCRINOLOGY
6899 LYMPHATIC PATH • NODINE, FL 32811 • 407-555-4661

PATIENT: ELLISON, TIFFANY
ACCOUNT/EHR #: ELLTI001
Date: 10/15/11

This 11-year-old Caucasian female was referred by her family doctor, Dr Frieda, with complaints of excessive facial hair and a deepening of her voice.

PAST MEDICAL HISTORY: At the age of 8 it was noted that she had a rather early appearance of pubic hair growth, showed evidence of acne on her forehead, had increased amounts of apocrine sweat gland activity, and yet had little evidence of breast development or signs of menarche. As part of her mild presenting symptoms of androgen excess, she had a DHEA-S blood level drawn at the time that was 600 ng/mL. She was in the 90th percentile for height and weight. The diagnostic impression at this time was precocious adrenarche. This was based on a mildly elevated DHEA-S level, normal serum estradiol and a bone age of 10½ years. Over the next 3 years, this young girl experienced progression of her facial acne and began to show increasing evidence of facial hair growth. Her acne manifestation prompted a dermatologic consultation that resulted in treatment with Retin-A and tetracycline. She also started to experience significant weight loss that reached 15 pounds by the time she was 11. This was partially attributed to an intense ballet program and her desire to lose weight at the suggestion of her ballet teacher. Her family physician, however, became concerned with her overt manifestations of virilism and referred her to me.

PHYSICAL EXAMINATION: Patient is a thin, white female with virilizing features including excessive facial hair, a deep voice, and considerable cystic acne. Her evaluation included an MRI of the adrenals and ovaries and an ACTH stimulation test. A diagnosis of delayed onset congenital adrenal hyperplasia was considered, but hormone analysis revealed a normal baseline cortisol and 17 hydroxyprogesterone and 11 deoxycortisol levels. The cortisol level, however, did not stimulate beyond the baseline level following Cortrosyn stimulation. She also has markedly elevated levels of DHEA-S for her age at 3,000 ng/mL and an elevated testosterone level at 218 ng/dL. Her bone age is 13, with a chronological age of 11. An MRI scan revealed a right adrenal mass with a normal left adrenal suggesting a right adrenal tumor.

DX: Virilizing tumors of the adrenal gland

PLAN: Treatment options are discussed with the patient and her parents. She will be scheduled for surgery to excise the right adrenal mass. It is expected that a successful outcome of the surgery will show her elevated androgen levels to return to normal for her age and pubertal status.

Derrick Alexander, MD

10/15/11 11:47:39

You Code It!

What are the best, most accurate codes?

Diagnosis Codes: _____

Procedure Codes: _____

Anesthesia Codes (when applicable): _____

HCPCS Level II codes (when applicable): _____

PATIENT: CRAIG, THEODORE
ACCOUNT/EHR #:   CRATH001
Date: 10/15/11

HISTORY OF PRESENT ILLNESS: This 50-year-old African-American male presents today because he has become quite cantankerous with his coworkers and family. He states these symptoms have been noted for approximately the past year or so. He states he has pain in his back, legs, and hands but has no clinical evidence of inflammatory arthritis, such as heat and redness.

PHYSICAL EXAMINATION: Middle-aged gentleman with erratic behavior, tenderness on his right index finger, as well as RT and LT hands. Augmented peristalsis.

LAB TEST RESULTS:
Hemoglobin 14.7 g
Hematocrit 48%
WBC 7430 nl diff.
Serum calcium 13 mg/dL (Nl 10.5)
PTH elevated to 3 SI units (Nl = 1)
Urine Nl.
Alkaline phosphatase 7 (nl 1–4 B units)

IMAGING STUDIES:
Thyroid scan, Normal
X-ray, HAND, RT, shows bony resorption of distal phalange of index finger

DX: Parathyroid adenoma

PLAN: Discussed surgical options with patient. Patient agrees and procedure is scheduled for 2 weeks.

Derrick Alexander, MD

10/15/11 11:47:39

You Code It!

What are the best, most accurate codes?

Diagnosis Codes: _____

Procedure Codes: _____

Anesthesia Codes (when applicable): _____

HCPCS Level II codes (when applicable): _____

Family Practice Cases and Patient Records

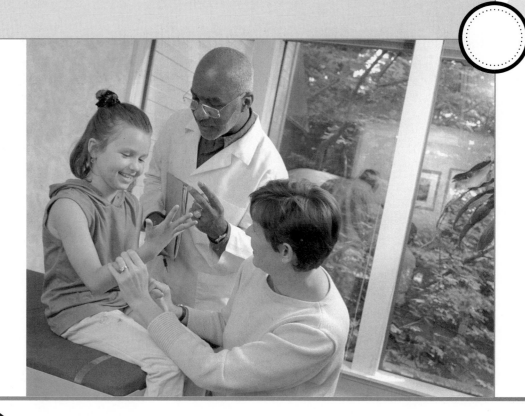

INTRODUCTION

The following case studies are from a family health practice. In a family health practice, a professional coding specialist is likely to handle many different kinds of health situations, especially preventive health care services.

Family medicine practices are health care facilities that specialize in the total health care of the individual and the family. These physicians diagnose and treat a variety of health conditions and diseases in patients of all ages and both sexes. In addition, they are primarily responsible for providing preventive health care advice and procedures, such as vaccinations, annual physical examinations, and age-appropriate screenings.

Family health care specialists may be board-certified by the American Board of Family Medicine, which is recognized by the American Board of Medical Specialties.

You can use these cases to practice coding diagnoses, E/M, procedures, DME, or other HCPCS Level II items, as applicable; code for the physician or the facility; code inpatient and outpatient services, as applicable:

1. Code for the physician.
2. Code for the anesthesiologist, when applicable.
3. Code for the hospital, when applicable.
4. Code for the pathology and laboratory, when applicable.
5. Code HCPCS Level II codes, when applicable.

Note: It is not unusual for family physicians to treat heart disease (cardiology), diabetes (endocrinology), infants (neonatology), children (pediatrics), etc. You can use the other chapters in this book to practice coding those conditions.

FAMILY DOCTORS ASSOCIATES
123 MAIN STREET • ANYTOWN, FL 32711 • 407-555-1234

PATIENT: KRAMDEN, RONALD
ACCOUNT/EHR #:   KRARO001
Date: 11/23/11

Attending Physician: James Healer, MD

This 35-year-old male was last seen by me in August. He presents today for a pre-employment health examination. Patient denies any symptoms or health-related concerns; states he quit smoking in September; drinks on occasion (socially).

Wt. 193 lb. B/P: 120/85, P 25, R reg. T 98.6 HEENT: unremarkable; Cardiopulmonary sounds within normal standards. Abdomen: unremarkable. UA, dipstick, nonautomated w/o microscopy and Gen Health panel normal. Circulation good at extremities.

Screening form completed and signed.

_____

James Healer, MD

JHW/mg   D: 011/23/11 09:50:16   T: 011/25/11 12:55:01

You Code It!

What are the best, most accurate codes?

Diagnosis Codes: _____

Procedure Codes: _____

Anesthesia Codes (when applicable): _____

HCPCS Level II codes (when applicable): _____

FAMILY DOCTORS ASSOCIATES
123 MAIN STREET • ANYTOWN, FL 32711 • 407-555-1234

PATIENT: FRANKLIN, FRANCES
ACCOUNT/EHR #:   FRAFR001
Date: 10/18/11

Attending Physician: Valerie R. Victors, MD

S: This 57-year-old female came for her routine physical exam. Pt does not smoke, drinks alcohol occasionally, and exercises three times per week. Pt states she has no specific health concerns at this time.

O: Ht 5'3" Wt. 145 lb. R 20. HEENT: unremarkable; Respiratory: unremarkable; Musculoskeletal: age-appropriate. No sign of osteoporosis. Bone density appropriate, as per test results. Discussed the importance of keeping up her exercise regimen.

A: Pt is in good health.

P: 1. Follow-up prn
    2. Comprehensive metabolic panel, awaiting results
    3. Schedule screening mammogram
    4. Schedule screening colonoscopy

_____

Valerie R. Victors, MD

VRV/mg   D: 10/18/11 09:50:16   T: 10/23/11 12:55:01

You Code It!

What are the best, most accurate codes?

Diagnosis Codes: _____

Procedure Codes: _____

Anesthesia Codes (when applicable): _____

HCPCS Level II codes (when applicable): _____

FAMILY DOCTORS ASSOCIATES
123 MAIN STREET • ANYTOWN, FL 32711 • 407-555-1234

PATIENT: KELLER, ANDRIENNE
ACCOUNT/EHR #: KELAN001
Date: 12/21/11

Attending Physician: James I. Cipher, MD

S: This Pt is a 35-year-old female who was here 6 months ago for her annual physical. Today, she presents with a cut in the palm of her right hand. Pt states that she was hanging ornaments on her tree and a glass ball broke in her hand. She is otherwise healthy and has no other stated health concerns.

O: Pt laid back on the examination table and her right hand was draped in a sterile fashion. A topical antiseptic is applied and the superficial laceration, measuring 2.0 cm in length, was checked for residual glass shards. None were found and the wound was cleansed and a simple repair was accomplished with a tissue adhesive.

A: Superficial laceration of the right hand, 2.0 cm

P: Follow-up in ten days.

James I. Cipher, MD

JIC/mg   D: 12/21/11 09:50:16   T: 12/22/11 12:55:01

You Code It!

What are the best, most accurate codes?

Diagnosis Codes: _____

Procedure Codes: _____

Anesthesia Codes (when applicable): _____

HCPCS Level II codes (when applicable): _____

FAMILY DOCTORS ASSOCIATES
123 MAIN STREET • ANYTOWN, FL 32711 • 407-555-1234

PATIENT: BURNHAM, KERRY
ACCOUNT/EHR #:   BURKE001
Date: 12/21/11

Attending Physician: Donald J. Peters, MD

S: This Pt is a 27-year-old female who was here two years ago. Today, she presents for a prophylactic vaccination required by her new job, working as a laboratory technician. She is otherwise healthy and has no other stated health concerns.

O: Vaccine was administered. I gave the patient a brochure with information about the vaccine and possible side effects.

A: Inoculation against smallpox, IM

P: Follow-up prn

_____

Donald J. Peters, MD

DJP/mg   D: 12/21/11 09:50:16 T: 12/22/11 12:55:01

You Code It!

What are the best, most accurate codes?

Diagnosis Codes: _____

Procedure Codes: _____

Anesthesia Codes (when applicable): _____

HCPCS Level II codes (when applicable): _____

FAMILY DOCTORS ASSOCIATES
123 MAIN STREET • ANYTOWN, FL 32711 • 407-555-1234

PATIENT: DAUPHINE, DOLORES
ACCOUNT/EHR #:   DAUDO001
Date: 02/05/11

Attending Physician: James Healer, MD

S: Pt is a 15-year-old female seen in our office for a physical exam as a requirement for her admission to the Marlberry School for Girls.

O: BP 130/95 P normal R normal Ht 5'0" Wt 165 lb. HEENT: unremarkable. Heart and lung sounds unremarkable. Pt is clinically obese. Elevated blood pressure noted. Extensive discussion with pt regarding her weight, the health risks associated with obesity, and the options available to her.

A: Obesity, benign essential hypertension

P: 1. Complete school admission form
     2. Referral to nutritionist for diet and exercise regime
     3. Return for check-up in 6 months

James Healer, MD

JH/mg   D: 02/05/11 09:50:16 T: 02/08/11 12:55:01

You Code It!

What are the best, most accurate codes?

Diagnosis Codes: _____

Procedure Codes: _____

Anesthesia Codes (when applicable): _____

HCPCS Level II codes (when applicable): _____

FAMILY DOCTORS ASSOCIATES
123 MAIN STREET • ANYTOWN, FL 32711 • 407-555-1234

PATIENT: TRENTON, BASIL
ACCOUNT/EHR #: TREBA001
Date: 02/05/11

S: Pt is a 43-year-old male who comes to the office today, accompanied by his wife, for a follow-up visit for his hypertension. After addressing the issues related to his hypertension, the patient says, "By the way doc, I am so tired. I've been having trouble sleeping. Are sleeping pills all right to take?" His wife states. "You need to do something about his sleeping. He snores so loud it is ridiculous. He keeps me up all night with that noise. When I finally get to sleep, he sometimes kicks me and wakes me up as he gasps for air."

PAST MEDICAL HISTORY: Significant only for obesity and hypertension.

FAMILY HISTORY: Noncontributory. Patient denies psychiatry history.

SOCIAL HISTORY: The patient denies any alcohol use or abuse, caffeine use, stimulants, or street drug abuse or history of it.

MEDICATIONS: Patient only takes thiazide diuretic for control of hypertension and denies nocturia.

Patient denies palpitations, diaphoresis, tremor, or any other signs of thyroid disease. When asked if he sleeps alone, pt states "I never sleep alone and my partner never has any complaints."

ROS: Pt denies arthritis, burning sensation when eating foods, and abdominal pain associated with meals, or angina. Pt denies leg weakness and pain when performing activities or at rest.

O: PHYSICAL EXAMINATION

VITAL SIGNS: Temp 38.1; blood pressure 150/80; pulse 80; respiration 16; weight 250 lb; height 5'3".

GENERAL: Obese male, generally awake/alert/oriented. Speech understandable and comprehensible, without slurring or hesitation. No infection identified; uvula, palate are midline, noninflamed, and normal in size. There are no masses palpable in the thyroid. Chest wall absent for deformities, breathing is deep with regular rate, good air exchange without wheezes or egophony. Heart exam within normal limits. Abdominal exam within normal limits. Neurologic exam is grossly intact.

TEST RESULTS: Labs come back with elevated hemoglobin & hematocrit, normal WBCs, normal renal function, normal thyroid panel. Polysomnogram is ordered.

A: Obstructive sleep apnea

P: 1. Rx: Continuous positive airway pressure (CPAP) equipment
   2. Recommend weight loss. Offer of referral to nutritionist.

_____

James Healer, MD

JHW/mg   D: 02/05/11 09:50:16   T: 02/08/11 12:55:01

You Code It!

What are the best, most accurate codes?

Diagnosis Codes: _____

Procedure Codes: _____

Anesthesia Codes (when applicable): _____

HCPCS Level II codes (when applicable): _____

FAMILY DOCTORS ASSOCIATES
123 MAIN STREET • ANYTOWN, FL 32711 • 407-555-1234

PATIENT: WITZKE, REBECCA
ACCOUNT/EHR #:   WITRE001
Date: 02/05/11

This patient is a 34-year-old Caucasian woman who presents complaining of headaches.

HISTORY OF PRESENT ILLNESS: She describes her current headaches as happening every day in mid-afternoon for the past month. The pain is steady, nonpulsatile, and starts in the occipital region with bilateral radiation to the frontal area. There is no associated aura or photophobia. She is not awakened from sleep with the headaches, and she does not wake up in the morning with a headache. Tylenol lessens the discomfort "sometimes."

When asked if there were any other complaints Mrs. Witzke wishes to discuss, she mentions significant stress at home regarding her 11-year-old son. Her concern centers on continued problems with discipline. "He just won't listen to me anymore—he's always beating up on his little brother and getting into fights at school. His grades have really dropped, and he might even be held back this year. I just don't know what to do." In reviewing Mrs. Witzke's chart I note she has been in to our office seven times over the past year.

SOCIAL HISTORY: Patient is a college graduate who works part-time as a nursery school teacher. She and her husband, an accountant, have two sons, ages 11 and 6. Further discussion reveals that Mrs. Witzke's husband has become increasingly controlling over the past few years. In fact, he often calls home up to ten times per day, making sure Mrs. Witzke comes home right after work or appointments and stays at home until he returns from work. Mrs. Witzke then discloses that he grabbed her around the neck once. "But it was only once . . . and that was a few weeks ago. It was probably my fault, because dinner wasn't ready when he got home, and he becomes kind of hypoglycemic."

The patient also states her husband shoved her a few months ago in the kitchen during a dispute over how she has been handling their son. The following day she went to the ED after work. X-rays of her lower extremities showed no fractures, but significant swelling persisted in her knees for a few weeks. Mrs. Witzke reassured me that she feels safe going back to her home, and that she in fact does not want to leave.

PERSONAL MEDICAL HISTORY: Hypothyroidism and headaches

MEDICATIONS: Synthroid l25 mcg each day, Tylenol 650 mg two or three times a day

VITAL SIGNS: Temp 98.1; BP 135/85; pulse 80; respiration 20; weight 145 lb; height 5'3".

GENERAL: Her physical exam is unremarkable with normal vital signs and neurological exam.

Continued

LABS:TSH from 6 months ago = 0.l5 mcg/mL and cholesterol 2 years ago= 172 mg/dL.

A: Stress headaches

P: I supplied the patient with the phone number for the National Domestic Violence Hotline (1-800-799-SAFE). I explained that they are available at all times and can give her the location of the nearest shelter. I called in a report to the Hotline at 3:42 p.m.

James Healer, MD

JHW/mg   D: 02/05/11 03:50:16   T: 02/08/11 12:55:01

You Code It!

What are the best, most accurate codes?

Diagnosis Codes: _____

Procedure Codes: _____

Anesthesia Codes (when applicable): _____

HCPCS Level II codes (when applicable): _____

FAMILY DOCTORS ASSOCIATES
123 MAIN STREET • ANYTOWN, FL 32711 • 407-555-1234

PATIENT: PRICE, JANICE
ACCOUNT/EHR #:   PRIJA001
Date: 02/05/11

S: This new patient is a 56-year-old white female with a 4-month history of increasing fatigue and frequent urination. She denies fever, chills, back pain, or hematuria. She denies any recent viral illnesses. Appetite is normal. Fatigue is chronic over the past few months, which has made it difficult for her to carry out her duties as a cashier at a local grocery store.

PAST MEDICAL HISTORY: Hypertension—well controlled; Menopause age 53

PAST SURGICAL HISTORY: Tonsillectomy age 6, Cholecystectomy age 51

FAMILY HISTORY:
- Father deceased, age 68 of myocardial infarction. History included HTN & AODM.
- Mother deceased, age 74 of ruptured aortic aneurysm. History included osteoarthritis and HTN.
- Brother alive age 61—AODM, HTN, BPH.
- Maternal grandmother deceased, age 54 of breast cancer
- Maternal grandfather deceased, age 31 of industrial accident
- Paternal grandmother deceased, age 70 of a stroke. History included HTN, AODM, obesity.
- Paternal grandfather deceased, age 45 of myocardial infarction.

SOCIAL HISTORY: Married, rare alcohol intake and has never smoked. Employed as a cashier in a local grocery store. Three grown children. Good relationship with her husband. Completed high school education.

MEDICATIONS: Hydrochlorothiazide 12.5 mg daily; Conjugated estrogen 0.625 mg daily, Medroxyprogesterone acetate 2.5 mg daily

O: Height 5'1" and weight is stable at 190 lb. B/P 146/88 Pulse 82 Resp. 16

OPTHALMOLOGIC EXAM: PERRLA, EOMI

FUNDUSCOPIC EXAM: Disc sharp, macula appears normal, vessels without nicking, no abnormalities noted

CARDIAC EXAM: Regular rate and rhythm, without murmur, rub, gallop PMI normal

PULSES: Femoral, popliteal, dorsalis pedis, posterior tibial normal. No bruits noted.

FOOT EXAM: Skin and nails free from breaks in the skin/ulcers, 6-mm callous plantar surface of L foot, monofilament testing reveals normal sensation. Proprioception intact R & L. Gait reveals pronation during walking.

THYROID: Smooth, not enlarged, no nodules palpated

Continued

SKIN EXAM: Multiple nevi (normal appearing), few seborrheic keratoses on back, no skin lesions or ulcers noted.

NEUROLOGIC EXAM: Grossly intact

DENTAL EXAM: Anodontia, upper and lower dentures removed—no ulcers or lesions noted. Well-fitted dentures.

A: Diabetes mellitus (type 2), hypertension, and obesity.

P: Rx: Lisinopril 10 mg daily for her blood pressure; atorvastatin (Lipitor) 10 mg each evening for her hypercholesterolemia, and aspirin 81 mg daily. Referral to a dietician and diabetes educator for diet and exercise guidance. Rx home blood glucose monitor, blood pressure monitor

James Healer, MD

JHW/mg   D: 02/05/11 03:50:16   T: 02/08/11 12:55:01

You Code It!

What are the best, most accurate codes?

Diagnosis Codes: _____

Procedure Codes: _____

Anesthesia Codes (when applicable): _____

HCPCS Level II codes (when applicable): _____

PATIENT: ESTRADA, DAWN
ACCOUNT/EHR #:   ESTDA001
Date: 02/05/11

S: This new patient is a 35-year-old African-American female complaining of pain when she urinates. She is a divorced mother of three children ages 3, 5, and 9. She admits to having multiple sexual partners. She has not used any form of birth control since undergoing tubal ligation after the birth of her last child. She is not sure when her last menstrual period was because her menses have always been irregular. She thinks it was six weeks ago. Other than a recent URI, she states that she has been in good health. She has no other complaints.

HISTORY OF PRESENT ILLNESS: Upon further questioning I learned that this patient has been experiencing mild pelvic pain. She also says that she feels like she "always has to go." She has been waking up four to five times at night to urinate for the last two nights. Although she has not taken her temperature, she has felt warm now and then over the past week, but she dismisses this as part of her recent cold symptoms. She denies blood in her urine, chills, or an increased sense of urgency to urinate. She has never had a urinary tract infection. She admits that she has been feeling fatigued and run down lately. Her job is becomingly increasingly stressful as she takes on more responsibility. When asked about her sexual history, she states that since the divorce she has been seeing a few guys she met in local clubs. She refers to this as "sowing her wild oats." She says she married and had children at such a young age that she missed out on a lot of the experiences other women her age have already enjoyed. She loves her children but finds them overwhelming when they "act like little devils."

PAST MEDICAL HISTORY: Asthma, allergic rhinitis

PAST SURGICAL HISTORY: Appendectomy age 13; Tubal ligation after the birth of her last child

MEDICATIONS: Albuterol inhaler and Claritin, as often as she can get samples from the city clinic

SOCIAL HISTORY: Patient works full-time as an assistant manager in a retail store. Only recently has she begun receiving health insurance benefits. She has not had regular annual gynecological exams or received any consistent health care. She drinks 2–3 beers per day, usually more on the weekends to help her deal with the stress of her children. She denies tobacco or illicit drug use.

FAMILY HISTORY: Mother—diabetes type 2, hypertension. Father died last year of an MI at age 60.

O: PHYSICAL EXAMINATION

VITALS: Temp 99.0F, Pulse 82, BP 127/84, Resp 16/min

HEENT: Head normocephalic. PERRL. EOMI. oropharynx and TMs clear.

NECK: Some nodal enlargement in the anterior cervical chain. Nontender.

CV: S1, S2, RRR. No murmurs, rubs, or gallops appreciated.

CHEST: Good air exchange. Slight expiratory wheezes over upper lung fields. No crackles. No CVA tenderness.

ABDOMEN: 1BS. soft, ND. Diffuse lower quadrant tenderness. Marked suprapubic tenderness. No rebound or guarding.

EXTREMITIES: Peripheral pulses strong and equal bilaterally. DTRs 2 upper and lower extremities.

RECTAL: Not performed

Continued

GYNECOLOGIC: Normal external genitalia without lesions. Cervix and vaginal wall appeared normal. No bacteria or fungus were seen on KOH prep and wet mount. GC and chlamydia cultures sent. Bimanual exam shows normal size uterus, no cervical motion tenderness, and no adnexal masses or tenderness.

TEST RESULTS: UA dipstick positive for UTI

DX: Urinary tract infection, pathogenic strains of E. coli

RX; Septra, p.o. one TAB b.i.d. x3

James Healer, MD

JHW/mg   D: 02/05/11 03:50:16   T: 02/08/11 12:55:01

You Code It!

What are the best, most accurate codes?

Diagnosis Codes: _____

Procedure Codes: _____

Anesthesia Codes (when applicable): _____

HCPCS Level II codes (when applicable): _____

FAMILY DOCTORS ASSOCIATES
123 MAIN STREET • ANYTOWN, FL 32711 • 407-555-1234

PATIENT: LYND, GORDON
ACCOUNT/EHR #:   LYNGO001
Date: 02/05/11

S: This patient is a 46-year-old, middle-aged, well-appearing male, slightly overweight, who comes to see me in the office for a physical exam before taking up a new exercise program he heard about on TV. I have not seen this patient in two years. He has no significant past medical history and is generally in good health. He works as a busy executive at an amusement park, and his wife thinks that he could stand to lose a few pounds.

FAMILY HISTORY: Both parents still living, although his father just had a triple bypass operation a year ago at age 72. He knows of no other history of heart disease or hypertension.

SOCIAL HISTORY: The patient explains that he currently has not been making the time for exercise in his busy schedule. He is interested in trying to walk at lunchtime 3-4 days a week for about a half hour. He drinks two cups of coffee in the morning at work every day. He does not smoke, and he drinks a glass of wine two nights a week with dinner.

PAST MEDICAL HISTORY: His past BPs have been running in the 130s–140s over 80s–90s.

MEDICATIONS: Multivitamin.

O: VITAL SIGNS: Ht 6 ft O in. Wt 210 lb. BP 156/94 P 82 R 12 T 98.3

ROS reveals no shortness of breath; no palpitations; no headache or sweats; no orthopnea, paroxysmal nocturnal dyspnea, or lower extremity edema.

MENTAL STATUS: Alert and oriented x 3.

CRANIAL NERVES: II–XII intact

FUNDI: No retinopathy, no AV nicking, no papilledema. No exophthalmos.

NECK: No thyromegaly, no carotid bruits, no JVD

HEART: PMI in the MCL, nondisplaced, nonenlarged. No sternal heave. S1 S2 present, regular, no S3 or S4, no murmurs, no rubs.

LUNGS: Chest is symmetric with equal breath sounds. No changes to percussion.

ABDOMEN: BS present, normoactive, no renal or aortic bruits. Soft, nondistended, nontender, no striae. No hepatosplenomegaly.

Continued

EXTREMITIES: Upper: radial pulses 2 bilateral. Lower: No edema, erythema. DP and femoral pulses 2+ bilateral.

LAB RESULTS: U/A, CBC, electrolytes, renals, glucose, cholesterol, and ECG are within normal limits.

A: Essential hypertension

P: Patient is told to come back in 6 weeks for a BP recheck.

Rx: Hydrochlorothiazide, 25 mg

James Healer, MD

JHW/mg   D: 02/05/11 03:50:16   T: 02/08/11 12:55:01

You Code It!

What are the best, most accurate codes?

Diagnosis Codes: _____

Procedure Codes: _____

Anesthesia Codes (when applicable): _____

HCPCS Level II codes (when applicable): _____

FAMILY DOCTORS ASSOCIATES
123 MAIN STREET • ANYTOWN, FL 32711 • 407-555-1234

PATIENT: LAFONE, MICHELLE
ACCOUNT/EHR #:   LAFMI001
Date: 02/05/11

This patient is a 56-year-old African-American woman who is well-known to me. Eight years ago I diagnosed her with type II diabetes mellitus, and she is here today for a regular check-up (including her feet) and to go over her most recent lab results.

PAST MEDICAL HISTORY: She is currently taking medications to control her blood sugars. She checks herself about once a day, sometimes forgetting, and usually runs around 130s to 160s. She is postmenopausal, overweight, and her blood pressure has been around 142/90 the past several visits. She has no other significant past medical history. She last visited her ophthalmologist 6 months ago and has not had any retinopathic changes yet.

SOCIAL HISTORY: She does not smoke or drink alcohol.

FAMILY HISTORY: Her father died at age 70 from renal failure from diabetes, but her mother is alive and well, having just had triple heart bypass surgery last year.

MEDICATIONS: Metformin, Rosiglitazone

LAB RESULTS: Her HbA1c is 8.1%, and she has some microalbuminuria (60 mg/d). A BUN and Cr are 35 and 1.3 respectively. A fasting lipid profile revealed total cholesterol 262, LDL 174, HDL 50, triglycerides 162.

A: Diabetes mellitus, type 2, essential hypertension

Rx: Captopril, 25 mg, t.i.d.

I explained to the patient the benefits this medication will have for her, emphasizing its importance in decreasing the progression of renal impairment. I also reiterated to her the importance of controlling her blood glucose levels. She seems to comprehend my advice and agrees to begin taking the Captopril as well as to pay closer attention to her glucose checks.

James Healer, MD

JHW/mg   D: 02/05/11 03:50:16   T: 02/08/11 12:55:01

You Code It!

What are the best, most accurate codes?

Diagnosis Codes: _____

Procedure Codes: _____

Anesthesia Codes (when applicable): _____

HCPCS Level II codes (when applicable): _____

FAMILY DOCTORS ASSOCIATES
123 MAIN STREET • ANYTOWN, FL 32711 • 407-555-1234

PATIENT: PICKARD, BARNEY
ACCOUNT/EHR #: PICBA001
Date: 02/05/11

This patient is a 74-year-old patient of mine for the past 20 years. He is a retired construction worker who now lives at home alone after his wife's recent death. He has COPD from years of smoking, but quit 12 years ago. I asked the patient how he is doing with the diuretic I had prescribed, and he good-naturedly responded that he hasn't been able to keep track of it real well now that his wife isn't there nagging him all the time. I explain to him that it is important for him to take his medication. He states, "Hey, doc, come on, I'm 74 already and haven't had any health problems! What's the big deal anyways?" I patiently stress further to Mr. Pickard the importance of this medication. He agrees to try harder to stay on schedule with his HCTZ. "It'll be just like punchin' the clock, doc; no problem."

PAST MEDICAL HISTORY: He had an appendectomy as a child and three inguinal hernia repairs during his working life. He has long-standing HTN, and that has never been well-controlled. We tried him on clonidine, methyldopa, and prazosin back when those were the choice drugs. I recently switched him to hydrochlorothiazide (25 mg) from clonidine to see if it couldn't make an impact on his BP.

FAMILY HISTORY: He can't remember what his parents died from, but thinks it was "old age."

VITAL SIGNS: BP 176/104.

DX: Essential hypertension

RX: Nifedipine

_____

James Healer, MD

JHW/mg   D: 02/05/11 03:50:16   T: 02/08/11 12:55:01

You Code It!

What are the best, most accurate codes?

Diagnosis Codes: _____

Procedure Codes: _____

Anesthesia Codes (when applicable): _____

HCPCS Level II codes (when applicable): _____

FAMILY DOCTORS ASSOCIATES
123 MAIN STREET • ANYTOWN, FL 32711 • 407-555-1234

PATIENT: CHASTEN, LORRAINE
ACCOUNT/EHR #:   CHALO001
Date: 02/13/11

This patient is a 45-year-old white female with complaints of abdominal pain. She sees me yearly for her gynecologic exam but does not regularly visit for any other reason. She states that her pain began about three weeks prior to her presentation and has gradually worsened. The pain is sharp in nature and located in the middle of her upper abdomen, just below her rib cage. It occurs most often between meals and is relieved with meals only to recur several hours later. She denies any weight loss, anorexia, dysphagia, diarrhea, or constipation. Her stools are a bit darker than usual but without any signs of bright red blood. She has never had pain like this in the past, is uncertain as to its cause, and has been using some over-the-counter antacid without relief. Her last menstrual period was three weeks prior to her presentation and was of the usual timing (q 28 days) and duration (five days). Her abdominal pain did not worsen during the time of her menses. She does not consider her periods heavy.

PAST MEDICAL HISTORY: She has three healthy children delivered by cesarean section but no other surgery. She has a history of seasonal allergies for which she takes over-the-counter antihistamines with good relief.

MEDICATIONS: None. She denies use of aspirin or nonsteroidal products.

ALLERGIES: Meperidine (Demerol) caused her to break out in a rash, her only medication allergy.

SOCIAL HISTORY: She is physically active, running two or three miles every other day. She uses condoms and spermicidal lubricant for birth control. She is sexually active with her boyfriend of the last 6 months, with whom she feels safe and supported; she has no history of domestic violence. She has never contracted a sexually transmitted disease. She has smoked one pack of cigarettes a day for 25 years, rarely drinks alcoholic beverages, and uses no other substances. She works as a legal secretary for a large law firm. Her oldest child, a son, is away at college; her two youngest children are at home, including a 12-year-old daughter recently diagnosed with a learning disability. She had all of her children by her former husband from whom she's been divorced for three years. She reports some stress related to being a single parent and sharing custody but does not believe that this is the cause of her abdominal pain.

FAMILY HISTORY: Her father is alive and well despite suffering a myocardial infarction at age 62. Her mother died from colon cancer at age 60. She has two sisters who are alive and well, ages 40 and 47.

PHYSICAL EXAMINATION: She is a thin white female, appearing her stated age. Her weight at this visit is 125 pounds. Her blood pressure is 110/67 mmHg supine and 105/60 mmHg standing. Her heart rate is 68/min supine and 72/min standing. Her conjunctiva are without pallor; mucus membranes are moist.

Continued

There are no oral lesions. Neck is without bruits or thyromegaly. Lungs are clear to auscultation and percussion. Heart is regular without murmurs rubs or gallops. Abdomen is soft and nondistended with normoactive bowel sounds. There is epigastric tenderness to palpation without rebound or guarding. Murphy's sign is positive. Stool is dark brown and tests guaiac negative for occult blood. Deep tendon reflexes are 2 and equal. Skin is without lesions.

LAB RESULTS: Evidence of infection with *H. pylori.* Her duodenal biopsy is negative for malignancy.

DX: Cholelithiasis

RECOMMENDATION: I recommend that the patient have a laparoscopic cholecystectomy. After explaining the benefits and dangers of this surgery, she agrees. Referral to general surgeon.

James Healer, MD

JHW/mg   D: 02/13/11 03:50:16   T: 02/18/11 12:55:01

You Code It!

What are the best, most accurate codes?

Diagnosis Codes: _____

Procedure Codes: _____

Anesthesia Codes (when applicable): _____

HCPCS Level II codes (when applicable): _____

Gastroenterology Cases and Patient Records

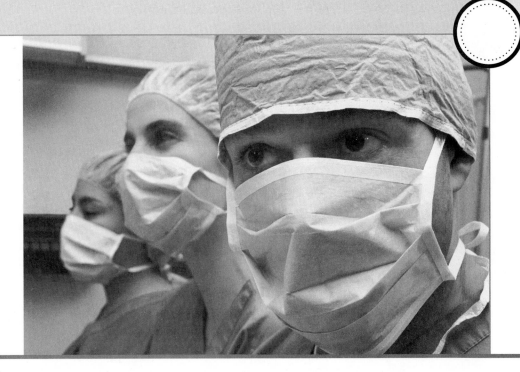

INTRODUCTION

The following case studies are from a gastroenterology practice. In a physician's office of this type, a professional coding specialist will have patients with signs, symptoms, and diagnoses involving the digestive system.

Gastroenterologists are physicians who specialize in the diagnosis and treatment of diseases of the digestive system, such as gastroesophageal reflux disease (GERD), hiatal hernia, peptic ulcers, irritable bowel syndrome, and colon or rectal cancer.

In their care of these patients, gastroenterologists may administer many specialized tests, such as sigmoidoscopy, esophagogastroduodenoscopy (EGD), and colonoscopy, to screen for diseases and disorders, as well as to accurately diagnose and/or treat diseases of the gastrointestinal system.

These specialists can be board-certified by the American Board of Internal Medicine, which is recognized by the American Board of Medical Specialties.

Within the specialty of gastroenterology, there is a subspecialty: colonrectal surgery. Colonrectal surgeons typically focus on the diagnosis and treatment of diseases such as colon cancer, Crohn's disease, ulcerative colitis, and conditions such as hemorrhoids.

Board certification for colon and rectal surgeons is awarded through the American Board of Colon and Rectal Surgery, which is also recognized by the American Board of Medical Specialties.

You can use these cases to practice coding diagnoses, E/M, procedures, DME, or other HCPCS Level II items, as applicable; code for the physician or the facility:

1. Code for the physician.
2. Code for the anesthesiologist, when applicable.
3. Code for the hospital, when applicable.
4. Code for the pathology and laboratory, when applicable.
5. Code HCPCS Level II codes, when applicable.

CARROLTON DIGESTIVE MEDICINE, PA
765 SWOLLOW PATH • PASSING, FL 32811 • 407-555-7985

PATIENT NAME: Friedman, Doris
MRN: FRIEDO001
Date: 23 September 2011

Procedure performed: Colonoscopy

Physician: Matthew Appellet, MD

Indications: History of inflammatory bowel disease

Procedure: The patient was given no premedication at her request and the Olympus PCF-130 colonoscope was used. The mucosa of the rectum was essentially normal apart from some mild nonspecific edema. Photographs and biopsies were obtained. The remainder of the rectum was normal. The sigmoid was normal as was the descending colon, splenic flexure, transverse colon, hepatic flexure, right colon, and cecum. No evidence of polyps, tumors, masses, or inflammation. The scope was then withdrawn, these findings confirmed. The procedure was terminated and the patient tolerated it well.

Impression: Normal colonic mucosa through the cecum.

Plan: Await results of rectal biopsies.

09/23/11 19:38:17

You Code It!

What are the best, most accurate codes?

Diagnosis Codes: _____

Procedure Codes: _____

Anesthesia Codes (when applicable): _____

HCPCS Level II codes (when applicable): _____

CARROLTON DIGESTIVE MEDICINE, PA
765 SWOLLOW PATH • PASSING, FL 32811 • 407-555-7985

PATIENT: BENJAMIN, DAVIDA
ACCOUNT/EHR #:   BENJDA001
Date: 09/16/11

Attending Physician: Suzanne R. Taylor, MD

S: Pt is a 49-year-old female complaining of abdominal pain. She states that the pain has been consistent since noon, and she has been vomiting since 2 p.m. She has been experiencing chills and weakness as well. No diarrhea. Last BM was a small one at 7 A.M. and again at 2 P.M. She was in good health prior to the symptoms at noon. She also has GERD.

   Patient had a total hysterectomy 3 years ago and a laparoscopic cholecystectomy 10 years ago. She quit smoking 10 years ago. Current meds: Evista, Prevacid p.r.n.

O: Wt 140 Ht 5′2″ T 99 P 90 R 18 BP 128/73. Abdomen distended, tympanic, tender. CT scan abd/pelvis: Dilated small bowel loop appears to contain semisolid material in RLQ, compatible with early small bowel obstruction. EKG: Sinus tachycardia, otherwise normal EKG. Bowel sounds are normal and hypoactive. Breathing pattern is nonlabored, breath sounds clear. Heart rhythm: Regular. Neck veins: Nondistended. Skin: warm, dry, intact. Peripheral pulses: Normal. CBC w/differential: WBC, RBC, HGB, and HCT are high; MCHC is low; all other results unremarkable. Glucose and BUN/Creat are high, anion gap is low, all other chemistry unremarkable. UA: UR is cloudy, glucose high.

A: Small bowel obstruction; pure hypercholesterolemia; diaphragmatic hernia; esophageal reflux

P: Admit to hospital for surgery

_____

Suzanne R. Taylor, MD

SRT/pw   D: 09/16/11 09:50:16   T: 09/18/11 12:55:01

You Code It!

What are the best, most accurate codes?

Diagnosis Codes: _____

Procedure Codes: _____

Anesthesia Codes (when applicable): _____

HCPCS Level II codes (when applicable): _____

CARROLTON DIGESTIVE MEDICINE, PA
765 SWOLLOW PATH • PASSING, FL 32811 • 407-555-7985

PATIENT NAME: CASTANO, FELICIA
ACCOUNT #:   CASTFEO1
Date: 3 November 2011

Attending Physician: Califf M. Mohammed, MD

DX: Rectal bleeding

PROCEDURE: After obtaining informed consent and explaining the risks and benefits of the procedure to the patient, a colonoscopy was performed with the patient's approval. Conscious sedation was obtained using 100 micrograms of fentanyl IV and 4 mg of Versed IV.

    The PCF-160AL colonoscope was advanced from the rectum up to and including the cecum without difficulty. The ileocecal value was visualized, as was the appendiceal orifice. The colonoscopy was notable for internal hemorrhoids, external hemorrhoids seen on rectal examination. Additionally, there was a 0.8-cm polyp in the rectum at approximately 15 cm. This was removed with the snare and sent to pathology. The specimen labeled #1, rectal polyp appears tan-pink, measuring 0.6x0.5x0.3 cm in greatest dimension. The polyp is bisected longitudinally and entirely submitted in one cassette.

ASSESSMENT: 1. Polyp
                2. Hemorrhoids

PLAN: Will check pathology. Assuming it is adenomatous, repeat colonoscopy in 3 years.

_____

Califf M. Mohammed, MD

CMM/mg   D: 11/03/11 10:57:00 T: 11/05/11 08:19:10

You Code It!

What are the best, most accurate codes?

Diagnosis Codes: _____

Procedure Codes: _____

Anesthesia Codes (when applicable): _____

HCPCS Level II codes (when applicable): _____

CARROLTON DIGESTIVE MEDICINE, PA
765 SWOLLOW PATH • PASSING, FL 32811 • 407-555-7985

PATIENT: MILLER, JUDITH
ACCOUNT/EHR #:   MILJU001
Date: 10/15/11

Admitting Diagnosis: Gastrointestinal hemorrhage

HISTORY OF PRESENT ILLNESS: The patient is a 71-year-old white female who presents with maroon stools.

The patient noticed several episodes of maroon stools with clot yesterday. She called on the phone, was told to come to the emergency room (ER). The patient did not come to the ER and instead came to the office. There, she was noted to have normal vital signs and maroon stools in the rectal vault. The patient is now admitted for further evaluation.

PAST MEDICAL HISTORY: The patient denies any previous history of gastrointestinal bleeding. She does have a history of arthritis and has been on Daypro.

ALLERGIES: Bactrim

SOCIAL HISTORY: Negative for smoking or drinking

FAMILY HISTORY: Noncontributory

REVIEW OF SYSTEMS: Notable for marked anxiety

PHYSICAL EXAMINATION

GENERAL: This is a well-developed, well-nourished, white female who was markedly anxious.

VITAL SIGNS: Pulse 80, BP 130/70

HEENT: Conjunctivae pink. Sclerae anicteric

NECK: Without jugular venous distention

LUNGS: Clear

HEART: Regular rhythm

ABDOMEN: Bowel sounds present, nontender, no rebound or guarding. NO masses or organomegaly.

EXTREMITIES: No cyanosis, clubbing or edema

Continued

RECTAL: Exam revealed maroon stools.

IMPRESSION: 1. Gastrointestinal bleeding, etiology to be determined
2. Anxiety
3. Allergy to Bactrim

SUGGESTIONS: 1. Follow vital signs closely
2. Colonoscopy
3. Gastroscopy if colonoscopy is negative
4. Transfuse p.r.n

Harold R. Carrolton, MD

HRC/fa 10/15/11 11:47:39

You Code It!

What are the best, most accurate codes?

Diagnosis Codes: _____

Procedure Codes: _____

Anesthesia Codes (when applicable): _____

HCPCS Level II codes (when applicable): _____

CARROLTON DIGESTIVE MEDICINE, PA
765 SWOLLOW PATH • PASSING, FL 32811 • 407-555-7985

PATIENT: MILLER, JUDITH
ACCOUNT/EHR #:   MILJU001
Date: 10/15/11

Procedure: Colonoscopy
Indications for Procedure: Gastrointestinal bleeding

DESCRIPTION OF OPERATION: The patient was placed in the left lateral decubitus position. She was gradually sedated with 10 mg of intravenous Versed and 50 mg of intravenous Demerol. Her perirectal area was inspected and no lesions noted. Digital examination revealed no masses or tenderness. The Olympus single channel colonoscope was introduced into the rectum and directed under visual control through the sigmoid, descending, transverse, and ascending colon to the cecum. Position of the cecum was confirmed by visualization of the ileocecal valve, ballottement, and transillumination. The mucosa throughout the colon was intact without evidence of edema, erythema, or friability. The patient had extensive diverticulosis with circular muscle hypertrophy. There were no masses or polyps. There was no bleeding in the lower GI tract. The colon was decompressed and the endoscope removed. The patient tolerated the procedure well.

IMPRESSIONS: 1. Uncomplicated diverticulosis
2. Internal hemorrhoids
3. No evidence of any bleeding in the colon

Harold R. Carrolton, MD

HRC/fa 10/15/11 11:47:39

You Code It!

What are the best, most accurate codes?

Diagnosis Codes: _____

Procedure Codes: _____

Anesthesia Codes (when applicable): _____

HCPCS Level II codes (when applicable): _____

CARROLTON DIGESTIVE MEDICINE, PA
765 SWOLLOW PATH • PASSING, FL 32811 • 407-555-7985

PATIENT: MILLER, JUDITH
ACCOUNT/EHR #:   MILJU001
Date: 10/15/11

Procedure: Gastroscopy and biopsy
Indications for Procedure: Gastrointestinal bleeding and negative colonoscopy

DESCRIPTION OF OPERATION: The patient had received 10 mg of intravenous Versed and 50 mg of intravenous Demerol for sedation. The oropharynx was anesthetized with Cetacaine spray. The Olympus video gastroscope was then passed through the cricopharyngeal muscle into the esophagus, stomach, and duodenum. The esophagus was unremarkable. The stomach was entered. There was evidence of multiple gastric ulcers involving the antrum and prepyloric area. There was some blood adherent to the ulcers along the anterior aspect of the antrum. There was no active bleeding noted. The duodenal bulb and duodenal sweep were unremarkable. The endoscope was returned to the stomach and retroflexed. The cardia was observed and no additional lesions identified. Biopsies were taken of the ulcers for histology. The patient tolerated the procedure well.

IMPRESSIONS: Multiple small gastric ulcers

Harold R. Carrolton, MD

HRC/fa 10/15/11 11:47:39

You Code It!

What are the best, most accurate codes?

Diagnosis Codes: _____

Procedure Codes: _____

Anesthesia Codes (when applicable): _____

HCPCS Level II codes (when applicable): _____

CARROLTON DIGESTIVE MEDICINE, PA
765 SWOLLOW PATH • PASSING, FL 32811 • 407-555-7985

PATIENT: PATCHMON, PETER
ACCOUNT/EHR #: PATPE001
Date: 10/15/11

Preop Diagnosis: Acute cholecystitis, cholelithiasis
Postop Diagnosis: Acute cholecystitis, cholelithiasis
Procedure: Laparoscopic cholecystectomy

Surgeon: Derick Marks, MD
Assistant: Frank Scottsboro, MD

Anesthesia: General endotracheal
Findings at Surgery: Pericholecystic adhesions, large gallstones

DESCRIPTION OF OPERATION: After the induction of general endotracheal anesthesia, the patient's abdomen was prepped and draped in the usual sterile manner and a small infraumbilical incision was made in the skin and carried down to the linea alba, which was grasped with a clamp and incised in a vertical manner. The peritoneum was entered under direct vision. Stay sutures were placed in the fascia. The Hasson introducer was placed. Pneumoperitoneum was established, and following this, three additional trocars were placed in the abdomen: one in the left epigastrium and two in the right upper quadrant, all 5.0 mm. Following this, the gallbladder was grasped with cephalad retraction of the gallbladder fundus and lateralward retraction of the gallbladder infundibulum. The dissector was employed to take down the peritoneum overlying the gallbladder infundibulum and cystic duct junction. When this was well delineated on both the anterior and posterior surfaces of the cystic duct, the 5-mm endoscopic clip applier was inserted and two clips were placed on the patient's side, on the gallbladder side of the cystic duct, which was transected. Further dissection in the triangle of Calot revealed the cystic artery, which was handled in an identical manner. The remainder of the dissection was performed by using the Bovie spatula cautery, and the liver bed was dry. A 10- to 15-mm camera change-out was performed, and the camera was inserted into the left epigastric port. A toothed clamp was passed through the umbilicus to grasp the gallbladder, which was then removed through the umbilicus in a standard manner. Following this, the operative field was copiously irrigated with saline and the return was clear. All three upper abdominal ports were seen to exit the abdomen under direct vision, and with the Hasson introducer removed, the fascial incision was closed with a 2-0 Vicryl figure-of-eight suture. The skin at the umbilicus was closed with a 4-0 Maxon subcuticular suture. Steri-strips were applied at all sites. The patient tolerated the procedure well.

ADDENDUM: There were three cystic artery branches; each was doubly clipped and transected.

Derick Marks, MD

DM/fa 10/15/11 11:47:39

You Code It!

What are the best, most accurate codes?

Diagnosis Codes: _____

Procedure Codes: _____

Anesthesia Codes (when applicable): _____

HCPCS Level II codes (when applicable): _____

CARROLTON DIGESTIVE MEDICINE, PA
765 SWOLLOW PATH • PASSING, FL 32811 • 407-555-7985

PATIENT: HART, LOUIS
ACCOUNT/EHR #:   HARLO001
Date: 09/15/11

Admission Diagnosis: 1. Abdominal pain with symptomatic cholelithiasis
                         2. History of depression
                         3. History of degenerative joint disease
Final Diagnosis: 1. Abdominal pain secondary to cholelithiasis, status post laparoscopic
                            cholecystectomy
                         2. History of depression
                         3. History of degenerative joint disease

DISCHARGE INSTRUCTIONS: Medications: Keflex 500 mg one tablet four times a day for one week,
Percocet 2.5/325 one tablet four times a day p.r.n for pain, Vicodin 5.0/500 one or two tablets p.o q4h
p.r.n for pain. Recommended follow-up in my office in about two weeks' time, and also recommended
to follow-up with the surgeon in about 7–10 days' time.

HOSPITAL COURSE: Patient is a pleasant 39-year-old Caucasian male with a past medical history of
degenerative joint disease and a history of depression. He presented to my office with a chief complaint
of right upper quadrant pain. The patient had been evaluated by the ER on August 31, 2011 with a
sonogram, which revealed multiple echogenic foci, consistent with stones. As the patient was not
getting any better and he was symptomatic, he was admitted electively for possible cholelithiasis and
evaluation of his abdominal pain for possible cholecystectomy.
    The patient was admitted to the surgical floor. We obtained a surgical consultation from Dr. Carter's
group. Following the surgical evaluation, the patient underwent laparoscopic cholecystectomy. The
patient's postoperative course was unremarkable. He was tolerating the pain better on pain medication.
Once the patient was advanced on his diet and clinically improved and he was afebrile, he was
discharged with the above discharge instructions, to be followed up on an outpatient basis.

Harold R. Carrolton, MD

HRC/fa 09/15/11 11:47:39

You Code It!

What are the best, most accurate codes?

Diagnosis Codes: _____

Procedure Codes: _____

Anesthesia Codes (when applicable): _____

HCPCS Level II codes (when applicable): _____

PATIENT: KINCAIDE, WENDY
ACCOUNT/EHR #:   KINWE001
Date: 09/19/11

HISTORY OF PRESENT ILLNESS: The patient, age 59, had been admitted to this medical center because of abdominal pain. She complained of lower abdominal pain starting on September 1. Since that time, she has had loose stools and complained of marked fatigue. Her appetite has been poor and she has been aware of a low-grade fever.

     The patient complained of similar symptoms about six months ago. At that time, studies included an upper GI series, barium enema and colonoscopy, which were reported as normal. She has continued to have some lower abdominal discomfort.

     Prior to this admission, CT scan of the abdomen revealed thickening of the cecal wall and proximal ascending colon. A ruptured appendix with perforation and abscess formation was suspected.

PAST MEDICAL HISTORY: Revealed known hypertension. She has a history of seizure disorder, her last seizure being 27 years ago. She stated she had tumors removed from her left inguinal area approximately 25-30 years ago, the nature of which she is not certain. She has been treated for hypertension for the past 3 or 4 years.

ALLERGIES: Dilantin

PHYSICAL EXAMINATION

VITAL SIGNS: BP 122/70, Wt 128, T 100.2

GENERAL: The patient appeared to be in moderate pain on admission.

SKIN/MUCOUS MEMBRANES: There was no cyanosis or venous distention.

HEART: Heart sounds were regular and normal.

LUNGS: Clear

BREASTS: Revealed no masses

ABDOMEN: Soft with tenderness in the lower abdomen to palpation. There were no masses or organomegaly detected. The tenderness was noted especially in the right lower quadrant.

RECTAL: Normal; stool negative for occult blood

PELVIC: Unremarkable

EXTREMITIES: There was no dependent edema. Weak pedal pulses were present bilaterally.

LABORATORY STUDIES: Hemoglobin 11.4, hematocrit 33, WBC 11.6. Comprehensive metabolic profile: normal. Urinalysis: normal. Chest x-ray revealed no evidence of cardiopulmonary disease. DEXA: The bones were noted to be osteopenic. EKG revealed normal sinus rhythm and nonspecific T wave changes.

SUMMARY: On September 13, Dr. Larry Garrett performed exploratory laparotomy, appendectomy, and right salpingo-oophorectomy. Patient had an uneventful postoperative course. She was discharged on September 18, 2011.

Continued

DISCHARGE DIAGNOSIS: 1. Acute and chronic appendicitis with perforation and abscess formation
                         2. Hypertension
                         3. Seizure disorder
                         4. Allergy to DILANTIN

DISCHARGE MEDICATIONS: 1. Ziac 5 mg daily
                         2. Mysoline 250 mg three times per day
                         3. Tylenol #3 one or two 3-4h, p.r.n for pain
                         4. Cefaclor 250 mg q8h for one week

DISCHARGE INSTRUCTIONS: Patient was instructed to restrict her activities and to contact myself and
Dr. Garrett after discharge for follow-up

_____

Harold R. Carrolton, MD

HRC/fa 09/19/11 11:47:39

You Code It!

What are the best, most accurate codes?

Diagnosis Codes: _____

Procedure Codes: _____

Anesthesia Codes (when applicable): _____

HCPCS Level II codes (when applicable): _____

CARROLTON DIGESTIVE MEDICINE, PA
765 SWOLLOW PATH • PASSING, FL 32811 • 407-555-7985

PATIENT: PHARMANE, CATHERINE
ACCOUNT/EHR #:   PHACA001
Date: 04/17/11

Preop Diagnosis: Chronic appendicitis with abscess
Postop Diagnosis: Same
Surgeon: Alma Beach, MD

Anesthesia: General
Operative Procedure: Laparotomy with appendectomy and right salpingo-oophorectomy

INDICATIONS: The patient is a 51-year-old female, admitted on April 17, 2008, with abdominal pain. The patient complained of lower abdominal pain starting on April 8. Since that time, she had loose stools and complained of marked fatigue. Her appetite was poor and she had been aware of a low-grade fever. The patient had similar complaints approximately six months ago. At that time, studies included an upper GI series, barium enema and colonoscopy, which were reported as normal. Prior to this admission, a CT scan of the abdomen was performed, which revealed a thickening of the cecal wall and proximal ascending colon. A ruptured appendix with perforation and abscess formation was suspected. Plans were made for surgery.

DESCRIPTION OF OPERATION: The patient was taken to the operating room and placed in the supine position. After general endotracheal anesthesia was administered, a Foley catheter was placed, and then her abdomen was prepped and draped in the usual sterile fashion.

A knife was used to make a right paramedian incision and dissection taken down through the subcutaneous tissues. The anterior rectus sheath was divided and blunt dissection accomplished through the rectus muscles. The posterior rectus sheath and peritoneum were then opened sharply as well. There was a large inflammatory mass noted in the right lower quadrant. There was an abscess cavity entered, and this was cultured. The cecum was identified, and the tinea were followed to where the appendiceal origin should be. However, there was a great deal of inflammation in this area. The right tube and ovary were involved as well.

There was a tubular structure heading into the retrocecal area, which appeared to be the remnant of the appendix. This was followed back to the appendix and a straight clamp placed across it. This was then doubly tied with 0-Vicryl ties. The structure was adherent to the tube and ovary, a large inflammatory mass. The tube and ovary were excised by clamping their blood supply and tying these off with 0-Vicryl ties as well. The specimen was passed off the table.

Continued

The area was irrigated with copious amounts of saline. Hemostasis was good. A 10-mm Blake drain was placed in the abscess cavity and taken out through a lateral stab incision. This was secured in place with a 2.0 nylon suture. Again, the abdomen and pelvis were irrigated and suctioned out. The posterior rectus sheath and peritoneum were closed with a running 0-Vicryl suture, and the anterior rectus sheath was closed with a running #1 PDS suture. The subcutaneous tissues were irrigated with saline and the skin closed with staples.

The patient tolerated the procedure well and there were no complications. She returned to recovery in stable condition.

Alma Beach, MD

AB/fa 04/17/11 21:47:39

You Code It!

What are the best, most accurate codes?

Diagnosis Codes: _____

Procedure Codes: _____

Anesthesia Codes (when applicable): _____

HCPCS Level II codes (when applicable): _____

PATIENT: ANATOLE, RENE
ACCOUNT/EHR #:   ANARE001
Date: 06/19/11

HISTORY OF PRESENT ILLNESS: This patient is a 43-year-old white male who has been having severe epigastric and right upper quadrant pains radiating to his right shoulder since June 13. This occurred after fatty food. He took Zantac over the counter and Gas-X, but this didn't help him. He has had intermittent episodes that are severe. He remains quite tender in the right upper quadrant. He has been belching quite a bit as well.

He presented to the ER early the morning of June 18 for evaluation of this. Yesterday, he underwent ultrasound of the abdomen and the PIPIDA scan, which showed some delay emptying into the duodenum but otherwise was normal. No stones were seen on the ultrasound.

Today, he underwent a biliary tract ejection fraction evaluation and a CT of the abdomen and pelvis. The gallbladder ejection fraction was 17%, which is markedly low, and the CT showed a minimally dilated distal common bile duct without any obvious mass effect, stones, etc., and no other pathology.

He will present to the hospital for purposes of esophagogastroduodenoscopy. He has had a *Helicobacter pylori* infection in the past, and the esophagogastroduodenoscopy is being performed to rule out any cause such as peptic ulcer disease, reflux esophagitis, etc. for his pain. If all this is negative, then he will undergo laparoscopic cholecystectomy. He was placed on Zantac yesterday, 150 mg bid, and was switched to Prilosec today.

PMH: Negative with the exception of the above.

PAST SURGICAL HISTORY: Appendectomy and multiple ear surgeries.

ALLERGIES: None known of.

SOCIAL HISTORY: No tobacco, minimal alcohol.

FAMILY HISTORY: The patient was adopted.

REVIEW OF SYSTEMS: Negative with the exception of the above.

PHYSICAL EXAMINATION

GENERAL: Reveals a well-developed, well-nourished white male in no acute distress

VITAL SIGNS: BP 126/80, T 98.1, P 80, R 16

HEENT: Head is atraumatic, normocephalic

NECK: Supple, trachea midline

CHEST: Clear

HEART: Regular rhythm

ABDOMEN: Tender in the epigastric and right upper quadrant region. There are no masses or organomegaly.

EXTREMITIES: No cyanosis, clubbing, or edema

NEUROLOGIC: Grossly intact

Continued

IMPRESSION: 1. R/O peptic ulcer disease, reflux esophagitis, etc.
               2. Biliary dyskinesia

PLAN: 1. Esophagogastroduodenoscopy
               2. Laparoscopic cholecystectomy if no obvious reason for this patient's discomfort is
                  found

Harold R. Carrolton, MD

HRC/fa 06/19/11 11:47:39

You Code It!

What are the best, most accurate codes?

Diagnosis Codes: _____

Procedure Codes: _____

Anesthesia Codes (when applicable): _____

HCPCS Level II codes (when applicable): _____

PATIENT: STEVENS, MARIBELLA
ACCOUNT/EHR #:   STEMA001
Date: 09/15/11

Preop Diagnosis: Severe abdominal pain, R/O peptic ulcer disease, esophagitis, etc.
Postop Diagnosis: Minimal duodenitis
Operation Performed: Esophagogastroduodenoscopy

Surgeon: Lawrence Garrett, MD

Anesthesia: Topical

PROCEDURE IN DETAIL: After an adequate topical anesthetic was achieved using viscous Xylocaine, the Olympus upper GI endoscope was passed interorally and advanced down the esophagus through the GE junction and then in through the stomach, in through the pylorus, into the duodenum.

This study revealed the presence of some minimal friability in the duodenum. Some minimal duodenitis could be seen. The remainder of the examination appeared to be within normal limits, including the remainder of the stomach and esophagus.

The GE junction was at 40 cm; there is no hiatus hernia, there is no evidence of reflux esophagitis, there was no clear-cut gastritis, there were no peptic ulcers, etc. No evidence of neoplasm.

The endoscope was withdrawn, the above findings were reconfirmed. The patient tolerated the procedure well. A biopsy of the antrum was taken for CLO-test.

Lawrence Garrett, MD

LG/fa 09/15/11 11:47:39

You Code It!

What are the best, most accurate codes?

Diagnosis Codes: _____

Procedure Codes: _____

Anesthesia Codes (when applicable): _____

HCPCS Level II codes (when applicable): _____

CARROLTON DIGESTIVE MEDICINE, PA
765 SWOLLOW PATH • PASSING, FL 32811 • 407-555-7985

PATIENT:	CHAMBERS, DUANE
ACCOUNT/EHR #:	CHADU001
Date:	09/15/11

Preop Diagnosis:	Colon Cancer Screening
Postop Diagnosis:	1. A 4-mm polyp in the proximal rectum, not biopsied
	2. Normal sigmoid, descending colon, transverse colon, ascending colon, cecum, and ileum

Procedure: Colonoscopy to the ileum with hot biopsy polypectomy

Physician: Albert Mathews, MD

Anesthesia: Conscious sedation

PROCEDURE IN DETAIL: The patient was identified in the endoscopy room, sedated with 4.0 mg of Versed and 100 mcg of Fentanyl. The colonoscope was advanced to the ileum. On the way out, the mucosa was examined thoroughly and hot biopsy done in the rectum. Once the procedure was completed, the patient was kept in the room for an EGD. Preparation was good.

IMPRESSION: Proximal rectal polyp, about 4 mm

PLAN: EGD now.

_____

Albert Mathews, MD

AM/fa 09/15/11 11:47:39

You Code It!

What are the best, most accurate codes?

Diagnosis Codes: _____

Procedure Codes: _____

Anesthesia Codes (when applicable): _____

HCPCS Level II codes (when applicable): _____

CARROLTON DIGESTIVE MEDICINE, PA
765 SWOLLOW PATH • PASSING, FL 32811 • 407-555-7985

PATIENT: WOODS, BRIAN
ACCOUNT/EHR #: WOOBR001
Date: 09/15/11

CHIEF COMPLAINT: This is a 33-year-old white male, referred by Dr. Hallowing, with complaints of abdominal pain. He states that his pain began about 5 weeks prior to this appointment and has gradually worsened. The pain is sharp in nature and located in the middle of his upper abdomen, just below the rib cage. It occurs most often between meals and is relieved temporarily when he has just eaten and his stomach is full. He denies any weight loss, anorexia, dysphagia, diarrhea, or constipation. He states that his stools are darker than usual but there is no indication of blood. He has never had anything like this pain in the past, and he states he has no idea what could be the cause. He has been using some over-the-counter antacid without relief. He is sexually active with his girlfriend who he has been with for more than one year. He has never been diagnosed with a sexually transmitted disease.

PAST MEDICAL HISTORY: He has had no surgeries and takes no other medications.

ALLERGIES: NKA

FAMILY HISTORY: Both of his parents are alive and in good health. He has one brother, aged 35 and one sister, age 27 who are alive and well.

SOCIAL HISTORY: He is physically active and states that he works out at the gym several times a week and sometimes plays touch football with his friends on Saturdays. He drinks beer but rarely drinks alcoholic beverages, and uses no other substances. He works as a roofer for a large construction firm. He reports some stress related to business being slow because of the economy, but does not believe that this is the cause of the abdominal pain.

PHYSICAL EXAMINATION: He is a well-appearing thin white male, appearing hisstated age. Wt 163 pounds, unchanged from the previous visit 6 months before. BP 120/79 mmHg supine and 112/70 mmHg standing. Heart rate: 68/min supine and 72/min standing. Respiratory rate is 12. T 98.8F. His conjunctiva are pale, sclerae are anicteric, mucus membranes are moist. Mouth shows no oral lesions. Neck is without bruits or thyromegaly. Lungs are clear to auscultation and percussion. Heart is regular without murmurs, rubs, or gallops. Abdomen is soft and nondistended with normoactive bowel sounds. There is epigastric tenderness to palpation without rebound or guarding. Murphy's sign is negative and there is no organomegaly. Stool is dark brown and tests guaiac positive for occult blood. Deep tendon reflexes are 2 and equal. Skin is without lesions. Rapid urease test positive for *H pylori*.

DIAGNOSIS: Infection with *H pylori*.

PLAN: RX: Antibiotics and a proton-pump inhibitor.

Albert Mathews, MD

AM/fa 09/15/11 11:47:39

You Code It!

What are the best, most accurate codes?

Diagnosis Codes: _____

Procedure Codes: _____

Anesthesia Codes (when applicable): _____

HCPCS Level II codes (when applicable): _____

CARROLTON DIGESTIVE MEDICINE, PA
765 SWOLLOW PATH • PASSING, FL 32811 • 407-555-7985

PATIENT: MONTANA, JOANNE
ACCOUNT/EHR #:   MONJO001
Date: 09/15/11

CHIEF COMPLAINT: Joanne is a 51-year-old female whom I have not seen in two years. She comes in complaining of abdominal pain. This pain is very different from abdominal pain that she suffered 1 year ago. Now her pain is sharp and stabbing, though still located in the midepigastrium. The pain occurs about 45 minutes after eating and lasts less than an hour. The pain occasionally radiates over her right shoulder. She notes the pain is the worst after her favorite meal, pizza.

PHYSICAL EXAMINATION: She is a thin white female, appearing her stated age. Wt 125 pounds. BP 110/67 mmHg supine and 105/60 mmHg standing. Heart rate: 68/min supine and 72/min standing. Her conjunctiva are without pallor, mucus membranes are moist. There are no oral lesions. Neck is without bruits or thyromegaly. Lungs are clear to auscultation and percussion. Heart is regular without murmurs rubs or gallops. Abdomen is soft and nondistended with normoactive bowel sounds. There is epigastric tenderness to palpation without rebound or guarding. Murphy's sign is positive. Stool is dark brown and tests guaiac negative for occult blood. Deep tendon reflexes are 2 and equal. Skin is without lesions.

TESTS: Sonogram performed in office reveals presence of gallstones.

DIAGNOSIS: Cholelithiasis

PLAN: Discussed the recommendation for a laparoscopic cholecystectomy. All benefits and risks are reviewed. Patient decides to go ahead with the procedure. Surgery scheduled for two weeks on Friday.

Albert Mathews, MD

AM/fa 09/15/11 11:47:39

You Code It!

What are the best, most accurate codes?

Diagnosis Codes: _____

Procedure Codes: _____

Anesthesia Codes (when applicable): _____

HCPCS Level II codes (when applicable): _____

CARROLTON DIGESTIVE MEDICINE, PA
765 SWOLLOW PATH • PASSING, FL 32811 • 407-555-7985

PATIENT: STEVENSON, CHRISTOPHER
ACCOUNT/EHR #:   STECH001
Date: 09/15/11

CHIEF COMPLAINT: This patient is a 41-year-old male, referred by Dr. Sherman, with complaints of abdominal pain. He states that the pain is intermittent and accompanied by bouts of diarrhea. Between bouts of pain with diarrhea (which predominate), he is constipated with small hard stools. He describes the pain as crampy without localization. Patient denies weight gain or loss but constantly feels bloated. Dairy products and caffeine exacerbate his diarrheal symptoms. His diet includes limited fiber intake. He remains with the same partner. They are considering marriage, and this is the source of some friction between him and his youngest child, now a sophomore in high school.

PHYSICAL EXAMINATION: He is mildly anxious but in no acute distress and is non–ill appearing. His weight is 162 pounds, blood pressure is normal, he is not tachycardic, and he is afebrile. His physical examination, including abdominal and rectal examinations, is unremarkable; stool is guaiac negative.

DIAGNOSIS: Irritable bowel syndrome (IBS)

PLAN: Rx psyllium to regulate bowel function and alleviate symptoms. Discuss with patient that the fact that his diarrheal symptoms are aggravated by dairy products suggests that he may have a component of lactose intolerance. We also discuss in detail dietary interventions for IBS, such as keeping a food diary to discover any associations of symptoms with specific dietary intake.

Albert Mathews, MD

AM/fa 09/15/11 11:47:39

You Code It!

What are the best, most accurate codes?

Diagnosis Codes: _____

Procedure Codes: _____

Anesthesia Codes (when applicable): _____

HCPCS Level II codes (when applicable): _____

CARROLTON DIGESTIVE MEDICINE, PA
765 SWOLLOW PATH • PASSING, FL 32811 • 407-555-7985

PATIENT: FINSTER, PETER
ACCOUNT/EHR #:   FINSPE001
Date: 11/08/11

Preop Diagnosis: Malignant polyp in sigmoid colon
Postop Diagnosis: Malignant polyp in sigmoid colon
Procedure: Laparotomy, intraoperative colonoscopy for polypectomy site
                            localization, sigmoid colectomy with colorectal anastomosis
Anesthesia: General endotracheal

INDICATIONS FOR OPERATION: This is a 57-year-old male who was found to have a malignant polyp in
the sigmoid colon. The pathology was reviewed and a colectomy was recommended. All risks, benefits,
and alternatives were explained, and he consented to surgery. He received a full mechanical and
antibiotic bowel preparation preoperatively. Deep venous thrombosis prophylaxis was accomplished
with the PAS stockings.

DESCRIPTION OF PROCEDURE: The patient was brought to the operating room and after the induction
of general endotracheal anesthesia, a Foley catheter was inserted. He was placed in the modified
lithotomy position in the Allen stirrups. Rectal irrigation was performed until clear with saline and
Betadine. The abdomen was shaved, prepped with Betadine solution, and draped in a sterile fashion.
An infraumbilical transverse incision was made and carried down through the anterior rectus sheath.
The rectus muscle on the right side was divided with electrocautery. The epigastric arteries were
individually clamped, divided, and ligated with #0 Vicryl. The incision was carried down across the
midline to the right rectus muscle, and this was partially divided. Exposure was then accomplished with
the Burke-Walter retractor. Palpation of the liver, gallbladder, and stomach was normal. The small bowel
was normal in appearance. The sigmoid colon had diverticulosis, but there was no palpable tumor
noted. At this point, I introduced the colonoscope transanally and localized an ulcer consistent with the
polypectomy site at the 25 cm level. This site was marked in the serosa with a Vicryl suture. I then
rescrubbed and regowned and gloved and proceeded with the operation. The sigmoid colon and
descending colon were mobilized and reflected medially, incising along with white line of Toldt. We
carried the mobilization until the distal descending colon was quite mobile. The left ureter was identified
and kept out of harm's way. We then divided the distal descending colon at its junction with the sigmoid
colon with the 75-mm linear stapler. The mesentery at the sigmoid at the point was then divided
between clamps, ligating with #0 Vicryl. The superior rectal artery was divided and was suture ligated
with #0 Vicryl. This allowed us access into the vasculature plane, and we carried this in a caudal
direction over the sacral promontory into the presacral space. Once we were below the marked site, we
divided the rectal mesentery between clamps, ligating with #0 Vicryl. Once we had achieved a good
margin, we came across the superior rectum with a TA-55 mm linear stapler. The specimen was then
excised and removed and sent off the field. The specimen was opened to make sure that we had
achieved a good margin and that we had the polypectomy site, and indeed we have achieved both. The
descending colon was then mobilized a little further until the anastomosis could be created to be
completely tension free. The end of the descending colon was then prepared by clearing some of the
mesentery, thereby exposing the serosa. We quarantined the peritoneal cavity with towels, exposing
the descending colon. The staple line was opened and a pursestring of #0 Prolene was created. The

Continued

detached head of the 29 mm ILS stapler was then secured in place with this pursestring suture. The descending colon was well vascularized. The ILS 29-mm stapler was then introduced transanally and advanced all the way up to the staple line of the rectum. The instrument was opened and the rod came out at the level of the staple line. We then connected the descending colon to the rectum via the stapler, closed the instrument, and fired. Two perfect donuts were retrieved and a circular anastomosis was created. The pelvis was then filled with saline. Air was insufflated transanally descending the descending colon to the anastomosis, and there was no air leak noted. We then irrigated the pelvis and the abdominal cavity with saline solution until clear. I changed my gown and gloves at this point and proceeded with draping the omentum over the small intestine. The posterior rectus sheath was closed with a running #1 PDS suture. The rectus muscle was irrigated and the anterior rectus sheath was then closed with a running double-stranded #1 PDS suture. The subcutaneous tissue was irrigated. The skin was infiltrated with 20 cc of 0.5% Marcaine. The skin was then closed with a running subcuticular #4-0 Vicryl. This was reinforced with Steri-Strips. A dressing was applied. The patient tolerated the procedure well and left the operating room in stable condition. The final sponge, needle, and instrument counts were correct times two. There were no Intraoperative complications.

Harold R. Carrolton, MD, surgeon
Sander Lawrence, assistant surgeon

HRC/fa 11/08/11 11:47:39

You Code It!

What are the best, most accurate codes?

Diagnosis Codes: _____

Procedure Codes: _____

Anesthesia Codes (when applicable): _____

HCPCS Level II codes (when applicable): _____

CARROLTON DIGESTIVE MEDICINE, PA
765 SWOLLOW PATH • PASSING, FL 32811 • 407-555-7985

PATIENT: LELAND, BELLA
ACCOUNT/EHR #:   LELABE001
Date: 10/13/11

This is a 61-year-old previously healthy black female who presented to her primary care physician, Dr. Ronald Block, complaining of fatigue, right upper quadrant (RUQ) fullness, fever, and nausea of three days duration. On physical examination, Dr. Block felt a pulsating mass in her RUQ and midepigastrium and referred her to me for consultation.

HISTORY: The patient denied any travel history and had no pets at home. She also denied diarrhea, shortness of breath, or palpitations. Her past medical history was significant for pernicious anemia and a hysterectomy in 1980.

EXAM: Upon arrival to this clinic, physical examination was significant for a temperature of 39.2 C orally, blood pressure was 155/84 mm Hg, pulse was 66 beats/minute, and respiratory rate was 15/minute. She had no murmurs, rubs, or gallops on her cardiac examination. Her abdominal examination was significant for a large midepigastric and RUQ mass that was pulsatile in nature. Peripheral pulses in her upper and lower extremities were symmetrical. Rectal examination revealed brown and guaiac negative stools. Physical examination was otherwise unremarkable. The patient was most comfortable when lying on her right side. Her white blood cell count was 14.5/mm^3 (normal 3.2–9.8) with 88% neutrophils and 3% bands. Hematocrit was 41% (normal 35–45) with a mean corpuscular volume (MCV) of 81 FL (normal 80–96), AST 15 IU/L (normal 10–60 IU/L), ALT 23 (normal 10–60 IU/L), alkaline phosphatase 54 IU/L (normal 30–135 IU/L), and bilirubin 0.6 IU/L (normal 0.2–1.2 IU/L). Serum electrolytes, creatinine, amylase, and lipase were all within normal limits.

Because of the concern about a possible abdominal aortic aneurysm, an abdominal computerized tomography scan was obtained; this revealed multiple low attenuation lesions in the liver compatible with cysts but a normal aorta and periaortic region. The largest cyst was 9 x 10 cm in the left lobe of the liver and was identified lying immediately adjacent to the aorta. Two small low-attenuation lesions were identified in the right kidney and another in the left kidney compatible with renal cysts. *Entameba Histolytica* serum antibody and echinococcal titers were negative. Parietal cell antibody serum titers were minimally elevated (1: 40). Blood cultures remained without growth. Intravenous ampicillin-sulbactam and metronidazole were initiated on admission to the hospital.

The patient underwent aspiration of the largest cyst under ultrasound guidance. Cyst fluid culture grew *Escherichia coli.* Giemsa stain of the fluid showed no parasites. Pathologic examination of the fine needle aspirate showed marked inflammation, histiocytes, and degenerating hepatocytes, consistent with infected material. The patient was then switched to intravenous ceftazidime and defervesced 48 hours after cyst drainage.

Continued

A colonoscopy was performed and revealed hemorrhoids. An upper gastrointestinal series and an upper endoscopy revealed a large (4.5 × 4.0 cm) duodenal diverticulum located lateral to the D2-D3 transition but no evidence of fistulous communication with the liver or biliary system. Because of the presence of multiple cysts and the concern that the patient might have an underlying malignancy, the patient was surgically explored and underwent resection of the duodenal diverticulum, a left lobectomy of the liver, and drainage of the other cysts. Pathology of the resected hepatic cyst was consistent with infected hepatic cyst and no malignancy.

DIAGNOSIS: Infected hepatic cyst masquerading as an abdominal aortic aneurysm

Harold R. Carrolton, MD

HRC/fa 10/13/11 11:47:39

You Code It!

What are the best, most accurate codes?

Diagnosis Codes: _____

Procedure Codes: _____

Anesthesia Codes (when applicable): _____

HCPCS Level II codes (when applicable): _____

CARROLTON DIGESTIVE MEDICINE, PA
765 SWOLLOW PATH • PASSING, FL 32811 • 407-555-7985

PATIENT:	CALLMAN, CAROLINE
ACCOUNT/EHR #:	CALLCA001
Date:	10/21/11

Preop Diagnosis:	Dysphagia, acute cerebrovascular accident in a diabetic patient, unable to eat and swallow
Postop Diagnosis:	1. Dysphagia, acute cerebrovascular accident in a diabetic patient, unable to eat and swallow 2. Gastric tear from a nasogastric tube 3. Gastric polyp 4. Hiatus hernia
Procedure:	Esophagogastroduodenoscopy with biopsies of gastric polyp followed by a percutaneous endoscopic gastrostomy placement
Preoperative Meds:	50 mg Demerol; 25 mg Vistaril; 0.4 mg Atropine
Monitoring:	Oximeter and cardiac monitor
Instrument:	Pentax video system and the Bard 20-French gastrostomy tube

INDICATIONS FOR ENDOSCOPY: A surveillance endoscopic procedure is performed to assist in percutaneous endoscopic gastrostomy tube placement.

DESCRIPTION OF PROCEDURE: With the patient in the left lateral decubitus position, the gastroscope was advanced under direct vision with the following findings.

The vocal cords and posterior pharynx are grossly normal.

The scope was advanced to the esophagus. The esophagus showed normal mucosa, no exudates, and no inflammation or varices or intrinsic lesions. The z-line was localized at 35 cm from the frontal incisors.

The scope was advanced in the stomach. There was a small sliding hiatus hernia noted. On retroversion, the gastroesophageal junction is normal. The scope was advanced to the body and fundus of the stomach, which showed normal mucosa and normal peristalsis. The scope was advanced to the antrum. The pyloric antrum is deformed. A tear approximately 1 cm $\times$ 0.2 cm is noted with cellulites. There are small erosions suggesting trauma from the previous nasogastric tube. This was photographed.

A gastric polyp, mucosal-like, approximately 0.5 cm, was noted on the anterior wall of the antrum and likely is a reaction to the inflammation in the posterior wall. A biopsy was obtained and submitted to pathology.

At this time, the scope was advanced through the duodenal bulb, which showed normal mucosa and no ulcerations or bleeding. The post bulb of the duodenum is normal.

The scope was withdrawn to the stomach as to assist with the percutaneous endoscopic gastrostomy tube. Using transillumination from the light and finger palpation, the localization of the gastrostomy tube was selected to the left anterior clavicular line and perpendicular to a point one-third of the distance between the left costal margin and the umbilicus.

The area was selected and using Betadine, the abdomen was cleaned. This was followed by injection of 1% lidocaine and followed with the insertion of a Seldinger needle intragastrically. This was observed via the video gastroscope. The stylet was removed and replaced with a guidewire. Using a polypectomy snare, the guidewire was secured and brought cephalad by pulling the scope out; the snare and guidewire followed in tandem.

With the guidewire outside the patient's mouth, this was secured to a gastrostomy assembly, 20-French Bard PEG. Using the Ponsky technique, the gastrostomy was placed, and this was followed again by the insertion of the gastroscope.

Continued

No ischemia in the skin nor ischemia of the mucosa was noted. The external bolster was applied under direct vision without any sign of ischemia.

The scope was withdrawn and the patient tolerated the procedure well.

GASTROENTEROLOGY ASSESSMENT:
1. Sliding hiatus hernia
2. Gastric tear with erosions and deformed pylorus, likely trauma from the nasogastric tube
3. Gastric polyp
4. Successful placement of a gastrostomy tube to start feedings in the morning. Orders are given.

Albert Mathews, MD

AM/fa 10/21/11 11:47:39

You Code It!

What are the best, most accurate codes?

Diagnosis Codes: _____

Procedure Codes: _____

Anesthesia Codes (when applicable): _____

HCPCS Level II codes (when applicable): _____

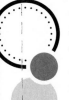

Gerontology Cases and Patient Records

10

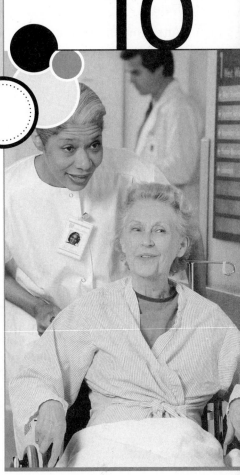

INTRODUCTION

The following case studies are from a gerontology practice. In a physician's office of this type, a professional coding specialist is likely to see many different kinds of health situations, especially preventive health care services.

Geriatric specialists, also known as geriatricians, are typically family medicine physicians or internists specializing in the diagnosis and treatment of conditions and diseases of older adults. As individuals get older, their health concerns become greater and more serious. For example, a 40-year-old diagnosed with the flu will usually be out of work for a few days; however, for an 80-year-old, a case of the flu can be life-threatening. These health care professionals may care for their patients in their office, in the patient's home, or in a nursing home or assisted living facility.

Geriatric medicine specialists may be board-certified in family medicine, internal medicine, or geriatric medicine by the American Board of Family Practice or the Board of Internal Medicine. Both of these boards are recognized by the American Board of Medical Specialties.

You can use these cases to practice coding diagnoses, E/M, procedures, DME, or other HCPCS Level II items, as applicable; code for the physician or the facility; code inpatient and outpatient services, as applicable:

1. Code for the physician.
2. Code for the anesthesiologist, when applicable.
3. Code for the hospital, when applicable.
4. Code for the pathology and laboratory, when applicable.
5. Code HCPCS Level II codes, when applicable.

ADULT HEALTH ASSOCIATES
720 LONG STREET • ETERNITY, FL 32711 • 407-555-7322

PATIENT:	ANDERSON, LAWRENCE
ACCOUNT/EHR #:	ANDELA01
Date:	04/22/11

Attending Physician: James Healer, MD

This 89-year-old male was seen in his room at the Sun City Nursing Home for his regular annual check-up. Pt is stable and doing well on his current regime of medications. PE shows age-appropriate condition. HEENT unremarkable. Coordination with resident medical director to review and affirm medical plan of care.

James Healer, MD

JHW/mg   D: 04/22/11 09:50:16   T: 04/25/11 12:55:01

You Code It!

What are the best, most accurate codes?

Diagnosis Codes: _____

Procedure Codes: _____

Anesthesia Codes (when applicable): _____

HCPCS Level II codes (when applicable): _____

ADULT HEALTH ASSOCIATES
720 LONG STREET • ETERNITY, FL 32711 • 407-555-7322

PATIENT: CARR, FAITH
ACCOUNT/EHR #:   CARRFA01
Date: 04/22/11

Attending Physician: James Healer, MD

This is a 79-year-old Native American female who lives in a very rural area about 30 miles outside the city. Her home is a crowded two-bedroom cottage in which three of her five children and six of her grandchildren reside. She does not speak or understand English very well and requires a translator when meeting with health care professionals. Her youngest daughter, Lantana, came to interpret for her today.

HPI: She has come to the office today because she is experiencing shortness of breath, upper bilateral chest pain, and difficulty swallowing solids and semisolids (but not liquids).

EXAM: T 101.5F, R 15, Ht 5ft 1 in. Wt. 180 lb. HEENT: Head—unremarkable; eyes—PERRLA; ears—unremarkable; nasal passages appear to be clear; throat—mucosa appears erythematic, and there are indications of edema. Chest sounds are raspy and difficult.

LAB/RADIOLOGY: Sputum cytology, CBC w/differential, chest x-ray, swallowing assessment, and laryngoscopy are performed during this visit.

DX: Advanced cancerous lesions in both lungs with metastasis to her larynx.

TX: Patient is admitted to the hospital for an emergency laryngectomy because her airway system was being compromised by the laryngeal tumor.
    Patient, along with her daughter, was seen by the consulting ENT, Dr. Fallana, and speech-language pathologist (SLP), Roxan Kinney pre- and postoperatively.
    Roxan Kinney, SLP, counseled the patient, via interpretation by her daughter, regarding the use and care of an electrolarynx (Servox brand). Written instructions (in English) were given to the daughter regarding the use and care of the electrolarynx, as well as a description of nonverbal communication strategies.

PLAN: Patient to undergo a short course of chemo- and radiotherapies intended to ease her chest pain. Long-term therapies are not recommended or implemented.

Prognosis: Poor

James Healer, MD

JHW/mg   D: 04/22/11 09:50:16 T: 04/25/11 12:55:01

You Code It!

What are the best, most accurate codes?

Diagnosis Codes: _____

Procedure Codes: _____

Anesthesia Codes (when applicable): _____

HCPCS Level II codes (when applicable): _____

ADULT HEALTH ASSOCIATES
720 LONG STREET • ETERNITY, FL 32711 • 407-555-7322

PATIENT: DOYLE, TODD
ACCOUNT/EHR #:   DOYLTO01
Date: 04/22/11

Attending Physician: James Healer, MD

Pt is brought into the ED unconscious, after being found in an alley by a neighbor. He smelled of alcohol. He had no personal identification. EMTs administered fluids IV and oxygen on site. Pt exhibited brief consciousness during the ambulance ride. He spoke only gibberish and was unable to provide a history. Consequently, there was no known previous or current medical history, his medications, his address, his next of kin, languages spoken, employment status, or marital status.

His behavior while in the ED was disruptive. He hallucinated and spoke gibberish to imaginary people and voices. He was an unreliable historian. He also was suspicious of hospital staff, which may have made him wary of sharing truthful information. The pt said, in rather forceful words (including foul language), that there was nothing wrong with him, that he did not want or need to be there (in the hospital), and that he wanted to leave.

PHYSICAL EXAMINATION: Pt appeared to be malnourished, was underweight, and was thought to suffer hearing problems (possibly deafness). His left ankle shows gangrene and tissue necrosis, evidence of frostbite.

LABS: CBC is abnormally low complete; vitamin B12 deficiency.

DX: Frostbite, left foot below ankle; suspicion of alcoholic dementia.

PLAN: Admission for BTA amputation of left foot; neuropsychology consult requested.

_____

James Healer, MD

JHW/mg   D: 04/22/11 09:50:16   T: 04/25/11 12:55:01

You Code It!

What are the best, most accurate codes?

Diagnosis Codes: _____

Procedure Codes: _____

Anesthesia Codes (when applicable): _____

HCPCS Level II codes (when applicable): _____

PATIENT: SALIERI, PHYLLIS
ACCOUNT/EHR #:   SALIPH01
Date: 04/22/11

Attending Physician: Amanda Christoper, MD

Pt. is a 73-year-old female who is a resident of the Aston Farrell Nursing Home for 12 years. She has a high school education and speaks both English and Italian. She was the manager of a distribution center for a supermarket chain for 15 years but took early retirement to go on a disability pension, about 9 years after being diagnosed with chronic progressive multiple sclerosis (MS). She was divorced over 25 years ago. She has no children or close family. She has a good relationship with some of the cleaning and kitchen staff, and with the recreation worker and several of the volunteers. She likes to participate in all recreation activities (e.g., bingo, movies, outings, etc.). She also likes to write poetry using her typewriter, which she keeps in her room.

PHYSICAL ASSESSMENT: Pt. demonstrates significant trunk and limb ataxia. She is right-handed and cannot write due to the ataxia but is still able to type using one hand to stabilize the other. Her voice is also affected (low volume and articulation problems), so she uses the typewriter to communicate, preparing notes for people who have difficulty understanding her. She demonstrates some subtle euphoria (often associated with multiple sclerosis) and is beginning to show limitations in her insight.

    Pt. propels her wheelchair independently but requires the assistance of one staff member to transfer into and out of the chair. She can feed herself finger foods but requires the assistance of a staff member for all other self-care activities. She has neurogenic bladder problems and has stress and spasm incontinence, for which she wears an incontinence garment.

CURRENT MEDS: Antispasticity medication to deal with elevated tone in skeletal muscle.

BEHAVIORAL ASSESSMENT: Nursing staff report that the patient has made sexual remarks during personal care and that she has apparently touched them inappropriately. In addition, she was discovered having sexual intercourse with a male patient with TBI. Gossip was rampant about this event. It is difficult to determine whether this was done consciously or whether it was a result of her ataxia. Staff is concerned that the pt.'s actions (the disinhibition) may be the result of cognitive impairment possibly emerging as a result of the multiple sclerosis. There has been discussion as to whether or not the pt. should undergo an assessment of her cognitive abilities.

TEAM CONFERENCE: In attendance are me, the attending physician, George Matheson; head nurse, Erica Maphumulo; primary care nurse—days; Father Gribbins, chaplain; Nicola Monssen, recreation director; and Maurica Randolph, dietitian. By special request, also present were Vusi Walthour, occupational therapist, and Dionne Pyle, physical therapist, who have worked with the pt. in the past. Given the unprecedented nature of the incident, Keith Anders, the administrator of the facility, also attended.

Continued

In the first moments of the discussion, very different issues and perspectives became clear. One team member thought the issue was the illicit sexual activity, another identified the potential health risks as the key concern, while another was most concerned by the breach of confidentiality shown in the widespread gossip about the incident. Proposed solutions ranged from discharging one or both residents to changing institutional policy to allow them privacy for future encounters. The discussions became quite heated. It was determined that a cognitive assessment should be done to get a clearer picture of the patient. The results may provide an indication of the best course to follow. The meeting was adjourned 45 minutes later.

Amanda Christoper, MD

AC/mg   D: 04/22/11 09:50:16   T: 04/25/11 12:55:01

You Code It!

What are the best, most accurate codes?

Diagnosis Codes: _____

Procedure Codes: _____

Anesthesia Codes (when applicable): _____

HCPCS Level II codes (when applicable): _____

PATIENT: ALDERS, STEFAN
ACCOUNT/EHR #:   ALDEST01
Date: 04/22/11

Attending Physician: Amanda Christoper, MD

This new patient is a 76-year-old male, referred to me by Dr. Theodore Lee, the family physician. He resides in his own two-story house where he enjoys listening to the radio and the occasional record and tending to his garden. He denies ever marrying and states that he does not have any children. He attended one year of community college, after which he obtained employment as a clerk in a lawyer's office. He kept this job for 40 years and retired when he was 67. He had an older brother, who was killed during World War II, and he has an older sister (80 years old) who resides in a nearby nursing home and whom he visits occasionally. His native language is French; however, he speaks and understands English very well. He still drives his own car for occasional trips but has expressed concern lately about getting lost when driving outside of his neighborhood.

The patient attends an Adult Day Program affiliated with a Senior Center twice a week. He has had several falls over the last six months and fractured a rib during the last fall incident, four months ago. Currently, he receives nursing service from Home Care once a week to monitor medications. He used to visit his sister once a week in a nearby nursing home, but the frequency of the visits has lessened over the past few months.

Over the past month or so, day program staff noticed the patient's personal appearance is deteriorating. There are days when he wears soiled clothes, and his hair is not always clean or even combed. Patient showed up at the Center on the wrong day for preplanned activities three times in the past 2 months. It appears that he is forgetting the names of staff and other members of the group whose names he knew. He appears more withdrawn and seems to have trouble following conversations. Maxine Shaw, MSW, the social worker at the adult day program recommended this geriatric assessment to Dr. Lee, who referred the patient to me.

ASSESSMENT: The patient has a history of being a highly anxious person; he has a history of benzodiazepine use, as well as a history of psychiatric admissions for depression and anxiety. He states he has been experiencing increased anxiety following a diagnosis of skin cancer 7 months ago. He has asthma and uses Ventolin for control of symptoms. He states that he frequently calls his family physician, Dr. Theodore Lee, regarding the asthma attacks.

VITAL SIGNS: Temp: Afebrile; Resp: 17—accessory muscle use unremarkable; BP: 125/85 supine, 128/80 sitting, and 125/85 standing; weight: 145 lb. relatively stable (according to patient records from Dr. Lee); P normal; pulse oximeter O2 sat: 80%

ATTITUDE: Patient is compliant and appears to be slightly resentful of the idea that something is wrong with him. He is slightly slow in some responses.

GAIT: Patient is mildly unstable. Movement is slow, unsteady, and purposeful. At times, it appears that he tries to move and his feet are not quite following.

FOLSTEIN MINI-MENTAL STATUS EXAM (MMSE): Score of 19 indicating possible depression and some cognitive impairment.

INTEGUMENTARY SYSTEM: Skin is slightly pale; some diminished elasticity; slightly dehydrated. No signs of skin cancer, decubitus ulcers, or other ulcerations or wounds. There is some bruising, mostly on extremities, all of which appear to be normal for a patient of this age. No lesions are evident. HEAD: No signs of head trauma; no signs of Paget's disease.

EYES: Screening funduscopic examination is negative for cataracts. Visual fields for glaucoma—mild bilateral cataract developing in left eye; Snellen Eye chart for rapid test of visual acuity is normal.

Continued

EARS: Bilateral hearing aids for SNHL in the left ear and a mixed hearing loss in the right ear as a result of a stapedectomy when he was a child, which caused a conductive hearing loss. Some cerumen impaction, which is normal for patients who wear hearing aids.

NOSE: No nasal obstruction

OROPHARYNX: Patient wears upper and lower dentures that appear to fit correctly. No evidence of leukoplakia, cancers, erosions. Throat examination results show no throat infections or airway obstruction.

NECK: ROM is unremarkable. Lymph nodes show no signs of malignancy. Cervical lymph nodes show no signs of infection, trachea is not deviated from midline, thyroid gland—no nodules indicating malignancy, thyromegaly is negative for hyperthyroidism. Carotid arteries—possible carotid occlusion. Thromboembolic risk is moderate, and auscultation for bruits is negative.

LYMPH NODES: Posterior auricular, preauricular, supramandibular, anterior and posterior cervical, supraclavicular, axillary, and inguinal lymph nodes are all unremarkable.

SPINAL/BACK: Evidence of moderate kyphosis. There is no spinal tenderness or any associated kyphos. There is some flank tenderness near the area of the previous rib fracture. Back mobility is limited.

CHEST/LUNG: No signs of pulmonary edema, obstructive lung disease, pneumonia, or TB.

HEART: PMI and character of apex beat—unremarkable; parasternal lifts and thrills—unremarkable; no added heart sounds (S3/S4) or murmurs; carotid beat during auscultation (for upstroke for AS)—unremarkable.

PERIPHERAL VASCULAR: Pulses checked: Bilateral temporal—OK, carotid—slow, brachial—OK, radial—OK, femoral—OK, popliteal—OK, dorsalis pedis—OK, posterior tibialis—OK.

ABDOMINAL: Unremarkable

MUSCULOSKELETAL/EXTREMITY: Cyanosis, clubbing, edema, capillary refill appear unremarkable; no deformities; patient's shoes seem to be too large, thereby affecting gait; muscle strength, and ROM is limited and not outside of age-appropriateness.

NEUROLOGIC: Gait/fall risk: "get up and go" test (coordination and strength), Tandem Romberg, retropulsion, 360 degree turn—slow, affected. Coordination is within age range; however, strength is a concern. Wasting (local and generalized) and stigmata of stroke and common motor diseases is somewhat apparent. Cerebellar exam: finger to nose, rapid alternating movements, heel-knee to shin, Romberg—all slow but functional.

GENITOURINARY EXAM: Digital rectal examination—unremarkable; patient denies fecal impaction or urinary frequency.

DX: Arteriosclerosis, rule out normal pressure hydrocephalous

PLAN: Screening for arthritides; Hemoccult test; MRI head; carotid artery angiography—bilateral

Amanda Christoper, MD

AC/mg   D: 04/22/11 09:50:16   T: 04/25/11 12:55:01

You Code It!

What are the best, most accurate codes?

Diagnosis Codes: _____

Procedure Codes: _____

Anesthesia Codes (when applicable): _____

HCPCS Level II codes (when applicable): _____

ADULT HEALTH ASSOCIATES
720 LONG STREET • ETERNITY, FL 32711 • 407-555-7322

PATIENT: WOLLENBERG, LINDSAY
ACCOUNT/EHR #:   WOLLLI01
Date: 04/22/11

Attending Physician: Louis R. Ferguson, MD

This new patient is a 77-year-old female, who has been referred to me by her internal medicine physician, Dr. King. Patient reports a sudden hearing loss following a month of fullness in both ears attributed to altitude changes (recent airplane trip across country) and swimming. She states that she experienced unilateral loss (on the left side), preceded by dizziness and rushing in left ear.

    Tympanometry testing completed in office during this visit.

    Right ear shows normal thresholds, tympanogram results, and reflexes.

    Left ear exhibits severe hearing loss (pure tone average (PTA) and speech recognition thresholds (SRT) 70 dB hearing level (HL)—masked right ear) and poor word recognition scores, normal ipsiand contralateral stapedial reflexes.

DX: Unilateral sensorineural hearing loss, left ear

PLAN: Follow-up with patient in two weeks for further evaluation of continued services.

_____

Louis R. Ferguson, MD

LRF/mg   D: 04/22/11 09:50:16   T: 04/25/11 12:55:01

You Code It!

What are the best, most accurate codes?

Diagnosis Codes: _____

Procedure Codes: _____

Anesthesia Codes (when applicable): _____

HCPCS Level II codes (when applicable): _____

ADULT HEALTH ASSOCIATES
720 LONG STREET • ETERNITY, FL 32711 • 407-555-7322

PATIENT: MAYOR, ROLLAND
ACCOUNT/EHR #:   MAYORO01
Date: 04/22/11

Attending Physician: James Healer, MD

This patient is a 75-year-old male who lived on his family-owned tree farm outside of the city for most of his adult life. I am seeing him for the first time today due to concerns by his daughter about his recent falls.

PATIENT/SOCIAL: In October, he moved into a townhouse located in the suburb of Geneva, retiring from the farm due to his declining ability to manage the business. His townhouse is a two-story, single-family home. The kitchen, living room, bathroom, laundry, and storage facilities are located downstairs, and the bedroom and main bathroom are on the second floor.

The patient has never learned to drive a car and has relied on public transportation or his children since his wife died six years ago.

He is a member of the Kiwanis Club and the local Farmer's Association. Patient states he enjoys gardening and fishing.

The patient has two adult children. His son, Raymond, took over management of the tree farm 8 years ago. He is in contact with him on a regular basis but rarely gets to see him because Raymond is busy with the farm. Raymond is married and has three children. Patient's daughter, Vanessa, lives in the area and provides most of the support for her father. It is Vanessa who encouraged the patient to move so that they could live closer and take advantage of various support services. Vanessa is married and has two young children.

HISTORY OF PRESENT PROBLEM: Patient is in good general health. He suffers from osteoarthritis in both hips and knees. He has cataracts and kyphosis, and he reported having "ringing in her ears" (tinnitus). The patient takes Metamucil daily and one 81-mg aspirin per day, and uses Clear Vision eye drops as needed. He is physically strong and was quite active until a fall that occurred February 5.

On February 13, his daughter noticed that he was limping as a result of bruising from the recent fall.

On March 15, the patient experienced a second fall, this time on the walkway outside his home. It appeared nothing was broken; however, there was severe bruising on his left side. On March 21st, the daughter took the patient to her own family physician, Dr. Fidele, because the patient's primary physician had recently retired. According to the daughter, Dr. Fidele assessed the bruising. During the session, he communicated primarily with the daughter who periodically explained to the patient what the doctor said. The doctor recommended physical therapy and wrote an order for home care services. The physical therapist first saw the patient at his home on April 8.

On April 15, the patient moved in with his daughter, son-in-law, and two grandchildren because he developed a fear of falling again and suffering a more debilitating injury. In addition, it is thought that the daughter can assist with his recovery from his last fall. The son-in-law is not pleased with this situation.

Continued

PE: T 98.1F; B/P 135/90; R 16; P normal.

HEENT: unremarkable;

CHEST: clear;

ABDOMEN: unremarkable;

EXTREMITIES: Patient states sharp pain is experienced during dorsiflexion of the left foot. Circulation good.

DX: Achilles tendon contracture

PLAN: Referral for physical therapy; Rx for specialized series of shoes

_____

James Healer, MD

JHW/mg   D: 04/22/11 09:50:16   T: 04/25/11 12:55:01

You Code It!

What are the best, most accurate codes?

Diagnosis Codes: _____

Procedure Codes: _____

Anesthesia Codes (when applicable): _____

HCPCS Level II codes (when applicable): _____

ADULT HEALTH ASSOCIATES
720 LONG STREET • ETERNITY, FL 32711 • 407-555-7322

PATIENT: FINN, WILMA
ACCOUNT/EHR #:   FINNWI01
Date: 04/22/11

Attending Physician: James Healer, MD

This patient is an 82-year-old female being evaluated for care plan oversight services.

She was admitted February 18 via the ED after suffering a fall. She sustained a fracture of her right dominant humerus and bruising along her right shoulder and hip. In the emergency room, she was reluctant to discuss how she fell and she also refused to answer questions about her family or her medical history. There was evidence of significant recent alcohol intake. She was admitted to acute care and underwent internal fixation of the fracture.

After three days in acute care, she was transferred to the nursing facility. It is expected that she will be discharged within the week.

MEDICAL HISTORY: Dr. Patel, her family physician, sent over her records that document a long-standing history of depression. Dr. Patel prescribed Prozac for the depression and Levothyroxine for hypothyroidism diagnosed 10 years ago. The record also indicates that the patient is suspected of having an alcohol abuse problem.

Social history documented by Dr. Patel states that the patient's husband divorced her approximately 20 years ago. Family history documented in the record identifies that the patient has a 41-year-old son who lives with her and who was diagnosed with schizophrenia in his middle 20s. The patient and her son have had periodic involvement with various municipal social service agencies over the past 15 years.

There is concern that her recent fall could be due to her being under the influence of alcohol. However, there is evidence that she may have been pushed by her son. There are reports of suspicious bruising in the past, identified by Dr. Patel during annual physicals. Hospital staff raised concerns about the patient's cognitive status because she is such a poor informant and her information is often inconsistent. Staff could not tell whether she could or would not provide information. She is bitter about her son's illness and was angry when questioned about it.

PLAN: After 45 minutes of evaluation and interviews with current and recent care givers, the best course of action at this time is for the patient to be admitted into an assisted living facility upon discharge from the nursing facility. In this environment, she can receive continued PT and be protected from any possible abuse at the hands of her son.

_____

James Healer, MD

JHW/mg   D: 04/22/11 09:50:16   T: 04/25/11 12:55:01

You Code It!

What are the best, most accurate codes?

Diagnosis Codes: _____

Procedure Codes: _____

Anesthesia Codes (when applicable): _____

HCPCS Level II codes (when applicable): _____

ADULT HEALTH ASSOCIATES
720 LONG STREET • ETERNITY, FL 32711 • 407-555-7322

PATIENT: ENGLISH, ARTHUR
ACCOUNT/EHR #:   ENGLAR01
Date: 07/22/11

Attending Physician: James Healer, MD

This 87-year-old male patient was brought into this ED by ambulance after he called 911. Patient stated he awoke and discovered that he was having difficulty walking and speaking.

FAMILY/SOCIAL HISTORY: This patient is a right-handed, 87-year-old, English-speaking widower who lives alone in his own home. His house is a ranch style, single-family home.

    The patient drives his own car. He enjoys reading and sports. He volunteers as a coach for the neighborhood softball league.

    The patient has two adult children. His daughter, Joellyn, lives about 45 minutes away and speaks, by phone, weekly with her father. The patient's son, Mark, lives in another state and is in touch about once or twice per month.

HISTORY OF PRESENT ILLNESS: Patient exhibits some confusion and loss of coordination. His motor and sensory functions appear to be impaired.

PE: Weakness and numbness in leg are evident. CT scan of brain and EEG are positive for CVA. CBC shows decreased RBC, elevated lactate dehydrogenase (LDH) levels.

DX: Left anterior occlusive cerebral vascular accident (CVA).

PLAN: Admit patient to acute care for additional care.

_____

James Healer, MD

JHW/mg   D: 07/22/11 09:50:16   T: 07/25/11 12:55:01

You Code It!

What are the best, most accurate codes?

Diagnosis Codes: _____

Procedure Codes: _____

Anesthesia Codes (when applicable): _____

HCPCS Level II codes (when applicable): _____

ADULT HEALTH ASSOCIATES
720 LONG STREET • ETERNITY, FL 32711 • 407-555-7322

PATIENT: TOWNSEND, MARISSA
ACCOUNT/EHR #:   TOWNMA01
Date: 10/22/11

Attending Physician: James Healer, MD

PATIENT HISTORY: This patient is a 75-year-old female who ran her own doll repair business for 32 years out of a converted garage behind her house. She has been married for over 51 years to Thomas, who is 77 years old. The Townsends have three adult children. The eldest daughter, Jacklyn, aged 49, is a family therapist who lives in Texas. Their other daughter, Laila, aged 45, suffers from developmental disabilities and lives in a group home in a nearby city. Their son, the middle child, Kevin, age 47, is a high school principal who lives in New York with his wife and two children.

MEDICAL HISTORY: The patient has a recent history of angina for which she takes nitroglycerine tablets sublingually as required. Her vision is deteriorating, and she wears bifocals, which were prescribed and fitted within the last four months. She suffers from presbycusis, which was identified three years ago in a full audiometric evaluation as a bilateral, mild-moderate sensorineural hearing loss. She was prescribed a behind-the-ear (BTE) hearing aid for the right ear but does not wear it.

PRESENTING PROBLEM: Currently the patient is suffering from recent memory problems and confusion, which, according to her husband, have been increasing slowly in severity over the past year or so. She wanders from her home, now more frequently than ever, especially during the late afternoon. She gets lost easily. Mr. Townsend has been spending more time watching out for his wife because of this increased wandering. He has not yet sought support from any outside agencies.

Two days ago, while the patient was wandering through the downtown shopping center, she was crossing the street when a car struck her. Her head hit the pavement quite hard. She was not wearing her hearing aid at the time. An ambulance took her to the hospital ED. An x-ray was performed to determine skull fracture, if any, as a result of the head injury. The patient was discharged home in the care of her husband with a diagnosis of multiple bruises and a mild concussion.

Her husband brought her in to our office today because he noted that she was behaving strangely. At first, he figured it was just due to the trauma of the event and was concussion-related. Overnight, the patient exhibited confusion. She wandered the house aimlessly, repeatedly searching through the drawers and closets and urinating in a garbage can. When asked by her husband about her behaviors (e.g., 'What are you searching for?'), the patient insisted that she wanted to go home but could not find her way there. She accused her husband of keeping her against her will and kept repeating that she wanted to go home. She became very agitated.

PE: Patient shows unequal papillary response, and decerebrate posturing. CT can shows ischemic tissue and hematoma with no skull fracture.

Continued

DX: Epidural hematoma

PLAN: Admit patient to hospital for further evaluation and treatment.

James Healer, MD

JHW/mg   D: 10/22/11 09:50:16   T: 10/25/11 12:55:01

You Code It!

What are the best, most accurate codes?

Diagnosis Codes: _____

Procedure Codes: _____

Anesthesia Codes (when applicable): _____

HCPCS Level II codes (when applicable): _____

ADULT HEALTH ASSOCIATES
720 LONG STREET • ETERNITY, FL 32711 • 407-555-7322

PATIENT: LYNDELL, JACOB
ACCOUNT/EHR #:   LYNDJA01
Date: 12/22/11

Attending Physician: James Healer, MD

This patient is a 75-year-old male diagnosed with insulin-dependent diabetes mellitus (IDDM), who was last seen by me almost two years ago. He is a retired fish wholesale worker, married, with 12 children, seven of whom still live in the area. He lives with his wife, Charlotte, in a retirement community.

HISTORY: Patient has peripheral neuropathy with paresthesias of his fingers and feet, diabetic retinopathy, bilateral sensorineural hearing loss (SNHL), and peripheral vascular disease. The patient admits that he still smokes, on average, one pack of cigarettes a day.

PRESENTING PROBLEM: The patient is grossly overweight and denies following the diet given to him by me at our last encounter. He was diagnosed with IDDM five years ago and admits that he occasionally forgets to take his insulin.

PE: Decubitus ulcers are evident on the left foot and ankle. Sights of necrotic tissue and the beginnings of gangrene are observed. Decubitus ulcers forming on the right foot require monitoring in hopes of avoiding amputation of the right leg. GTT is abnormal.

DX: IDDM, uncontrolled, with peripheral angiopathy and gangrene.

PLAN: Admit to hospital for below-the-knee (BTK) amputation of left leg.

_____

James Healer, MD

JHW/mg   D: 12/22/11 09:50:16 T: 12/25/11 12:55:01

You Code It!

What are the best, most accurate codes?

Diagnosis Codes: _____

Procedure Codes: _____

Anesthesia Codes (when applicable): _____

HCPCS Level II codes (when applicable): _____

ADULT HEALTH ASSOCIATES
720 LONG STREET • ETERNITY, FL 32711 • 407-555-7322

PATIENT: COLLINS, ANDREA
ACCOUNT/EHR #:   COLLAN01
Date: 04/13/011

Attending Physician: James Healer, MD

This patient is an 81-year-old white female that I am meeting for the first time in the hospital, where she was admitted following a visit to the ED.

Prior to this hospital admission, she has been living independently in her own suburban house several houses down from her grandson, who is very attentive, helping her with yard care and grocery shopping in which she is limited by arthritic pain. The patient is otherwise independent, with ADLs (Activities of Daily Living) and other IADLs (Instrumental Activities of Daily Living).

PATIENT HISTORY: The patient lost her husband to cancer two years ago and takes pride in maintaining her independence. She has been relatively healthy throughout her life but did smoke for 35 years. She stopped smoking 10 years ago.

She takes hydrochlorothiazide 25 mg daily for hypertension and has an albuterol inhaler that she uses prn for mild emphysema and bronchitis. She needs the inhaler only occasionally, usually in the spring and fall, when pollen is in the air, or if she catches a cold. She also takes regular Tylenol about five days out of the week for "arthritis" of her knees. She has never been hospitalized for any reason, other than the birth of her children.

The patient was brought to our office by her grandson, Barney, with a report of maroon stools, which she has been experiencing for the last three days. He states that she has also exhibited a recent onset of dizziness. Patient denies pain or loss of appetite and states she feels well otherwise.

PE: She is a well-developed, well-nourished female who looks younger than her stated age. Her skin looks somewhat pale. Her BP lying down is 130/78 with a pulse of 84. On standing, her BP is 100/63 with a pulse of 124.

Patient is prepped, and I performed a flexible sigmoidoscopy to the splenic flexure. A bleeding polyp is identified in the descending colon. The polyp was removed by snare technique. Tissue sent to lab.

DX: Intestinal neoplasm, pending lab report for malignancy.

James Healer, MD

JHW/mg   D: 04/13/11 09:50:16   T: 04/15/11 12:55:01

You Code It!

What are the best, most accurate codes?

Diagnosis Codes: _____

Procedure Codes: _____

Anesthesia Codes (when applicable): _____

HCPCS Level II codes (when applicable): _____

ADULT HEALTH ASSOCIATES
720 LONG STREET • ETERNITY, FL 32711 • 407-555-7322

PATIENT: MCLAUGHLIN, RYAN
ACCOUNT/EHR #:   MCLARY01
Date: 04/22/11

Attending Physician: James Healer, MD

It has been 8 months since the last time I saw this 67-year-old male. He states that he has been experiencing terrible "knee pain" in both legs.

    Patient states that he is taking extra-strength Tylenol around the clock (two tablets every 4 hours) with little or no relief. He has thought about trying Aleve, which his neighbor swears by, but he remembers that the doctors at the hospital told him he should not take those types of pills.

PE: He has Heberden's and Bouchard's nodes and deformity of the knee joints with decreased range of motion. On the basis of the patient's history and this examination, osteoarthritis is suspected. Patient is taken down the hall to our imaging department.

    AP/Lat X-rays of each knee confirms diagnosis of osteoarthritis. There are no other findings to suggest other diagnoses.

DX: Osteoarthritis, bilateral

Rx: Tripod cane
    Patient is advised to begin taking OTC glucosamine plus chondroitin sulfate.
    Patient to return prn.

_____

James Healer, MD

JHW/mg   D: 04/22/11 09:50:16 T: 04/25/11 12:55:01

You Code It!

What are the best, most accurate codes?

Diagnosis Codes: _____

Procedure Codes: _____

Anesthesia Codes (when applicable): _____

HCPCS Level II codes (when applicable): _____

ADULT HEALTH ASSOCIATES
720 LONG STREET • ETERNITY, FL 32711 • 407-555-7322

PATIENT: EDWARDS, DEACON
ACCOUNT/EHR #: EDWADE01
Date: 04/22/011

Attending Physician: James Healer, MD

This is a 75-year-old male who recently moved back to the area to be closer to family. He presents to our office for the first time today for his regular annual check-up. He inquires about health prevention and screening. Throughout the years he has remained relatively healthy.

He reports that his current medications consist of 0.15 mg of levothyroxine for treatment of hypothyroidism and a multivitamin. His only surgeries consist of nonmalignant mole removals.

After retiring from his job as an office manager two years ago, he maintains a very active lifestyle, watching his two preschool age grandchildren, volunteering at the local library and working in his garden. Every morning he and his wife of 42 years go for a three-mile walk in the local park. He has never smoked, limits his alcohol consumption to a glass of wine on special occasions, and drinks two cups of coffee a day.

Patient states that his parents are still independent and live locally. His father, age 94, takes medication for HTN; and his mother, age 92, has been on Alendronate for treatment of osteoporosis. Both of his children, a son, aged 41, and a daughter, aged 37, are in perfect health. Unfortunately his sister, age 70, was just diagnosed with breast cancer.

Patient states that neither he nor his wife, Alma, suffers from depression and that Alma's only medical problem was a gallbladder attack five years ago when she was 64.

PE: Patient is a thin, Caucasian male. He is 5'6" and weighs 121 lb. His BP is 120/70. Heart, lung, chest, and abdominal exam are all within normal limits.

DX: Annual exam—no concerns highlighted

PLAN: Patient to return prn.

_____

James Healer, MD

JHW/mg   D: 04/22/11 09:50:16   T: 04/25/11 12:55:01

You Code It!

What are the best, most accurate codes?

Diagnosis Codes: _____

Procedure Codes: _____

Anesthesia Codes (when applicable): _____

HCPCS Level II codes (when applicable): _____

ADULT HEALTH ASSOCIATES
720 LONG STREET • ETERNITY, FL 32711 • 407-555-7322

PATIENT: ARCHER, PENELOPE
ACCOUNT/EHR #: ARCHPE01
Date: 06/22/11

Attending Physician: James Healer, MD

This 77-year-old female presents with significant memory problems and deficits in functional ability. She is a retired bookkeeper/executive secretary being evaluated for memory loss. As per the referral from her family physician, Dr. Fraiser, her physical examination is normal.

HISTORY OF PRESENT ILLNESS: The patient's husband mentions that her memory problems have been occurring for about three years; the patient thinks it has been only one year. According to the husband, the patient's memory loss has been "slow and gradually getting worse." She is having trouble remembering the names of familiar people and misplaces personal belongings such as keys or her glasses. She sets the table for five or six people when there are only two who will be eating. She is mildly depressed and is being treated for her depression by Dr. Fraiser. She does not smoke or drink significant amounts of alcohol. There is a family history of heart disease.

NEUROLOGIC ASSESSMENT: The patient's physical exam is normal. During the neurologic examination, the patient scores 25 out of 30 on the Functional Activity Questionnaire (FAQ)26, showing difficulty in almost all areas, including financial tasks, preparing meals, driving, current events, and ability to follow and understand books, movies or TV programs. Her Mini-Mental State Examination (MMSE) 27 score is 21; she is unable to copy a cube.

NEUROPSYCHOLOGIC TESTING: Neuropsychologic testing finds moderately severe memory impairment, mild impairment of language comprehension, and borderline impairment in orientation and attention.

LABORATORY EVALUATION: CT scan shows the brain is slightly atrophied. A complete laboratory workup shows no correctable cause for dementia.

DX: Senile dementia of the Alzheimer's type.

TREATMENT: The patient is started on a cholinesterase inhibitor—EXELON (rivastigmine tartrate) 1.5 mg twice daily with full meals. Based on good tolerability, she will be increased to 3 mg of EXELON twice daily with full meals. She is also started on vitamin E 1000 IU twice daily. She is currently being treated for comorbid conditions including depression, hypertension, and hypercholesterolemia, and has been placed on estrogen replacement therapy.

James Healer, MD

JHW/mg   D: 06/22/11 09:50:16   T: 06/25/11 12:55:01

You Code It!

What are the best, most accurate codes?

Diagnosis Codes: _____

Procedure Codes: _____

Anesthesia Codes (when applicable): _____

HCPCS Level II codes (when applicable): _____

ADULT HEALTH ASSOCIATES
720 LONG STREET • ETERNITY, FL 32711 • 407-555-7322

PATIENT: ARCHER, PENELOPE
ACCOUNT/EHR #: ARCHPE01
Date: 09/30/11

Attending Physician: James Healer, MD

This 77-year-old female comes to the office today for a 3-month reassessment.

Both she and her husband feel that she has "significantly improved." She is much more active and feels that "things seem clearer." Her MMSE score has improved to 24. Her FAQ score is 14, and there are dramatic improvements in her ability to shop alone, prepare a meal, and understand her favorite TV shows. She is having much less difficulty with orientation. Up to this point, she has not experienced gastrointestinal side effects or any other difficulties with Exelon treatment.

DX: Senile dementia of the Alzheimer's type.

TREATMENT: The Exelon dose is increased to 4.5 mg twice daily with full meals. Return in 4 months for follow-up.

_____

James Healer, MD

JHW/mg   D: 09/30/11 09:50:16   T: 09/30/11 12:55:01

You Code It!

What are the best, most accurate codes?

Diagnosis Codes: _____

Procedure Codes: _____

Anesthesia Codes (when applicable): _____

HCPCS Level II codes (when applicable): _____

Neonatal and Pediatrics Cases and Patient Records

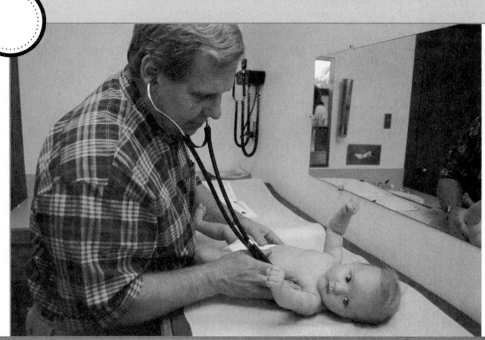

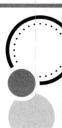

INTRODUCTION

The following case studies are from a neonatology and pediatric practice. In a physician's office of this type, a professional coding specialist is likely to see many different kinds of health situations, especially preventive health care services, relating to the care of children from birth up through the age of 18.

Neonatology is a pediatric subspecialty that deals with the diagnosis and treatment of disorders in newborns. A neonatologist typically consults with neonatal intensive care units (NICU) in hospitals and cares for babies born prematurely; with infections, such as neonatal streptococcal infections; and those born with congenital conditions and concerns, such as heart defects, genetic diseases, and malformations.

Neonatologists are board-certified through the Board of Pediatrics, which is recognized by the American Board of Medical Specialties.

Pediatricians also specialize in caring for children, from birth through 18 years of age. Pediatricians provide preventive health care, as well as treatment of childhood illnesses and diseases. Pediatrics has several sub-specialties in addition to neonatology, including:

- Adolescent medicine—health care specifically for teenagers
- Pediatric cardiology—heart problems in children
- Developmental disorders—behavior, communication, and mental disorders
- Pediatric endocrinology—endocrine glands and hormonal difficulties
- Pediatric gastroenterology—digestive system disorders
- Pediatric infectious disease—complex infections, which can include HIV/AIDS and hepatitis
- Pediatric nephrology—malfunction of the urinary system
- Pediatric oncology—treating children diagnosed with malignancy

The Board of Pediatrics certifies pediatricians, and this board certification is recognized by the American Board of Medical Specialties.

You can use these cases to practice coding diagnoses, E/M, procedures, DME, or other HCPCS Level II items, as applicable; code for the physician or the facility; inpatient or outpatient, as applicable:

1. Code for the physician.
2. Code for the anesthesiologist, when applicable.
3. Code for the hospital, when applicable.
4. Code for the pathology and laboratory, when applicable.
5. Code HCPCS Level II codes, when applicable.

PEDIATRIC COMPLETE CARE CENTER
123 BORNE PATH •YOUNGSTOWN, FL 32811 • 407-555-ABCD

PATIENT: THORNSON, BRITTA
MRN: THORBR001
Procedure Performed: Newborn Evaluation

Attending Physician: Pravdah H. Jeppard, MD

The patient is a female, gestational age 37 weeks, 4 days, born vaginally in this facility, 09/01/11, 04:15.

IMPRESSION: Neonate was of a single birth, BWT 2857 grams without significant OR procedures with a normal newborn diagnosis. 18.5" long. Head circumference: 33 cm. Amniotic fluid: clear, Cord: 3 vessels. Evidence of a benign tumor of blood vessels due to malformed angioblastic tissues (vascular hamartomas) at right groin. Appears pale, has poor skin turgor, is mucousy, and has transitional stool

APGAR SCORE: 1 min.= 9; 5 min.= 9. Heart rate: >100; Respiratory Effort: Good; Muscle tone: Active; Response to catheter in nostril: Cough; Color: Body pink, extremities blue

MATERNAL HISTORY: 29 year old, G1, blood type O+, spontaneous labor, 16 hr, 24 min., Epidural anesthesia, HIV-tested during pregnancy: neg

ADMINISTRATIONS: Hepatitis B, Peds, Vaccine (Recomb) 5 mcg/0.5 ml, given: 09/03/11

NEWBORN HEARING SCREENING: passed.

RECOMMENDATIONS: Follow-up in office two days

Pravdah H. Jeppard, MD

PHJ/mg   D: 09/03/11 09:50:16   T: 09/05/11 12:55:01

You Code It!

What are the best, most accurate codes?

Diagnosis Codes: _____

Procedure Codes: _____

Anesthesia Codes (when applicable): _____

HCPCS Level II codes (when applicable): _____

PEDIATRIC COMPLETE CARE CENTER
123 BORNE PATH • YOUNGSTOWN, FL 32811 • 407-555-ABCD

PATIENT: GEMISONN, PHILLIP
ACCOUNT/EHR #:   GEMIPH001
Date: 10/11/11

Attending Physician: Pravdah H. Jeppard, MD

S: Pt is a 3-day-old male who comes in for his first office visit after birth. He was a full-term infant, vaginally delivered. Mother provides prenatal history and family history including the paternal Rh factor and information regarding inherited red cell defects.

O: Wt. 6 lb. 3 ounces, T 98.6. Skin has yellowish skin coloration, including sclerae. Tests, including direct and indirect bilirubin levels, reveal gram-negative bacterial infection and serum bilirubin levels at 7 mg/dL. Blood tests are also performed to test infant and mother both for blood group incompatibilities, hemoglobin level, direct Coombs' test, and hematocrit.

A: Hyperbilirubinemia, due to gram-negative bacterial infection

P: 1. Rx albumin administration (1.0 g/kg of 25% salt-poor albumin)
    2. Rx antibiotics for infection
    3. Follow-up appointment in four days

Pravdah H. Jeppard, MD

PHJ/mg   D: 10/11/11 09:50:16   T: 10/13/11 12:55:01

You Code It!

What are the best, most accurate codes?

Diagnosis Codes: _____

Procedure Codes: _____

Anesthesia Codes (when applicable): _____

HCPCS Level II codes (when applicable): _____

PEDIATRIC COMPLETE CARE CENTER
123 BORNE PATH •YOUNGSTOWN, FL 32811 • 407-555-ABCD

PATIENT: ISAACSON, MARLO
MRN: ISAAMA001
Procedure Performed: Newborn Re-evaluation

Attending Physician: Pravdah H. Jeppard, MD

The patient is a female, gestational age 37 weeks, 15 days, born vaginally in this facility, 07/10/11, 17:45.

IMPRESSION: Neonate was of a single birth, BWT 2927 grams without significant OR procedures with a normal newborn diagnosis. 17.5" long. Head circumference: 32 cm. Amniotic fluid: clear, Cord: 3 vessels. PKU test normal at 48 hours.

APGAR SCORE: 1 min.= 9; 5 min.= 9. Heart rate: 100; respiratory effort: good, muscle tone: sctive; response to catheter in nostril: cough, Color: body pink, extremities blue

MATERNAL HISTORY: 31 year old, G2P2, blood type AB+, spontaneous labor 13 hrs, 55 min., epidural anesthesia, HIV-tested during pregnancy: neg; Scottish heritage with family history of phenylketonuria.

ADMINISTRATIONS: Hepatitis B, Peds, Vaccine (Recomb) 5 mcg/0.5 ml, given: 7/10/11

NEWBORN HEARING SCREENING: passed.
    At 35 hours of age, Guthrie screening test on capillary blood sample is positive for PKU.

RECOMMENDATIONS: Restricting dietary intake of amino acid phenylalanine to keep phenylalanine blood levels between 3 and 9 mg/dL. Referral to nutritionist for dietary standards. Follow-up in office 2 days.

Pravdah H. Jeppard, MD

PHJ/mg   D: 07/13/11 09:50:16 T: 07/15/11 12:55:01

You Code It!

What are the best, most accurate codes?

Diagnosis Codes: _____

Procedure Codes: _____

Anesthesia Codes (when applicable): _____

HCPCS Level II codes (when applicable): _____

PEDIATRIC COMPLETE CARE CENTER
123 BORNE PATH •YOUNGSTOWN, FL 32811 • 407-555-ABCD

PATIENT: TYSON, BROCK
ACCOUNT/EHR #:   TYSOBR001
Date: 05/15/11

Attending Physician: Pravdah H. Jeppard, MD

S: Pt is a 11-day-old male who is brought in by his father because it appears to him that the child had some kind of seizure the day before, and again last night. He states that this is frightening to his wife, and he admits, he is worried, too.

O: Wt. 7 lb. 9 ounces, T 98.6. Complete blood work, EEG, and ECG ordered.

PE reveals no anomalies.

A: Convulsions in newborn

P: 1. Follow-up appointment once test results are received
    2. Instructions on care given to father

_____

Pravdah H. Jeppard, MD

PHJ/mg   D: 05/15/11 09:50:16   T: 05/20/11 12:55:01

You Code It!

What are the best, most accurate codes?

Diagnosis Codes: _____

Procedure Codes: _____

Anesthesia Codes (when applicable): _____

HCPCS Level II codes (when applicable): _____

PEDIATRIC COMPLETE CARE CENTER
123 BORNE PATH •YOUNGSTOWN, FL 32811 • 407-555-ABCD

PATIENT: BECKMAN, WILLIAM

ACCOUNT/EHR #:   BECKWI001

Date: 10/11/11

Attending Physician: Pravdah H. Jeppard, MD

The patient is a male, gestational age 41 weeks, 6 days, born by cesarean section in this facility, 10/10/11, 27:37.

IMPRESSION: Neonate was of a single birth, BWT 2857 grams without significant OR procedures with a normal newborn diagnosis. 21" long. Head circumference: 31 cm. Amniotic fluid: clear. Cord: 3 vessels. Head is acrocephalitic, and there is evidence of premature cranial suture fusion. The fingers of the right hand are syndactylic, as well.

APGAR SCORE: 1 min.= 7; 5 min.= 8. Heart rate: 100; respiratory effort: good; muscle tone: active; response to catheter in nostril: cough; color: body pink, extremities blue

MATERNAL HISTORY: 41 year old, G2P2, blood type B+, planned c-section due to previous c-section birth 3 years ago. General anesthesia. HIV-tested during pregnancy: neg

ADMINISTRATIONS: Hepatitis B, Peds, Vaccine (Recomb) 5 mcg/0.5 ml, given: 10/12/11

NEWBORN HEARING SCREENING: passed.

RECOMMENDATIONS: Newborn has acrocephalosyndactyly. Consultation with neonatologist requested.

___

Pravdah H. Jeppard, MD

PHJ/mg   D: 10/11/11 09:50:16   T: 10/13/11 12:55:01

You Code It!

What are the best, most accurate codes?

Diagnosis Codes: _____

Procedure Codes: _____

Anesthesia Codes (when applicable): _____

HCPCS Level II codes (when applicable): _____

PEDIATRIC COMPLETE CARE CENTER
123 BORNE PATH • YOUNGSTOWN, FL 32811 • 407-555-ABCD

PATIENT: MALENNA, MORRIS
ACCOUNT/EHR #:   MALEMO001
Date: 09/16/11

Attending Physician: Suzanne R. Taylor, MD

Pt is a 7-month-old male brought in by his mother. She states that she picked the child up from their babysitter's house, and he has been listless and unresponsive since. There has been no loss of consciousness.

Eyes are glazed and unfocused with petechia showing in sclera. MRI brain confirms shaken infant syndrome with intracranial contusion of brainstem.

Child is admitted to hospital NICU for observation.

Authorities notified of suspected abuse.

_____

Suzanne R. Taylor, MD

SRT/pw   D: 09/16/11 09:50:16 T: 09/18/11 12:55:01

You Code It!

What are the best, most accurate codes?

Diagnosis Codes: _____

Procedure Codes: _____

Anesthesia Codes (when applicable): _____

HCPCS Level II codes (when applicable): _____

PEDIATRIC COMPLETE CARE CENTER
123 BORNE PATH • YOUNGSTOWN, FL 32811 • 407-555-ABCD

PATIENT: CRANSTON, TYLER
ACCOUNT/EHR #:   CRANTY001
Date: 09/16/11

Attending Physician: Suzanne R. Taylor, MD

S: This Pt is a 5-month-old male brought in by his father because of severe rash on his buttocks. This infant was seen in this office three months ago for a routine well-baby check-up.

O: Ht 37" Wt. 19.75 lbs. T 98.6 Pt appears in minor distress; however, examination shows nothing out of the ordinary.

A: Diaper rash

P: 1. Rx A&D ointment to be applied after each diaper change
    2. Return prn

_____

Suzanne R. Taylor, MD

SRT/pw   D: 09/16/11 09:50:16   T: 09/18/11 12:55:01

You Code It!

What are the best, most accurate codes?

Diagnosis Codes: _____

Procedure Codes: _____

Anesthesia Codes (when applicable): _____

HCPCS Level II codes (when applicable): _____

PEDIATRIC COMPLETE CARE CENTER
123 BORNE PATH • YOUNGSTOWN, FL 32811 • 407-555-ABCD

PATIENT: FREDERLANE, PENNY
ACCOUNT/EHR #:   FREDPE002
Date: 07/22/11

Attending Physician: James Healer, MD

S: Pt is a 5-year-old female brought in by her mother for her school vaccinations. She will be starting kindergarten in three weeks, and the vaccinations are required by the school for admission.

O: Ht 2'3" Wt. 37 lbs. R 16. Child is visibly small for her age. Her teeth show signs of calcification loss and neglect. Her hair is very thin and falls out easily. Eye orbits appear to be slightly sunken. Skin is pale. Complete CBC and urinalysis (dipstick) performed. MMR vaccine, live, sub q and IPV sub q, administered. Her language skills appear to be normal for her age; however, her activity level is low. She is friendly but quiet and responds when spoken to.

    I discussed with the mother my concern about Penny's nutritional health. She nodded in agreement and said she would "do her best."

A: Nutritional neglect by mother

P: 1. Nutritional guidelines reviewed with mother
      2. School certificate signed
      3. Authorities notified of suspected abuse

James Healer, MD

JHW/mg   D: 07/22/11 09:50:16 T: 07/25/11 12:55:01

You Code It!

What are the best, most accurate codes?

Diagnosis Codes: _____

Procedure Codes: _____

Anesthesia Codes (when applicable): _____

HCPCS Level II codes (when applicable): _____

PEDIATRIC COMPLETE CARE CENTER
123 BORNE PATH • YOUNGSTOWN, FL 32811 • 407-555-ABCD

PATIENT: WEIGNER, JULIAN
ACCOUNT/EHR #: WEIGJU001
Date: 10/17/11

Attending Physician: James I. Cipher, MD

S: Karl is a 13-month-old male brought in today by his grandmother. She cares for the child during the day while his mother is at work. She reports that he has been irritable and has been tugging at his left ear. For the past two days, he has been running a low-grade fever. There has been a slight cough with no discharge. Pt has a history of problems with his ears and sinuses. Pt is teething.

O: Ht 2'5" Wt. 27 lb. R 17. T 101.3. HEENT: Purulent nasal discharge, yellow-green in color, is noted. TM is erythematous unilaterally left, bulging and with purulent effusions. Oropharynx is nonerythematous without lesions. Two teeth on the bottom. Tonsils are unremarkable. Neck: Neck is supple with good ROM. Positive cervical adenopathy. Lungs: Clear. Heart: Regular rate and rhythm without murmurs.

A: Acute suppurative otitis media, left side.

P: 1. Rx Augmentin 40 mg/kg divided t.i.d. 10 days
    2. Bed rest, lots of fluids.
    3. Follow-up prn or if no improvement in 10 days

James I. Cipher, MD

JIC/mg   D: 10/17/11 09:50:16   T: 10/23/11 12:55:01

You Code It!

What are the best, most accurate codes?

Diagnosis Codes: _____

Procedure Codes: _____

Anesthesia Codes (when applicable): _____

HCPCS Level II codes (when applicable): _____

PEDIATRIC COMPLETE CARE CENTER
123 BORNE PATH • YOUNGSTOWN, FL 32811 • 407-555-ABCD

PATIENT: VONN, VANESSA
ACCOUNT/EHR #: VONNVA001
Date: 10/13/11

S: This is a 5 years, 7 months-old female, brought in by her parents with a stated persistent fever. I last saw this child at her annual well-child check-up four months ago. The father states that she has been lacking energy and has a decreased appetite. She was noted to be in her normal state of health until one week ago, at which time she developed conjunctival infection, fever to 103° F, and sore throat. Her parents attributed these symptoms to a recent viral upper respiratory infection that affected several children in Vanessa's class. Vanessa's mother noted an erythematous rash in her perianal region while bathing her last night and noted peeling of the skin near her fingernails. Vanessa has begun to complain of joint pain, as well. Her parents note they initially did not give her any antipyretics, but when they gave acetaminophen yesterday, it did not seem to have any effect. They are worried that a fever of 103° F could be dangerous and cause harm to the child.

O: Vanessa does not look "well." She appears tired and disinterested in playing with the toys in the waiting room. She appears to move slowly, saying that it hurts her knees to walk around. At this age, she is expected to be able to carry on a conversation, but she seems too exhausted to talk for long. She is noted to be an ill-appearing, febrile child. Erythema of the tongue gives it a "strawberry" appearance. Her lips are dry and cracked. Erythema and edema of the feet are noted, and she walks with a slight limp. She has a 1.7 cm palpable cervical lymph node and an erythematous rash of her lower trunk and perineum. Concerned about the possibility of serious illness, the parents and I make the decision to admit Vanessa to the pediatric floor of the hospital for possible Kawasaki syndrome.

A: Kawasaki syndrome

P: Admit child into the hospital for further tests and treatment. Parents are upset that they may have waited too long to bring her in and worry they may have done something to cause the illness. They are concerned that Vanessa's playmates will get the disease as well. I reassure them that this is not contagious and is a vasculitis seen in children.

Robert M. Katzman, MD

10/13/11 11:47:39

You Code It!

What are the best, most accurate codes?

Diagnosis Codes: _____

Procedure Codes: _____

Anesthesia Codes (when applicable): _____

HCPCS Level II codes (when applicable): _____

PEDIATRIC COMPLETE CARE CENTER
123 BORNE PATH • YOUNGSTOWN, FL 32811 • 407-555-ABCD

PATIENT: MARKOVICH, LISETTE
ACCOUNT/EHR #: MARLI001
Date: 10/15/11

HPI: Patient is a 2-month-old Caucasian female, here with her mother for a Well Child Exam. Her mother is a 25-year-old G1P1 woman whose past medical history is negative. Her mother, Andrea, appears relaxed and states that the baby has been doing well. She is eating and seems to be growing. Mother does state that she is concerned that Lisette may not be getting enough breast milk. She will be returning to work next week and wants to know if she should change to formula feeding. Also she wants to know when she should introduce other foods.

Lisette is at the 50th percentile for both weight and length; head circumference is at the 60th percentile. She has been following these growth parameters since birth without dropping off "the curve." Andrea is concerned with how much her baby should be eating and when it is ok to advance her diet. Andrea asks what developmental milestones are expected for a 2-month-old infant and what to expect over the next 10 months. We discuss key developmental milestones (gross motor, language, fine motor, social) in a 2–3 month old infant. I reassure the mother that rolling over is achieved between 3–6 months. She should expect to begin to bear weight on her legs and grasp a rattle in the next two months.

PHYSICAL EXAM: Lisette is smiling, playing with her hands, following objects past midline, laughing, and cooing. She holds her head up when placed her on her belly. Her exam is normal including primitive reflexes.

IMMUNIZATIONS: The mother would like her to receive vaccines on schedule and would like more information on vaccine safety and necessity. Lisette received Hep B #1 in the nursery. Handouts on each of the vaccines administered today are given to the mother.

ADMINISTERED TODAY: HIB, PCV, and Pediarix (DtAP, IPV and Hep B)

Robert M. Katzman, MD

10/15/11 11:47:39

You Code It!

What are the best, most accurate codes?

Diagnosis Codes: _____

Procedure Codes: _____

Anesthesia Codes (when applicable): _____

HCPCS Level II codes (when applicable): _____

PEDIATRIC COMPLETE CARE CENTER
123 BORNE PATH • YOUNGSTOWN, FL 32811 • 407-555-ABCD

PATIENT: DELVANEY, TODD
ACCOUNT/EHR #:   DELTO001
Date: 10/13/11

S: Patient is brought in by his mother and father for a Well Child Exam. He is an active 2-year-old male, adopted two weeks ago from Thailand. His parents do not have any of his medical records and are not sure if he has had any immunizations. They do know that his birth mother had some limited prenatal care and had a normal delivery at 38 weeks gestation. Todd has been healthy to date, living in a shelter in Thailand. They are concerned because they are not sure if he ever went to a doctor while in Thailand. His parents state that they want to know more about his immunization status and developmental status and how best to childproof their home. They would also like to be sure his physical exam is normal and that he does not have any underlying medical conditions of which they are not aware. Todd's parents are concerned about him receiving three shots in one day. They are also worried about side effects and wonder if there is any reason he should not receive a vaccine. Mrs. Delvaney notes that she had a sore arm and fever after receiving a flu shot at work—she wonders if this will happen to Todd.

SOCIAL HISTORY: The parents state that their home water supply does not contain fluoride. There is no smoking, alcohol, or drug use in the home. The mother, Lorraine, will care for him during the day for the next year before returning to her job as a nurse. His father, Calvin, is a local high school teacher. While at the shelter, Todd was consuming a diet of soy milk and table foods (predominately rice, meats, and beans). Since coming to the U.S., his diet has expanded and he drinks whole milk and fruit juice. Parents state that the child has a voracious appetite and particularly enjoys cheese, chicken, apples, and carrots. They do note he eats only when he wants, not necessarily at standard family meal times. They say he seems to have adjusted well over the past 2 weeks.

O: Todd is sitting nervously on his mother's lap. Though he appears thin, he is not believed to be malnourished. When asked, he states his name is "Toddy."

PHYSICAL EXAM: There is a noticeable 3/6 systolic murmur over the child's left lower sternal border (LLSB). There is no way to know if this murmur has been present since birth or changed at all as the boy has been growing. I reassured the parents that I believe this to be a benign murmur, but to be cautious I am going to refer them to a pediatric cardiologist to obtain a proper work-up. The remainder of this physical exam is within normal limits. Although he is thin, the child does not appear emaciated or malnourished. He is interactive during the exam and developmentally appears on target, meeting the proper 2-year-old milestones.

PLAN: Refer to Dr. Feld, Pediatric Cardiology Associates. Child to return p.r.n. or for next well child exam.

Robert M. Katzman, MD

10/13/11 11:47:39

You Code It!

What are the best, most accurate codes?

Diagnosis Codes: _____

Procedure Codes: _____

Anesthesia Codes (when applicable): _____

HCPCS Level II codes (when applicable): _____

PEDIATRIC COMPLETE CARE CENTER
123 BORNE PATH •YOUNGSTOWN, FL 32811 • 407-555-ABCD

PATIENT: MASSADA, CARTER
ACCOUNT/EHR #: MASCA001
Date: 09/16/11

This 3-year-old male is brought in by his mother with a chief complaint of delayed speech. Mother states that he started to babble at about nine months of age and then learned a few words such as "Dada" and "boo" at two years of age. She claims that she and her husband have tried to stimulate the boy's language development by reading to him, interacting with him during television watching, and teaching him to mimic others' speech. They became more concerned as he grew older, noting his speech was less than the other children in his playgroup. They try to engage him in interactive activities, but he does not seem interested. They note that he is very independent and that he is very serious. He likes to play by himself rather than talking with or singing with other children. They worry that he has no playmates or friends because of his speech delay. He has been generally healthy and has had a few ear infections.

PAST MEDICAL HISTORY: Prenatal and past medical histories are otherwise unremarkable, and he has not had any serious infections or need for hospitalization.

PHYSICAL EXAM: Vital signs are normal. Height, weight, and head circumference are between the 25th and 50th percentiles. His HEENT, heart, lung, abdominal, skin, and neuromuscular portions of the physical exam show no abnormalities. While talking with his parents, it is noted that the child separates from them easily and wanders about the room. He does not seem to notice that everyone is talking about him. He finds some blocks in the corner and sits down to play with them. He does not respond when called to. He starts to sort the blocks by color into groups and lines them up. He seems content playing by himself. I went over to him in the corner and sat down by him. He did not appear to notice that I am there. He continues to line up the blocks (very neatly) and my attempts to interrupt him are unsuccessful. Although he seems content, I notice that he does not laugh or even smile much. Also noted is that he does not look at me or check back to his parents. During the session, he did not say any words.

On developmental screening, his motor development is normal. He is delayed in his language, social, and self-help skills. I administered an audiology evaluation, which shows his hearing to be normal and conducive to speech development. Further evaluation reveals:

1) Social disturbance: Lack of eye contact, poor attachments, and shows a general lack of social interest.
2) Communicative disturbance: Failure to develop semantics (word use), failure to develop reciprocity in dialogue, and failure to use language for social interaction.
3) Behavioral features: Shows a particular attachment to objects. Parents have noted both hand flapping and toe walking.

ASSESSMENT: Autistic disorder

Robert M. Katzman, MD

09/16/11 11:47:39

You Code It!

What are the best, most accurate codes?

Diagnosis Codes: _____

Procedure Codes: _____

Anesthesia Codes (when applicable): _____

HCPCS Level II codes (when applicable): _____

PEDIATRIC COMPLETE CARE CENTER
123 BORNE PATH •YOUNGSTOWN, FL 32811 • 407-555-ABCD

PATIENT: WIRRMAN, BRUCE
ACCOUNT/EHR #: WIRBR001
Date: 11/15/11

This is a 3,640-gram newborn male infant born at 37 weeks gestation via normal spontaneous vaginal delivery (NSVD) at Harris Medical Center to an 18-year-old G3P0 mother who is A+, VDRL NR, Hepatitis B surface antigen (HBsAg) positive, rubella immune, group B streptococcus (GBS) negative, and HIV negative. Artificial rupture of membranes (AROM) occurred 15 hours prior to delivery with clear fluid. Apgar scores were 8 and 9 at 1 and 5 minutes respectively.

Maternal history is remarkable for one prenatal visit 3 months ago. An ultrasound performed at that time was consistent with 31 weeks gestation. Toxicology screening at that visit and on admission were negative. Mother is reportedly healthy, with no chronic medical problems and no significant family history. She reports no difficulty during the pregnancy. She denies alcohol, cigarette, medication, or drug use. Social history reveals that the mother's support system includes the father of the baby (FOB) and both maternal and paternal grandparents.

EXAM: VST 37.0 rectal, P 141, R48, BP 49/35. Weight 3640 grams (8 pounds) (75th%), 51 cm (20 inches) (75th%); head circumference 34 cm (13.5 inches) (50th%). This infant is term in appearance, pink and active. Anterior fontanelle is soft and flat. Caput succedaneum is present. Corneas are clear. Ears are normally placed. Nares are patent. Oral mucosa is pink and the palate is intact. Neck is supple without masses. Clavicles are intact. His chest is symmetric and mature breast buds are present. Lungs are clear with equal aeration. Heart is regular with no murmurs heard. Abdomen is flat and soft with no masses. Three vessels are visible within the umbilical cord. Femoral and brachial pulses are symmetric and 2. Hips demonstrate full range of motion, no tightness, no clicks. Ortolani and Barlow signs are negative. Perineal creases are symmetric. Anus is patent. Male genitalia are normal, with both testes descended. His skin is pink with a few facial petechiae. He moves all extremities well. His Moro reflex is intact. His grasp response is symmetrical. His suck reflex is strong.

By 7 hours of age, he has passed meconium once, has had no urine output, and has nippled 15 cc of infant formula from a bottle. His mother does not want to breastfeed because she says she has no milk and will be returning to school soon. Besides, she read that formula makes your baby grow just as well as breast milk.

Robert M. Katzman, MD

11/15/11 11:47:39

You Code It!

What are the best, most accurate codes?

Diagnosis Codes: _____

Procedure Codes: _____

Anesthesia Codes (when applicable): _____

HCPCS Level II codes (when applicable): _____

PEDIATRIC COMPLETE CARE CENTER
123 BORNE PATH •YOUNGSTOWN, FL 32811 • 407-555-ABCD

PATIENT: SIZEMORE, KYLE
ACCOUNT/EHR #: SIZKY001
Date: 06/13/11

This two-day-old male infant was referred from a community hospital for bilious vomiting and a heart murmur. The baby was born at 37 weeks gestation to a G4P3 39-year-old woman who had no prenatal care.

EXAM: VS T 37.1 (ax), P 150, R 45, BP 75/50, oxygen saturation 99% in room air. Height, weight, and head circumference are at the 50th percentile. He appears jaundiced, and has a flat facial profile; short, upslanting palpebal fissures; a flat nasal bridge with epicanthal folds; a small mouth with protruding tongue; and single palmar creases. His lungs are clear to auscultation. His heart is tachycardic with a loud holosystolic murmur. His abdomen is nondistended. Generalized hypotonia is present.

Abdominal radiograph shows a "double-bubble sign." Duodenal atresia is suspected. A nasogastric tube is placed and IV fluids are administered. A duodenostomy is performed. An echocardiogram demonstrates a ventricular septal defect, which is medically managed. A chromosomal abnormality is suspected and a karyotype is done. Trisomy 21 is diagnosed.

DX: Trisomy 21 (Down syndrome)

PLAN: Discuss details of condition with both parents. Informational brochures are provided, along with contact information for a local support group.

Robert M. Katzman, MD

06/13/11 11:47:39

You Code It!

What are the best, most accurate codes?

Diagnosis Codes: _____

Procedure Codes: _____

Anesthesia Codes (when applicable): _____

HCPCS Level II codes (when applicable): _____

PEDIATRIC COMPLETE CARE CENTER
123 BORNE PATH • YOUNGSTOWN, FL 32811 • 407-555-ABCD

PATIENT: NEWBERRY, DANIEL
ACCOUNT/EHR #:   NEWDA001
Date: 05/02/11

This is a 14-month-old male infant who is brought in by his parents with a chief complaint of high fever and no response to antipyretic therapy. This illness started suddenly with the abrupt onset of fever early yesterday morning. He then developed a severe cough and increased work of breathing. No other symptoms are noted. The patient was born in a refugee camp and lived in Texas before moving here three months ago. The mother reports that he is frequently ill. No reports from earlier health care visits are available, but his mother reports he was also seen as an outpatient frequently and he was hospitalized at least once in Texas. He was hospitalized two months ago for pneumococcal pneumonia (right upper lobe consolidation and pneumococcal bacteremia).

EXAM: VS T 40.3, P 145, R 55, BP 100/60, oxygen saturation 98%, weight 7 kg (5th percentile). He is listless, tired, and small for age. He is lying on the examination table, moving little, and whimpering slightly to stimulation with tachypnea and chest retractions. His head is normocephalic, without signs of trauma. Both ear canals contain purulent drainage. Mouth exam is unremarkable. His heart is tachycardic with no murmurs heard. His chest shows mild retractions, tachypnea, dullness to percussion over the posterior upper chest, and decreased breath sounds in the area of dullness with occasional fine crackles. His abdomen is scaphoid and soft, with active bowel sounds, no masses, and no hepatosplenomegaly. His extremities are slender and wasted with decreased muscle mass and strength. Neurologic exam is normal.

A blood culture is positive for pneumococcus. Because of his recurrent infections and the failure to meet normal growth expectations, an immunologic work-up is done. He is found to have markedly elevated IgM, undetectable IgG and IgA, with diminished total B lymphocytes (CD19). His clinical picture is consistent with hypogammaglobulinemia with high IgM or Hyper-IgM syndrome.

DX: Pneumocystis carinii pneumonia (PCP)

PLAN: Admit into hospital for intravenous antibiotics and IVIG replacement therapy with trimethoprim-sulfamethoxazole prophylaxis for Pneumocystis carinii pneumonia (PCP).

Robert M. Katzman, MD

05/02/11 11:47:39

You Code It!

What are the best, most accurate codes?

Diagnosis Codes: _____

Procedure Codes: _____

Anesthesia Codes (when applicable): _____

HCPCS Level II codes (when applicable): _____

PEDIATRIC COMPLETE CARE CENTER
123 BORNE PATH •YOUNGSTOWN, FL 32811 • 407-555-ABCD

PATIENT: WASHINGTON, JERMAINE
ACCOUNT/EHR #:   WASJE001
Date: 11/17/11

This is a 4-week-old male who has been brought in by his father and mother with a one-week history of "noisy breathing." His parents note that his noisy breathing is worse when they lay him down or with crying. It is most noticeable when he takes a breath in. There has been no history of fever, coughing, runny nose, change in his cry, apnea, or feeding difficulties. He has been gaining weight appropriately. Prenatal course was uneventful, and he was delivered at 38 weeks gestation by spontaneous vaginal delivery without complications. Family history is unremarkable.

EXAM: VS T 37.0, P 120, R 48, oxygen saturation 98% in room air. Weight and height are at the 50%ile. He is alert, active, in no acute distress. There is audible inspiratory stridor noted in the supine position, which is improved with extension of his neck. His anterior fontanel is soft and flat. His eyes and ears are normal. No nasal flaring is visible, and his nares appear patent. His throat shows no erythema or lesions. His lips are moist and pink. There are no retractions or pectus abnormalities. His lungs are clear to auscultation throughout once the stridor clears with airway repositioning (no wheezes or rales). Aeration is good. He has noisy referred upper airway sounds when he is supine with his neck flexed. His heart is regular without murmurs. His color, perfusion, capillary refill and pulses are good.
    A flexible fiberoptic laryngoscopy confirms the diagnosis of mild laryngomalacia.

DX: Mild laryngomalacia

PLAN: Come back in 2 weeks for recheck

Robert M. Katzman, MD

11/17/11 08:47:39

You Code It!

What are the best, most accurate codes?

Diagnosis Codes: _____

Procedure Codes: _____

Anesthesia Codes (when applicable): _____

HCPCS Level II codes (when applicable): _____

PEDIATRIC COMPLETE CARE CENTER
123 BORNE PATH • YOUNGSTOWN, FL 32811 • 407-555-ABCD

PATIENT: EVERSON, ADIN
ACCOUNT/EHR #:   EVEAD001
Date: 12/19/11

This is a newborn male infant born at 0415 on this date to a 23-year-old G2P1 mother at 39 weeks gestation via NSVD (normal spontaneous vaginal delivery).

Appropriate antenatal care and monitoring occurred throughout the pregnancy. As there were no significant antenatal problems, no prenatal ultrasonography was done. Immediately following delivery, the baby looks "normal." He cries immediately; however, at 1 minute of age, he remains very cyanotic. The neonatal resuscitation team is called to the delivery room. At 5 minutes of age, the baby remains very cyanotic, tachypneic, and dyspneic, despite 100% oxygen via mask. The resuscitation team starts bag-mask positive pressure ventilation with 100% oxygen, but the baby becomes bradycardic; therefore he is intubated and ventilated. Auscultation of the lungs reveals good breath sounds in the right chest, but no breath sounds in the left. The heart sounds seemed loudest in the right chest, and the abdomen appears scaphoid. Ventilation is continued through the endotracheal tube while an NG tube is inserted and suction is applied. A STAT chest x-ray is done, which reveals bowel (and the NG tube tip) in the left chest cavity.

DX: Congenital diaphragmatic hernia presenting in the delivery room
    The baby is transferred to the NICU.

Robert M. Katzman, MD

12/19/11 08:47:39

You Code It!

What are the best, most accurate codes?

Diagnosis Codes: _____

Procedure Codes: _____

Anesthesia Codes (when applicable): _____

HCPCS Level II codes (when applicable): _____

PEDIATRIC COMPLETE CARE CENTER
123 BORNE PATH • YOUNGSTOWN, FL 32811 • 407-555-ABCD

PATIENT: ABBOTT, JALEEL
ACCOUNT/EHR #:   ABBJA001
Date: 10/23/11

This is a 3-month-old male brought to this clinic by his parents with a chief complaint of decreased activity, poor feeding, and constipation.

PAST MEDICAL HISTORY: The infant was born at 39 weeks gestation, with no complications during the pregnancy or birth. The infant is exclusively breast fed, up-to-date on immunizations, and has suffered from no previous illness. On further questioning, his mother reports her son has not been himself for the past week. He has had no fever, and there are no sick contacts. He has been less active, with a weak cry during this time. His mother also notes the infant has not been as interested in feeding and has suffered from constipation. His urine output is decreased with only four wet diapers in the last 24 hours. Typically, he has three to four soft stools per day, usually after feeds, but has had no bowel movement in the past 5 days.

EXAM: VS 37.0, P 114, R 22, BP 98/62, Wt. 5.3 kg (75%), Ht. 57 cm (50%). He is awake and nontoxic appearing, with expressionless facies and a weak cry. His anterior fontanel is flat and soft. He has poor head control. He has diminished pupillary reflexes, absent corneal reflexes, bilateral ptosis, and decreased tearing. He has a weak suck and gag reflexes with increased oral secretions. His neck is supple without adenopathy. Heart and lungs are normal. Aeration is good. His abdomen is soft, full, and nontender, with decreased bowel sounds throughout. No hepatosplenomegaly. Rectal exam shows no stool in the rectal vault and decreased anal sphincter tone. His extremities are slightly cool, with delayed capillary refill. His skin shows no rash or petechiae. He has decreased muscle tone throughout and diminished deep tendon reflexes.

   A sepsis work-up is done, and he is started on IV fluids and empiric antibiotics for sepsis. Stool samples are sent for *Clostridium botulinum* toxin assays. His cultures are subsequently negative. His clinical condition worsens such that he cannot feed, and he eventually develops hypoventilation and respiratory insufficiency requiring mechanical ventilation. An electromyography study is done which shows brief, small, abundant, motor unit potentials, known by the acronym BSAP, a characteristic pattern associated with infant botulism. His stool assay returns positive for botulism toxin.

   He is hospitalized for infant botulism.

_____

Robert M. Katzman, MD

10/23/11 11:47:39

You Code It!

What are the best, most accurate codes?

Diagnosis Codes: _____

Procedure Codes: _____

Anesthesia Codes (when applicable): _____

HCPCS Level II codes (when applicable): _____

PEDIATRIC COMPLETE CARE CENTER
123 BORNE PATH •YOUNGSTOWN, FL 32811 • 407-555-ABCD

PATIENT: CARDONE, DAPHNE
ACCOUNT/EHR #: CARDA001
Date: 12/15/11

This is a 16-year-old female brought in by her father, with the chief complaint that he thinks his daughter is using drugs and wants her to get treatment. The father reports that she has often been acting "high," with sleeplessness for several days in a row, unusual euphoria, pressured speech, increased activity (e.g., cleaning the bathroom), suspiciousness, and some aggressive behaviors.

HPI: After requesting that the father wait outside, she admits that she uses "ice," or "batu," roughly two to three times per week, smoking it by pipe. She obtains the drug from her friends. She admits to occasional marijuana use and weekend drinking of alcohol, without any history of blackouts, hallucinations, or incapacitating withdrawal symptoms. Although previously an above-average student, she has, for the past year, been truant from school and is failing most of her classes. She has also run away from home on several occasions. She gives vague answers when asked about sexual history.

Her past medical history is otherwise negative. Family history is significant for a history of alcoholism and a possible psychotic illness. Her parents are divorced. There is no history of abuse or domestic violence.

EXAM: VS T 37.5, P 110, R 18, BP 130/80. She is somewhat restless and guarded, with poor eye contact and brief answers. HEENT significant for slightly dilated pupils. Heart shows regular rhythm and elevated rate. Pelvic examination is performed, although she has agreed reluctantly. The remainder of physical examination is normal.

LABS: Urine toxicology positive for methamphetamine, negative for others, including alcohol. Electrocardiogram is significant for sinus tachycardia, otherwise normal.

DX: Methamphetamine dependence and Chlamydia cervicitis.

PLAN: Pt is referred for admission to an adolescent substance abuse treatment program.

Robert M. Katzman, MD

12/15/11 11:47:39

You Code It!

What are the best, most accurate codes?

Diagnosis Codes: _____

Procedure Codes: _____

Anesthesia Codes (when applicable): _____

HCPCS Level II codes (when applicable): _____

12 Neurology Cases and Patient Records

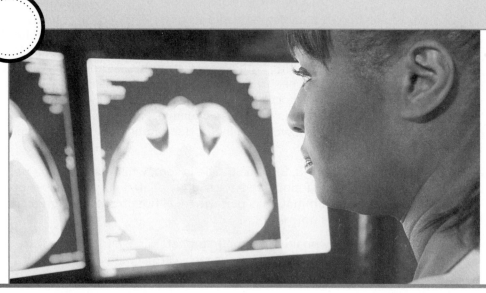

INTRODUCTION

The following case studies are from a neurologist's practice. In a neurologist's office, a professional coding specialist is likely to see many different types of health situations.

Physicians who specialize in the diagnosis and treatment of conditions of the nervous system including the brain and the spinal cord are called neurologists. These health care professionals identify, diagnose, and treat such diseases as Parkinson's disease, Alzheimer's disease, meningitis, and stroke. Neurosurgery is a subspecialty for physicians, who diagnose and treat conditions affecting the neurologic system, such as brain tumors or hydrocephalus. These professionals may also work with patients for pain management.

The Board of Psychiatry and Neurology bestows board certification to neurologists who qualify. The certification is recognized by the American Board of Medical Specialties.

You can use these cases to practice coding diagnoses, E/M, procedures, DME, or other HCPCS Level II items, as applicable; code for the physician or the facility; code inpatient and outpatient services, as applicable:

1. Code for the physician.
2. Code for the anesthesiologist, when applicable.
3. Code for the hospital, when applicable.
4. Code for the pathology and laboratory, when applicable.
5. Code HCPCS Level II codes, when applicable.

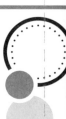

FRAISER, HARROLD, & YAWZI, Neurology
81 BAYER BOULEVARD • SENSATION, FL 32811 • 407-555-5852

PATIENT: SAMI, KAREN
ACCOUNT/EHR #:   SAMIKA001
Date: 09/16/11

Attending Physician: Suzanne R. Taylor, MD

The patient is a 29-year-old female with a history of recurrent sinus infections who was well until six days ago. She presents with fever, severe frontal headache, facial pain, and runny nose. Patient states she has been having difficulty concentrating.

Wt. 145 lbs. B/P: 120/85 T 101.5° HEENT: Tenderness over frontal and left maxillary sinuses. Nasal congestions visible.

    CT scan reveals opacification of both frontal and left maxillary, sphenoid sinuses and a possible large nonenhanced lesion in the brain.

    Parasagittal MRI and axial MRI show a large (7cm) well-circumscribed epidural collection compressing the left frontal lobe.

DX: Epidural abscess with frontal lobe lesions caused by significant compression on frontal lobe
    Recommendation for surgery to evacuate the abscess
    RX: antibiotics and pseudoephedrine

Suzanne R. Taylor, MD

SRT/pw   D: 09/16/11 09:50:16 T: 09/18/11 12:55:01

You Code It!

What are the best, most accurate codes?

Diagnosis Codes: _____

Procedure Codes: _____

Anesthesia Codes (when applicable): _____

HCPCS Level II codes (when applicable): _____

PATIENT NAME: JOHNSON, KELVIN
ADMISSION DATE: 11/09/11

Attending Physician: Carrie L. Sutton, MD

HPI: This is a male patient who was recently in the hospital. He was diagnosed at the time with a malignancy in the cerebral area. Patient has been undergoing outpatient radiation. The son called me and told me that the patient was having some difficulty breathing and his mental status seemed to have deteriorated in a rather rapid nature. I discussed this with the nurse at the extended care facility where he resides, and we did give him a Lasix injection 40 mg. He did not respond very much, and they brought him to the emergency room (ER). Initial tests basically were negative, but after discussion with this internist, it was decided to go ahead and admit patient for further neurologic evaluation.

PMH: Significant for the malignancy in the cerebral area, hypertension, gastritis, diabetes, secondary to steroids. He also has osteoarthritis.

MEDICATIONS: Patient has been maintained on Prevacid 30 mg po bid, Bumex 0.5 mg po q day prn, Captopril 100 mg q 12, Norvasc 10 mg po q day, insulin siding scale. He has been on Decadron per the radiation/oncologist. Depakote 250 mg qid and Diflucan recently 150 mg po q day. He received Phenergan on prn basis for nausea, Tylenol grains 10 q 4-6 prn pain, Darvocet one q 4-6 prn pain. Chloraseptic spray to the mouth. His diet is thick and liquid as tolerated, diabetic diet.

SOCIAL HISTORY: Noncontributory at this time.

FAMILY HISTORY: Noncontributory at this time.

VITAL SIGNS: Stable

GENERAL APPEARANCE: Somewhat lethargic-appearing white male, he has always been somewhat quiet with a flat affect.

HEENT: Normal

CERVICAL AND CARDIOPULMONARY EXAM: Unchanged

LUNGS: Clear

HEART: Heart rate regular

ABDOMEN: No obvious pain, normal bowel sounds

EXTREMITIES: Trace edema bilaterally

Continued

IMPRESSION: The patient is admitted with a known brain tumor, he has been undergoing radiation, he has an oncologist, and he is admitted at this time by the neurologist for further evaluation regarding his mental changes.

Carrie L. Sutton, MD

CLS/pw   D: 11/09/11 09:50:16   T: 11/15/11 12:55:01

You Code It!

What are the best, most accurate codes?

Diagnosis Codes: _____

Procedure Codes: _____

Anesthesia Codes (when applicable): _____

HCPCS Level II codes (when applicable): _____

PATIENT NAME: GARRAWAY, LUCAS
ADMISSION DATE: 11/10/11

Attending Physician: Carrie L. Sutton, MD

Findings & recommendations of consultant: Pt is an 84-year-old male who is known to have brain tumor, which I believe is a glioblastoma multiforme. Apparently he has been receiving radiation therapy but has begun to go downhill and was admitted with pneumonia several days ago. Despite treatment, because of his obtundation, the patient's pneumonia has progressed. He is having respiratory distress, apparently more yesterday than today. A chest x-ray today has shown a small, approximately 10% right pneumothorax. Today the patient has not evidenced any respiratory distress and in fact has been either sleeping or obtunded and apparently only slightly responding. He is no code and is receiving palliative therapy only with no intubation or CPR to be given in the case of an arrest. The family's intentions are that he be made comfortable and not to try to prolong his life. He has apparently not been complaining of any pain when he was able to state his complaints. His temperature is 100.0F at maximum, respirations are currently very unlabored at approximately 18 per minute, blood pressure 174/104, heart rate 116 with regular rhythm. His O2 saturations on a nonrebreather mask are in the mid 90s. The patient's most recent chest x-ray today shows the pneumonia to be worsening and the development of a small pneumothorax, as previously mentioned.

PMH: Discloses that he has hypertension and has glucose intolerance, apparently provoked at least partly by corticosteroids. An echogram was within normal limits. He apparently has been in reasonably good health. He has had hand surgery before and has history of enlarged prostate.

FAMILY HISTORY: Noncontributory

SOCIAL HISTORY: Noncontributory

ROS: Unobtainable

PE: Reveals an elderly gentleman who appears to be sleeping, and I did not try to rouse him. His vital signs show that he is afebrile. His blood pressure is 162/95, respirations are unlabored at 16–18, heart rate is 116, and temperature is currently 99.2. Head and neck examination: I do not find any acute abnormality, no JVD is seen, no palpable abnormal lymphadenopathy. His chest reveals a few coarse breath sounds and a few rhonchi, no wheezes, no rubs. Breath sounds are fairly good on both sides. Heart reveals a tachycardia with a regular rhythm, no rub, murmur, gallop. Abdomen is soft, nontender. Normal bowel sounds. No hepatosplenomegaly. GU/Rectal: Not done. Extremities show no acute changes. The patient's chest x-ray, as described previously.

Continued

OVERALL IMPRESSION: Pt appears to be quite comfortable at this time. The patient is not having any distress that I can observe, and I think that his prognosis is probably terminal. At this point in time, I would not recommend putting in a chest tube as he does not seem to be having any respiratory compromise or discomfort from having the pneumothorax, and given its small size, I suspect that a chest tube would be unlikely to afford him any improvement in symptoms. However, the pneumothorax is something that we could monitor, and should it progress or his symptoms become worse, this could always be re-evaluated. I discussed this in detail with the patient's son, who I believe understands all of the options and is in agreement with taking this course at this time. I also discussed this with Dr. Moore so he is informed.

Carrie L. Sutton, MD

CLS/pw   D: 11/10/11 09:50:16   T: 11/17/11 12:55:01

You Code It!

What are the best, most accurate codes?

Diagnosis Codes: _____

Procedure Codes: _____

Anesthesia Codes (when applicable): _____

HCPCS Level II codes (when applicable): _____

FRAISER, HARROLD, & YAWZI, Neurology
81 BAYER BOULEVARD • SENSATION, FL 32811 • 407-555-5852

PATIENT NAME: HARPER, VAN
ADMISSION DATE: 12/08/11

Attending Physician: Carrie L. Sutton, MD

This is the first visit for this 89-year-old, right-handed male who comes for evaluation of possible normal pressure hydrocephalus.

    The patient's family has been noting that the patient has symptoms consistent with normal pressure hydrocephalus and apparently were made aware of this in recent publications. The patient has had mental deterioration. He has a history of urinary urgency and has been seen by Dr. Reine for this. He has problems with his gait, which he describes as "vertigo in his legs," and he "minces his steps." His primary care physician is Dr. Torman.

    The patient has allergies to pollen and hay fever. His medications include Plavix, Aspirin, Lipitor, Avodart, Uroxatral, Hyzaar, Calcium 600 + Vitamin D and multivitamins.

PERTINENT MEDICAL HISTORY: The patient does not smoke cigarettes or drink alcohol.

SOCIAL HISTORY: He is married and is a retired optometrist.

FAMILY HISTORY: His mother died at the age of 96 of "dementia" and possible stroke. His father died at the age of 96 of an unknown cause.

REVIEW OF SYSTEMS: The patient has had several transient ischemic attacks in January, April, and July 2004. He is status post cataract surgery. He is status post a syncopal episode in January of 2004. He has a history of hypertension, asthma, and bronchitis, and a history of bilateral inguinal hernia repairs 45 years ago. In January of 2004, he had a urinary tract infection and also had a cardiac evaluation, which was negative. Otherwise, his review of systems is negative for cardiac, pulmonary, gastrointestinal, genitourinary, or musculoskeletal disease.

PHYSICAL EXAMINATION: This is a well-developed, well-nourished elderly white male in no acute distress who appears to be awake, alert, and oriented. His blood pressure is 170/70. His pulse is 70. His respiration is 16. His head is atraumatic, normocephalic. He is status post cataracts. He has dentures. His neck is subtle without jugular venous distention or bruits. His lungs are clear to auscultation. His heart is regular rhythm. His abdomen is soft. His extremities are without clubbing, cyanosis, or edema. Examination of his spine does not demonstrate any direct cervical spine tenderness. The patient has kyphoscoliosis of the thoracolumbar spine. Neurologic examination of cranial nerves II–XII demonstrate a decrease in upward gaze and a decrease in hearing. He wears hearing aids. Motor function is 5/5 = in all major motor groups. Sensory examination appears to be grossly intact in all extremities. Deep tendon reflexes are 0 = for the biceps, triceps, and brachioradialis. In the lower extremities, the patellas, suprapatellars, and hamstrings are 0 =. The right Achilles is 2 +; the left is absent. The toes are downgoing bilaterally. The patient's cerebellar testing is intact for finger to nose function. On regular gait testing, the patient has a magnetic/shuffling gait. Station testing does not demonstrate any drift or Romberg's sign.

Continued

REVIEW: There are no x-rays available for review.

IMPRESSION: The patient has possible normal pressure hydrocephalus versus ischemic cerebrovascular disease.

RECOMMENDATIONS: The patient should have an MRI scan, MR Angiogram of the brain, and MR Angiogram of the carotid and vertebral arteries and then return to see me in the office.

Carrie L. Sutton, MD

CLS/pw   D: 12/08/11 09:50:16   T: 12/13/11 12:55:01

You Code It!

What are the best, most accurate codes?

Diagnosis Codes: _____

Procedure Codes: _____

Anesthesia Codes (when applicable): _____

HCPCS Level II codes (when applicable): _____

FRAISER, HARROLD, & YAWZI, Neurology
81 BAYER BOULEVARD • SENSATION, FL 32811 • 407-555-5852

PATIENT NAME: WANG, JUI LI
ADMISSION DATE: 12/15/11

Attending Physician: Carrie L. Sutton, MD

The patient was last seen on November 10. The MRI scan of the brain demonstrates that the patient has hydrocephalus with transependymal edema.

IMPRESSION: The patient has either normal pressure hydrocephalus or a low pressure communicating hydrocephalus.

RECOMMENDATIONS: In either case, he requires a ventricular shunt placement. I have explained to the patient and his family the shunt procedure, its indications, risks, benefits, and alternatives in detail, including the risk of bleeding, infection, injury to the brain tissue with hemorrhages, stroke, paralysis, blindness, coma, or even death. All of their questions have been answered. No guarantees have been given. I have advised that the patient will need to have medical clearance from his primary care physician, Dr. Torman. Once we have the medical clearance, we can schedule him for surgery.

Carrie L. Sutton, MD

CLS/pw   D: 12/15/11 09:50:16   T: 12/21/11 12:55:01

You Code It!

What are the best, most accurate codes?

Diagnosis Codes: _____

Procedure Codes: _____

Anesthesia Codes (when applicable): _____

HCPCS Level II codes (when applicable): _____

PATIENT NAME:	TULLMAN, CLARISSA
Attending Physician:	Carrie L. Sutton, MD
Admission Date:	11 January 2012
Discharge Date:	15 January 2012

Operative Report:

Preoperative diagnosis:	Normal pressure hydrocephalus
Postoperative diagnosis:	Normal pressure hydrocephalus
Operation:	Right parieto-occipital ventriculoperitoneal shunt placement with cerebrospinal fluid manometry and Hakim valve programming.
Surgeon:	Carrie L. Sutton, MD
ANESTHESIA:	General endotracheal
ANESTHESIOLOGIST:	Carter H. Beauman, MD
ESTIMATED BLOOD LOSS:	Less than 10 cc.
COMPLICATIONS:	None

PROCEDURE: This 89-year-old female had progressive urinary, gait, and memory problems with MRI study demonstrating significant ventriculomegaly consistent with normal pressure hydrocephalus. Because of the patient's deterioration, she was offered the option of ventriculoperitoneal shunt placement to try to stop the downward deterioration of her mental faculties.

Following the obtaining of informed consent, the patient was taken to the operating table for the procedure. The patient was placed supine on the operating table, inducted under general anesthesia and intubated. Her right parieto-occipital scalp was shaved, and then the scalp, neck, chest, and abdomen on the right side were washed with alcohol and prepped with DuraPrep solution and then draped with sterile drapes with additional loban dressing. The skin incision was marked out with a skin marker for the right parieto-occipital scalp, centered on a point approximately 3 cm lateral to and 8 to 9 cm rostral to the inion, and in the right upper quadrant of the abdomen at the midcostal line. These incisions were then infiltrated with 0.5% lidocaine with 1:200,000 epinephrine solution. The skin incision was then made in the scalp with a #10 blade, and hemostasis was obtained with Bovie cauterization. A pneumatic perforator was used to drill a hole in the cranium, and then the margins of the bur hole were waxed with bone wax for hemostasis. Blunt dissection of the occipital scalp was used to create a subcutaneous cul-de-sac for placement of the value system, and following this, a subcutaneous passer was used to create a track for passing the distal Bactocill peritoneal catheter between the two incisions. The abdominal incision was also opened with a #10 blade to facilitate passage.

Once the distal catheter was in place, the dura was cauterized by using the Bovie cautery bayonet technique, and then a ventricular catheter was passed into the ventricles without difficulty. The cerebrospinal fluid pressure was measured to be approximately 9 cm of water, and cerebrospinal fluid was also sent for routine culture and Gram stain. Once the cerebrospinal fluid pressure had been measured, the Hakim valve was programmed to a pressure resistance of 60 mm of water. The valve was then connected to the ventriculostomy catheter, which was 10 cm in length. A Bactocill catheter was used for this also. The connection was made with a 2-0 silk ligature. The valve was also connected to the distal peritoneal catheter with a 2-0 silk ligature. The valve was then pulled underneath the scalp and anchored to the pericranium with 3-0 Prolene anchoring sutures to prevent migration of the valve. There was good spontaneous flow of cerebrospinal fluid from the distal portion of the peritoneal catheter. Excess length of the peritoneal cavity was removed and then several slits were made in the sides of the peritoneal catheter to provide additional egress points for cerebrospinal fluid as needed.

Continued

Once this was done, the abdominal incision was opened further with a Bovie cautery and cutting current. The anterior abdominal fascia was divided with a Bovie cautery, and then blunt dissection with a hemostat was used to split the fibers of the rectus abdominus muscles. The posterior abdominal fascia was then identified and lifted up with hemostats and then divided with Metzenbaum scissors. The peritoneum was then identified, lifted up with hemostats, and again divided with Metzenbaum scissors. Following this, the peritoneal cavity was easily visualized. A hemostat and then a peritoneal trocar were able to be passed into the peritoneal cavity without difficulty. Following this, the distal portion of the ventriculoperitoneal shunt was passed into the peritoneal cavity without difficulty, after it had once again been ascertained that there was spontaneous flow of spinal fluid. Once the catheter was in the peritoneal cavity, #0 Vicryl sutures were used to reapproximate the posterior abdominal fascia and then the anterior abdominal fascia. The Scarpa's fascia was then closed with #0 Vicryl interrupted sutures with inverted knots. Gelfoam soaked in Thrombin was placed overlying the point of insertion of the ventriculostomy catheter, and then the galea was closed with #0 Vicryl interrupted sutures with inverted knots. The areas were irrigated with Bacitracin irrigation solution during the closure process, and then the skin incisions were closed with 3-0 nylon simple running sutures with good skin approximation. The skin incisions were then washed again with Bacitracin irrigation solution and then dressed with triple antibiotic ointment and coverlet dressings. The patient was awakened from general anesthesia, extubated, and taken to the recovery room for further observation. Estimated blood loss from the entire procedure was less than 10 cc. The patient appeared to have tolerated the procedure well.

Carrie L. Sutton, MD

CLS/pw   D: 01/11/12 09:50:16   T: 01/27/12 12:55:01

You Code It!

What are the best, most accurate codes?

Diagnosis Codes: _____

Procedure Codes: _____

Anesthesia Codes (when applicable): _____

HCPCS Level II codes (when applicable): _____

FRAISER, HARROLD, & YAWZI, Neurology
81 BAYER BOULEVARD • SENSATION, FL 32811 • 407-555-5852

PATIENT NAME: KELLOGG, LAMONTE
MRN: KELLLA001

Attending Physician: Carrie L. Sutton, MD
Admission Date: 08 January 2012
Discharge Date: 13 January 2012

FINAL DIAGNOSIS: Normal pressure hydrocephalus. History of hypertension. History of benign prostatic hypertrophy. History of asthma. History of hypercholesterolemia.

HISTORY OF PRESENT ILLNESS: This 89-year-old male developed symptoms of normal pressure hydrocephalus, including gait problems and urinary problems as well as decreased mentation. The patient had outside studies, which demonstrated that he had large ventricles consistent with normal pressure hydrocephalus. and the patient was offered the option of ventricular shunt procedure. The patient agreed and was admitted for surgery.

    The patient has a history of allergies to pollen. His medications: the patient had home medications delineated in the order sheets. His social history: he did not smoke cigarettes or drink alcohol. He was a retired optometrist. Family history was positive for dementia and stroke. Review of systems was positive for transient ischemic attacks, hypertension, history of asthma and bronchitis, history of cataract surgery, and history of hernia repairs.

PHYSICAL EXAMINATION: On physical examination, this was a well-developed, well-nourished, elderly white male who was awake, alert, and in no acute distress. His head was atraumatic and normocephalic. His heart was regular rhythm. Lungs were clear to auscultation. Abdomen was soft and nontender. On neurologic examination, he had a magnetic gait. Extremities without clubbing, cyanosis, or edema.

HOSPITAL COURSE: The patient was admitted for surgery on January 08, 2012, and underwent a right parietooccipital ventricular peritoneal shunt placement with a Hakim valve, which was programmed to 60 mm after CSF manometry demonstrated higher pressures. The procedure was uneventful. Postoperatively, the patient was seen in consultation by Internal Medicine. He was awake, alert, and conversant. His postoperative CT scan demonstrated excellent position of the ventriculostomy catheter and the ventricles without the evidence of hemorrhage. The patient was noted to have a marked improvement in his gait according to his family within 48 hours of surgery. He had no headaches, and by January 13, 2012, he was felt to be sufficiently stable. He was able to be discharged home for outpatient follow-up. His condition at discharge was stable/improved.

Carrie L. Sutton, MD

CLS/pw   D: 01/13/12 09:50:16 T: 01/27/12 12:55:01

You Code It!

What are the best, most accurate codes?

Diagnosis Codes: _____

Procedure Codes: _____

Anesthesia Codes (when applicable): _____

HCPCS Level II codes (when applicable): _____

PATIENT NAME: MARKOV, SCOTT

MRN: MARKSC001

Attending Physician: Carrie L. Sutton, MD

Admission Date: 02/15/11

This is a left-handed male admitted for sudden onset of memory loss.

HISTORY OF PRESENT ILLNESS: At 5:15 p.m., pt took a nap. When he woke up, he could not remember anything, according to his wife. No loss of consciousness. No slurred speech. No motor or sensory loss in limbs. Presented to the ER.

PAST MEDICAL HISTORY: Two CVAs 1998 and 2005. Right hand weakness persisted. TIA 12/95. Syncope 6/95. Cardiac pacemaker. Seizure disorder. On Dilantin and Neurontin for a while, then discontinued by neurologist last several months (Dr. Promat). Penile implant. Inguinal herniorrhaphy. Hay fever.

SOCIAL HISTORY: Married. Nonsmoker for years.

FAMILY HISTORY: Noncontributory

MEDICATIONS: Tylenol 250 mg bid

ALLERGIES: Sulfa

ROS: As per HPI

EXAM: Afebrile, BP 163/86, HR: 71 (paced)

HEENT: Atraumatic. No lesions.

NECK: Without carotid bruits, supple

CHEST: Clean

HEART: No arrhythmia, Pacer

ABDOMEN: Soft, nontender

EXTREMITIES: No swelling, 4+ pedal pulses

NEURO: Awake, alert, but not oriented. He answers questions glibly and tangentially. Can't tell date but knows his name and address. Does not know MD's name. Does not seem to retain new information. Speech fluent.

    CN: II – VII intact
    MOTOR: Diminished dexterity, right hand and fingers
    SENSORY: No deficiency
    COORDINATION: No limb dysmetria

Continued

CAT SCAN (No C): Old left hemisphere infarct frontal, parietal and posterior temporal lobes. No mass effect. Atrophy diffuse.

EKG: Paced rhythm

LAB: Chol 242

IMPRESSIONS: Admit to observation.

Carrie L. Sutton, MD

CLS/pw   D: 02/15/11 09:50:16   T: 02/22/11 12:55:01

You Code It!

What are the best, most accurate codes?

Diagnosis Codes: _____

Procedure Codes: _____

Anesthesia Codes (when applicable): _____

HCPCS Level II codes (when applicable): _____

FRAISER, HARROLD, & YAWZI, Neurology
81 BAYER BOULEVARD • SENSATION, FL 32811 • 407-555-5852

PATIENT NAME: FLETCHER, LACY
MRN: FLELA001

Attending Physician: Carrie L. Sutton, MD
Admission Date: 08/16/11

This is a 2-year-old female who appeared to be recovering from an upper respiratory infection when she developed vomiting. Her grandmother may have given her aspirin, but she was supposed to have taken acetaminophen. She initially presents to the emergency department with irritability and restlessness. She subsequently develops convulsions, which are treated with anticonvulsants, and she is admitted to the PICU.

EXAM: VS T 37.8, P 100, R 50, BP 110/70, oxygen saturation 99% in room air. Height, weight, head circumference are at the 50th percentile. She is agitated and not cooperative. Head shows no signs of external trauma. Pupils are equal and reactive to light. Conjunctiva are clear, sclera nonicteric. EOMs cannot be fully tested, but they are conjugate. TMs are normal. Mouth is not easily examined. Neck reveals no adenopathy. She is agitated, so it is not possible to be certain that her neck is supple. Heart regular without murmurs. Lungs are clear. Abdomen is flat with normal bowel sounds. It is difficult to tell if she has any hepatosplenomegaly. No definite tenderness. No inguinal hernias are present. She moves all extremities. Reflexes are not testable because of her agitation.

LABS: Serum bilirubin: Normal. Serum AST and ALT: increased. Serum ammonia: increased. Prothrombin time: prolonged. A CT scan of the brain is obtained, which shows cerebral edema.
    Her neurologic symptoms rapidly worsen and she becomes unresponsive. She is intubated and put on mechanical ventilation. Reye's syndrome is suspected. A confirmatory liver biopsy reveals diffuse, small lipid deposits in the hepatocytes (microvesicular steatosis) without significant necrosis or inflammation. These findings are consistent with the diagnosis of Reye's syndrome.

_____

Carrie L. Sutton, MD

CLS/pw   D: 08/16/11 09:50:16   T: 08/23/11 12:55:01

You Code It!

What are the best, most accurate codes?

Diagnosis Codes: _____

Procedure Codes: _____

Anesthesia Codes (when applicable): _____

HCPCS Level II codes (when applicable): _____

FRAISER, HARROLD, & YAWZI, Neurology
81 BAYER BOULEVARD • SENSATION, FL 32811 • 407-555-5852

PATIENT NAME: YANGLER, BRUCE
MRN: YANGBR001

Attending Physician: Carrie L. Sutton, MD
Admission Date: 07/30/11

HISTORY OF PRESENT ILLNESS: This is a 6-year old male, referred by his pediatrician, Dr. Raul Boles, with an abnormal gait. He was adopted from another country about a year ago, and his adopting parents have noticed that he is clumsy when he runs and that he falls often. He runs on his tiptoes, which has occurred since they started taking care of him. Otherwise, he has no other problems. He is doing well in kindergarten despite his language difficulty. His teacher notes that he has trouble getting up from a sitting position at school. His parents deny any chronic fevers, leg pain, weight loss, seizures, skin rash, urinary or bowel incontinence, or frequent colds.

PAST MEDICAL HISTORY, DEVELOPMENTAL HISTORY, FAMILY HISTORY, BIRTH HISTORY are unknown. His immunizations are up-to-date, and his PPD this year has been negative.

EXAM: His vital signs are normal. His height, weight and head circumference are at the 50th percentile. He is alert, active, shy, well-nourished, slim, and in no distress. His skin shows no neurocutaneous stigmata. His head is normocephalic and atraumatic. His pupils are equal, round, reactive to light. No nystagmus is evident. His fundi are normal with sharp disk margins. His TMs are clear. His throat is normal with a uvula midline. His lungs, heart, and abdomen are normal. His back shows no sacral dimples.

NEUROLOGIC EXAM: A standard cranial nerve exam reveals no deficits. His strength is +4/5 in his deltoids, knee flexors, and extensors; +5/5 in his biceps and triceps. His calves are visibly enlarged with a firm, rubbery feeling. He gets up to a standing position using a Gowers' maneuver. No dysdiadochokinesia. Negative Romberg sign. Sensation to light touch is intact. His reflexes are +2/4 in his biceps, triceps, brachioradialis, patella, and ankle. His plantar reflex is downgoing (negative Babinski sign). No clonus is elicited. Normal anal wink and abdominal reflexes are present. His gait is best described as a wide-based waddling. When running, he tends to run on his toes. He is unable to jump.

LABS: CBC w/differential

PROCEDURES: Muscle biopsy to be performed.

DX: Duchenne muscular dystrophy (DMD)

Carrie L. Sutton, MD

CLS/pw   D: 07/30/11 09:50:16   T: 08/16/11 12:55:01

You Code It!

What are the best, most accurate codes?

Diagnosis Codes: _____

Procedure Codes: _____

Anesthesia Codes (when applicable): _____

HCPCS Level II codes (when applicable): _____

FRAISER, HARROLD, & YAWZI, Neurology
81 BAYER BOULEVARD • SENSATION, FL 32811 • 407-555-5852

PATIENT NAME: GREENE, JEFFREY

MRN: GREJE001

Attending Physician: Carrie L. Sutton, MD

Admission Date: 09/03/11

HISTORY OF PRESENT ILLNESS: Two days ago, this 6-month old male infant was sitting in an infant carrier, which was placed on top of a stroller. The carrier accidentally fell approximately three feet onto the ground. He hit his head on the plastic portion of the car seat. There was an immediate cry and no loss of consciousness. His behavior, activity, and feeding pattern are reported as normal. Two days later (today) his mother notes a boggy swelling in the right temporal area of the head, and because of this, she brought him to the ER for evaluation. He continues to have normal activity and no vomiting.

PAST MEDICAL HISTORY: He has been previously healthy. There is no history of substance use, or child protective services (CPS) involvement in the family.

EXAM: VS T 36.9, P 120, R 18, BP 92/50, oxygen saturation 100% in room air. Height, weight and head circumference at the 25th to 50th percentiles. He is alert, active, easily arousable on exam, and clean in appearance. He has a 9-by-7 cm swelling over the right temporal/parietal region that is soft, possibly tender, with no palpable bony deformity. No lacerations or wounds are noted. His anterior fontanel is soft and flat. Pupils are 3 mm bilaterally and reactive to light. EOMs are conjugate. There is no hemotympanum, no nasal discharge, and his mucus membranes are moist. His heart, lung, and abdomen exams are normal. Neurologic and extremity exams are normal.

A head CT scan shows a subgaleal hematoma (hematoma under the aponeurosis of Galen), a nondepressed linear skull fracture, and a normal brain.

He is discharged home to the care of his parents. He followed up with his pediatrician the next day without sequelae.

Carrie L. Sutton, MD

CLS/pw   D: 09/03/11 09:50:16   T: 09/11/11 12:55:01

You Code It!

What are the best, most accurate codes?

Diagnosis Codes: _____

Procedure Codes: _____

Anesthesia Codes (when applicable): _____

HCPCS Level II codes (when applicable): _____

FRAISER, HARROLD, & YAWZI, Neurology
81 BAYER BOULEVARD • SENSATION, FL 32811 • 407-555-5852

PATIENT NAME: ROMERO, ANGELA
MRN: ROMAN001

Attending Physician: Carrie L. Sutton, MD
Admission Date: 08/15/11

HISTORY OF PRESENT ILLNESS: This is a 10-month-old girl whose parents bring her into the ER for tonic-clonic seizures lasting a few minutes. This baby girl is a product of a normal pregnancy and was delivered full-term by normal spontaneous vaginal delivery. There were no postnatal complications, and this infant was discharged from the hospital at 48 hours of life. Her history is significant for jerking movements (onset at five months of age) described as sudden flexion of the neck, arms, and legs onto the trunk preceded by a cry. Her parents were not too worried about this behavior since the child would return back to normal and they attributed it to colic or "gas." There is no history of fever, coughing, vomiting, or diarrhea. She has been gaining weight appropriately and eating normally. She is on solid foods and formula, which the parents prepare correctly. Her immunizations are up to date. She is on no medications and her development has been normal. She is able to sit up, crawl, cruise with both hands, and combines syllables.

FAMILY HISTORY: Unremarkable in that there is no history of seizures, mental retardation, or consanguinity.

EXAM: VST 37.0, P 100, R 26, BP 90/60, O2 sat 100% on RA, weight 9.0 kg (50 %ile), length 73 cm (50 %tile), HC 44.5 cm (50 %tile). She is alert, active, and in no distress. She is not toxic. She tracks well. She has good bonding with her mother. She has multiple small 1–2 cm oval, irregular hypopigmented macules on her trunk and extremities. HEENT is normal. Her neck is supple without lymphadenopathy. Heart, lungs and abdomen are normal.

NEURO: She has no facial asymmetry. She moves all her extremities well. There are no focal deficits. She does not exhibit cortical thumbing or scissoring of her lower extremities. She tracks well. She has good head control and is able to support herself on her legs.

    A head CT scan revealing cortical tubers in the cerebral cortex and multiple subependymal nodules in the lateral ventricles. She is admitted to the floor, where an EEG shows "hypsarrhythmia." A complete echocardiogram and a complete renal ultrasound are also done showing tumors in both the heart and kidneys. A diagnosis of tuberous sclerosis is made. She is started on ACTH. Unfortunately her condition fails to improve, and she continues to have intractable seizures in addition to being mentally retarded.

Carrie L. Sutton, MD

CLS/pw   D: 08/15/11 09:50:16   T: 08/21/11 12:55:01

You Code It!

What are the best, most accurate codes?

Diagnosis Codes: _____

Procedure Codes: _____

Anesthesia Codes (when applicable): _____

HCPCS Level II codes (when applicable): _____

FRAISER, HARROLD, & YAWZI, Neurology
81 BAYER BOULEVARD • SENSATION, FL 32811 • 407-555-5852

PATIENT NAME: BINYON, ROSE
MRN: BINRO001

Attending Physician: Carrie L. Sutton, MD
Admission Date: 11/21/11

HISTORY OF PRESENT ILLNESS: This patient is a 6-month old female brought into the office as a new patient for a well baby visit. Her family moved here recently from Asia, where she was born. There were no prenatal or postnatal complications, and she has had no significant medical problems since birth.

FAMILY HISTORY: Positive for her father, who has a condition in which his body is covered with fleshy small growths, similar to skin tags, and on the father's side, there are several family members with the same warty growths, seizures, and high blood pressure.

EXAM: VS are normal. Her growth parameters are in the 25th to 50th percentiles. Her examination is otherwise unremarkable except for multiple coffee-colored spots on her trunk and abdomen.

DIAGNOSIS: Neurofibromatosis.
Schedule parents for a follow-up visit tomorrow to discuss this further.

Carrie L. Sutton, MD

CLS/pw   D: 11/21/11 09:50:16   T: 11/25/11 12:55:01

You Code It!

What are the best, most accurate codes?

Diagnosis Codes: _____

Procedure Codes: _____

Anesthesia Codes (when applicable): _____

HCPCS Level II codes (when applicable): _____

FRAISER, HARROLD, & YAWZI, Neurology
81 BAYER BOULEVARD • SENSATION, FL 32811 • 407-555-5852

PATIENT NAME: TINDER, JENNIFER
MRN: TINJE001

Attending Physician: Carrie L. Sutton, MD
Admission Date: 11/19/11

HISTORY OF PRESENT ILLNESS: The patient is a 16-year-old female, G1P0 mother at 37 weeks, scheduled for a C-section. Prenatal care was not sought until 32 weeks gestation. Mother did not take any vitamins or folate supplements prior to that time. Initial prenatal lab studies were significant for an elevated alpha fetoprotein. A prenatal ultrasound done at 34 weeks demonstrated a meningomyelocele. No hydrocephalus was noted at that time. A neurosurgeon was consulted. A C-section was scheduled to deliver the infant as nontraumatically as possible with the availability of the neurosurgeon close by.

    At delivery, the infant is delivered with Apgar scores of 7 and 8. Birthweight is 3.2 kg. A translucent membrane sac overlying the midlumbar region is noted. It is leaking xanthochromic fluid. Upper extremity movement is noted to be good, but lower extremity movement is not as vigorous. The infant is transferred to the NICU where vascular access is obtained and initial stabilization measures are performed. Five hours later, the infant is taken to the operating room where a neurosurgeon closes the meningomyelocele defect over the lower back. Postoperative recovery in the NICU is unremarkable. Lower extremity movement is moderate. A head ultrasound study shows mild hydrocephalus.

Carrie L. Sutton, MD

CLS/pw   D: 11/19/11 09:50:16 T: 11/29/11 12:55:01

You Code It!

What are the best, most accurate codes?

Diagnosis Codes: _____

Procedure Codes: _____

Anesthesia Codes (when applicable): _____

HCPCS Level II codes (when applicable): _____

FRAISER, HARROLD, & YAWZI, Neurology
81 BAYER BOULEVARD • SENSATION, FL 32811 • 407-555-5852

PATIENT NAME: LEWIS, COLLETTE
MRN: LEWCO001

Attending Physician: Carrie L. Sutton, MD
Admission Date: 12/27/11

HISTORY OF PRESENT ILLNESS: This is a 10-year-old female who is brought into the office by her parents with a chief complaint of clumsiness and blurred vision. She had been well until approximately two weeks ago, when she noticed a loss of sensation and strength in her left leg, a rapid deterioration in vision, and a decrease in coordination. There is no history of fever, vomiting, or seizures. One year prior to this event, she presented to the hospital with poor coordination, dizziness, and headaches. A left hemiplegia was noted as well as an asymmetric gait. A full recovery was made five days later, and she was discharged from the hospital without further treatment or a definite diagnosis.

EXAM: VS are normal. Her weight, height, and head circumference are all at the 50th percentile. She is alert but subdued. Her HEENT exam is notable for severe visual loss and pale optic discs on funduscopy. Her heart, lungs, and abdomen are normal. She is noted to have a hyporeflexive paraparesis noted on the left.

    I admitted her into the hospital. A CT scan shows slightly enlarged ventricles, and an MRI scan shows multiple lesions in the periventricular white matter and cerebellum. Pattern visual evoked responses showed markedly delayed latencies. She is treated with corticosteroids, and a full recovery within a few weeks is expected.

DIAGNOSIS: Multiple sclerosis (MS)

_____

Carrie L. Sutton, MD

CLS/pw   D: 12/27/11 09:50:16   T: 01/09/12 12:55:01

You Code It!

What are the best, most accurate codes?

Diagnosis Codes: _____

Procedure Codes: _____

Anesthesia Codes (when applicable): _____

HCPCS Level II codes (when applicable): _____

FRAISER, HARROLD, & YAWZI, Neurology
81 BAYER BOULEVARD • SENSATION, FL 32811 • 407-555-5852

PATIENT NAME: MILLER, NATASHA
MRN: MILNA001

Attending Physician: Carrie L. Sutton, MD
Admission Date: 10/07/11

HISTORY OF PRESENT ILLNESS: This is a 12-year-old Caucasian female brought to the ER by her mother with a chief complaint of leg weakness. One week prior, she had a fever of 101.4F with vomiting and diarrhea. After three days, the vomiting and diarrhea resolved. She was doing well until this morning when she fell while trying to get out of bed and could not stand or walk without support. She denies headache, blurred vision, tinnitus, vertigo, dysphagia, or incontinence. No history of toxic ingestion. Her immunizations are up to date. While in the ER, she complains that her arms feel weak.

EXAM: VST 37.0, P 84, R 24, BP 102/64. Height and weight are at the 25th percentile. She is alert, slightly fearful, but cooperative. HEENT: She has no nystagmus and no papilledema. Her extraocular movements are intact. Pupils are equal and reactive to light. No facial weakness or asymmetry is present. Heart, lung and abdomen exams are normal.

NEURO: Strength 4/5 in the upper extremities, 3/5 in the lower extremities. DTRs 1-2+ in the upper extremities and absent in the lower extremities. Sensation is intact in all extremities. Cerebellar function is normal except for the weakness. No cranial nerve abnormalities are noted. She refuses to walk.

    CBC, electrolytes, BUN, creatinine, glucose, calcium and liver function tests are normal. Urine toxicology screen is negative. A lumbar puncture is performed. Opening pressure is normal. CSF analysis shows protein 146 mg/dL (high), glucose 70 mg/dL, 5 WBC per cu-mm, 1 RBC per cu-mm, and gram stain shows no WBCs and no organisms.

    An MRI of the brain and spinal cord is normal. She is started on IVIG and over the next few days, she slowly regains strength in her arms and legs. However, she still requires assistance with walking at the time of discharge.

DX: Guillain-Barre syndrome (GBS)

She is referred to a rehabilitation hospital to continue outpatient physical therapy.

_____

Carrie L. Sutton, MD

CLS/pw   D: 10/07/11 09:50:16   T: 10/15/11 12:55:01

You Code It!

What are the best, most accurate codes?

Diagnosis Codes: _____

Procedure Codes: _____

Anesthesia Codes (when applicable): _____

HCPCS Level II codes (when applicable): _____

Obstetrics and Gynecology Cases and Patient Records

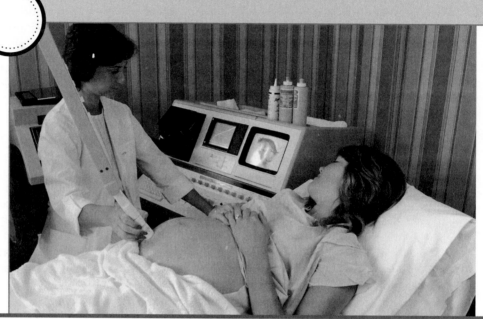

INTRODUCTION

The following case studies are from an obstetrics and gynecology practice. In a physician's office of this type, a professional coding specialist is likely to see many different kinds of health situations, including preventive health care services.

Gynecologists are physicians who specialize in women's health. These health care professionals provide routine care for women, including Pap smears and breast examinations, as well as help patients with such age-appropriate concerns as the onset of menses, birth control, family planning, and menopause. Subspecialties of gynecology include gynecologic oncology (the care and treatment of women with cancers of the reproductive organs), reproductive endocrinology (the care and treatment of women and men who have infertility problems), and surgery (diagnostic and therapeutic procedures such as hysterectomy or oophorectomy).

Gynecologists may also practice obstetrics, which is a subspecialty focusing on the care of women during pregnancy—from conception to labor and delivery and through the postpartum period. An obstetrician may further specialize in perinatology (maternal-fetal medicine), caring for women with high-risk pregnancies.

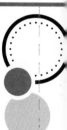

Gynecologists and obstetricians can be board-certified through the Board of Obstetrics and Gynecology, which is recognized by the American Board of Medical Specialties.

You can use these cases to practice coding diagnoses, E/M, procedures, DME, or other HCPCS Level II items, as applicable; code for the physician or the facility; code inpatient and outpatient services, as applicable:

1. Code for the physician.
2. Code for the anesthesiologist, when applicable.
3. Code for the hospital, when applicable.
4. Code for the pathology and laboratory, when applicable.
5. Code HCPCS Level II codes, when applicable.

THE WOMEN'S HEALTH CENTER
671 SENORA LANE • LOVELAND, FL 32772 • 407-555-8541

PATIENT NAME: REMARNI, SOPHIA
MRN: REMSO01
Admission Date: 13 September 2011
Discharge Date: 13 September 2011

Operative Report
Date: 13 September 2011

Preoperative Dx: Status post delivery, undesired fertility, multiparity
Postoperative Dx: Same
Operation: Laparoscopic bilateral tubal cauterization using Kleppingers

Surgeon: Rodney L. Cohen, MD
Assistant: None
Anesthesia: General endotracheal per Dr. Morrison Complications: None
Findings: See body of dictation Specimens: None
Disposition: See body of dictation

PROCEDURE: The patient was taken to the operating room (OR), was placed in the dorsal lithotomy position, and was prepped and draped in a sterile manner. A speculum was inserted into the vagina and a single-tooth tenaculum used to grasp the anterior lip of the cervix. A Hulka tenaculum was used to grasp the cervical lip and manipulate the uterus. Once this was done, an infraumbilical incision was made with the knife and a Veress needle inserted through the incision site. CO_2 gas was instilled after saline via syringe was checked for position. CO_2 gas, approximately 2 L, was instilled into the abdominal cavity. Once this was done, the Veress was removed, and a 5-mm trocar was inserted through the incision site. The laparoscopic camera was then placed through the sleeve.

Under direct visualization and transillumination, after Trendelenburg position, a second incision site was made with the knife suprapubically in the midline, and a 5-mm trocar was inserted through the incision site. First, a blunt probe was used to identify the fallopian tubes. They were easily visible, so the Kleppingers were then used to cauterize full thickness burns on each fallopian tube approximately five to six adjacent times until good cautery and using the monitor to perform this was done. Once this was finished and thought to be satisfactory, the instruments were removed. The CO_2 gas was allowed to passively escape. The incision sites were closed with 4-0 Vicryl in an interrupted manner. Approximately 10 cc total of 1.25% Marcaine was injected subcutaneously for pain relief. The Hulka tenaculum was removed, and a silver nitrate stick was used to cauterize one of the puncture sites on the cervix. This was the end of the procedure. The patient tolerated it well and went to the recovery room in good condition.

09/13/11 10:37:10

You Code It!

What are the best, most accurate codes?

Diagnosis Codes: _____

Procedure Codes: _____

Anesthesia Codes (when applicable): _____

HCPCS Level II codes (when applicable): _____

THE WOMEN'S HEALTH CENTER - AMBULATORY SURGICAL CENTER
671 SENORA LANE • LOVELAND, FL 32772 • 407-555-8541

PATIENT: SANDERS, MARLENE
MRN: SANMA01
Admission Date: 19 September 2011
Discharge Date: 19 September 2011
Date: 19 September 2011

Preoperative Dx: High-grade squamous intraepithelial lesion of the cervix
Postoperative Dx: Same
Operation: Loop electrosurgical excision procedure (LEEP) and ECC (endocervical curettage)

Surgeon: Rodney L. Cohen, MD
Assistant: None
Anesthesia: General by LMA
Findings: Large ectropion, large nonstaining active cervix essentially encompassing the entire active cervix
Specimens: To pathology
Disposition: Stable to recovery room

PROCEDURE: The patient was taken to the OR, where she was placed in the supine position and administered general anesthesia. She was then placed in cane stirrups and prepped and draped in the usual fashion. Her vaginal vault was not prepped. The coated speculum was then placed and the cervix exposed. It was then painted with Lugol, and the entire active cervix was nonstaining with the clearly defined margins where the stain began to be picked up. The cervix was injected with approximately 7 cc of lidocaine with 1% epinephrine. Using a large loop, the anterior cervix was excised, and then the posterior loop was excised in separate specimens. Because of the size of the lesion one piece in total was not accomplished. Prior to the excision, the endocervical curettage was performed and specimen collected. All specimens sent to pathology. The remaining cervical bed was cauterized and then painted with Monsel for hemostasis. The case was concluded with this. Instruments were removed. The patient was taken down from candy cane stirrups, awakened from the anesthesia, and taken to the recovery room in stable condition.

09/19/11 19:38:17

You Code It!

What are the best, most accurate codes?

Diagnosis Codes: _____

Procedure Codes: _____

Anesthesia Codes (when applicable): _____

HCPCS Level II codes (when applicable): _____

THE WOMEN'S HEALTH CENTER
671 SENORA LANE • LOVELAND, FL 32772 • 407-555-8541

PATIENT: CALLMAN, LOUISE
MRN: CALLO01
Admission Date: 7 September 2011
Discharge Date: 8 September 2011
Date: 7 September 2011

Preoperative Dx: Stenotic cervical os with hematometrium
Postoperative Dx: Same
Operation: Cervical dilatation with release of old blood. This was done under ultrasound guidance followed by endometrial curettage.

Surgeon: Rodney L. Cohen, MD
Assistant: None
Anesthesia: General by LMA
Complications: None
Findings: See body of dictation
Specimens: Endometrial curettings to pathology Disposition: Stable to recovery room

PROCEDURE: The patient was taken to the OR, where she was placed in the supine position and administered general anesthesia per LMA. She was then placed in candy-cane stirrups and prepped and draped in the usual sterile fashion. A weighted speculum was placed in the vagina, and with the aid of a Deaver retractor, the anterior portion of the cervix was grasped with single-toothed tenaculum. There were no evident holes or dimples or scenes suggestive of where the external cervical os might be, as the cervix had completely agglutinated across the entire surface. Using lacrimal ducts and gentle tension, the area of suspicion was gently poked until a perforation gave way. This tract was followed with serial dilators until ultimately brown old blood was released, ensuring that I was in the right place. This was done with the aid of abdominal ultrasound guidance, for the risk of false tracking and missing the endocervical canal uterus was real. The uterus was emptied. The cervix was dilated up to approximate 8 mm. This allowed for free flow of the contained old blood. This was followed by sharp curette of all the uterine lining surfaces. This specimen was captured and sent to pathology. Lastly, a small 7 size suction catheter was inserted to ensure the remainder of any old captured blood that may be sitting in the deep recesses of this severely retroverted uterus was obtained, and this concluded the case. The instruments were removed. The patient was taken down from cane stirrups. The patient was awakened from anesthesia and taken to the recovery room in stable condition.

09/7/11 15:47:39

You Code It!

What are the best, most accurate codes?

Diagnosis Codes: _____

Procedure Codes: _____

Anesthesia Codes (when applicable): _____

HCPCS Level II codes (when applicable): _____

PATIENT NAME: CAVELLI, JUDY
MRN: CAVJU01
Admission Date: 4 September 2011
Discharge Date: 5 September 2011

Operative Report
Date: 4 September 2011

Preoperative Dx: 1. Chronic pelvic pain;
                      2. History of endometriosis;
                      3. Right adnexal mass, probable endometrioma
Postoperative Dx: Same
Operation: Total abdominal hysterectomy with bilateral salpingo-oophorectomy
                      and lysis of pelvic adhesions with procedure of unusual difficulty,
                      secondary to endometriosis

Surgeon: Rodney L. Cohen, MD
Assistant: none
Anesthesia: General endotracheal intubation by Dr. Kastorman
Complications: None
Findings: See body of dictation
Specimens: Uterus, cervix, and portions of adnexa
Disposition: See body of dictation

PROCEDURE: The patient was taken to the OR and placed supine on the table. Underwent general anesthesia with endotracheal intubation without complication. The patient had Foley catheter inserted. Was prepped and draped in a sterile fashion for abdominal procedure. Scalpel was used to make a vertical midline incision in elliptical fashion, removing the previously noted dense abdominal scar, taken down through subcutaneous tissue to the level of the anterior rectus sheath, nicked in its midline, and extended the length of the incision. Blunt dissection through the midline rectus muscles exposed the peritoneum, sharply entered the midline, and extended the length of the incision down to the bladder. Balfour self-retaining retractor was put into place, elevated with blue towels with care taken to avoid posterior nervous injury. Initial attempts to pack the bowel off the field were difficult as there were significant adhesions between the colon and the previous area of the left adnexectomy and the endometrioma that was on the right side. Through an extensive and lengthy dissection, the bowel was carefully dissected from the pelvis with both blunt and sharp dissection with care to avoid bowel injury. The right adnexa was then carefully dissected by both blunt and sharp dissection off the side wall to avoid ureteral injury. After freeing up all tissue, the packing was removed from the abdomen, and the bowel was again repacked away from the operative site and then the hysterectomy was proceeded with in the usual fashion. Bilaterally, the utero-ovarian ligaments were cross-clamped with Kelly clamp for traction. The uterus was elevated. Bilaterally, the round ligaments were identified, cross-clamped with Heaney clamps, severed with pelvic scissors, and ligated with 0-Vicryl suture in a Heaney ligature type fashion. The bladder was sharply dissected from the lower uterine segment. Bilaterally, the uterine arteries were skeletonized, cross-clamped with Heaney clamps, severed with pelvic scissors, and then ligated with 0-Vicryl suture. The remaining portion of the cardinal ligaments were then cross-clamped with Heaney clamp, severed with pelvic scissors, and ligated with 0-Vicryl suture in Heaney ligature type fashion. At the upper most portion of the vagina, the angles were cross-clamped with Heaney clamp and severed with pelvic scissors, and the uterus, cervix, and remaining right adnexa were then removed from the vaginal cuff.

    Bilaterally, the angles were ligated with 0-Vicryl suture in Heaney ligature type fashion, and the central portion of the vaginal cuff was closed with a 0-Vicryl suture in a running interlocking fashion.

Continued

The pelvis was copiously irrigated and inspected and noted to be clean and dry with the exception of some small bleeding sites overlying the region of the right ureter in the region of the extensive dissection. These were cauterized and clipped with care taken to avoid a ureteral injury. There was a small tissue ooze due to the extensive dissection and Gelfoam was placed in the site. Prior to this, the pelvis was copiously irrigated and inspected and noted to be clean and dry. Prior to this, a look at all operative sites revealed good hemostasis. All pedicles revealed good hemostasis. All instrumentation was removed. The fascia and peritoneum were closed in a bulk fashion using 0-PDS suture in a running mixed simple interlocking fashion starting from the superior margin of the incision and running to the midline, starting from the inferior margin of the incision and running to the midline.

Subcutaneous tissue was irrigated and inspected and noted to be clean and dry. It was drawn together in the midline with 3-0 plain suture in a running simple fashion and then the skin was reapproximated with a 4-0 Vicryl suture in subcuticular fashion. Steri-Strips and overlying pressure dressing was applied. The patient was awakened on her own, breathing on her own in good condition and transferred to the recovery room.

09/04/11 12:43:45

You Code It!

What are the best, most accurate codes?

Diagnosis Codes: _____

Procedure Codes: _____

Anesthesia Codes (when applicable): _____

HCPCS Level II codes (when applicable): _____

PATIENT NAME: OPPENHEIM, OLIVIA
MRN: OPPOL01
Admission Date: 9 September 2011
Discharge Date: 10 September 2011

Operative report
Date: 10 September 2011

Preoperative Dx: 1. Menometrorrhagia refractory to medical treatment;
                              2. Endometrial mass; 3. Adnexal masses with normal CA-125
Postoperative Dx: Same
Operation: Supracervical hysterectomy, bilateral salpingo-oophorectomy

Surgeon: Rodney L. Cohen, MD
Assistant: None
Anesthesia: General endotracheal Complications: None
Findings: See body of dictation
Specimens: Uterus and cervix
Disposition: See body of dictation

PROCEDURE: The patient was taken to the OR, was placed supine position, and was prepped and draped in the usual sterile manner. A Foley catheter was inserted into the bladder to drain the urine. A Pfannenstiel skin incision was made with a knife and carried down to the fascia. The fascia was nicked in the midline and extended bilaterally. Kochers were used to grasp the superior portion of the fascia that was separated sharply and bluntly in the midline. Kochers were then used to grasp the inferior portion of the fascia that was separated sharply and bluntly. The rectus muscles were separated. Hemostats were used to grasp the peritoneum and extend superiorly under direct visualization and inferiorly under translumination. The bladder flap was developed and pushed away of the low uterine segment. The Balfour self-retaining retractor was placed and the bowel packed with warm moist laps. Two curved Kelly clamps were placed across the corneal area of the uterus on each side. The right round ligament was placed on stretch. A 0-Vicryl was used to suture ligate this ligament. The anterior and posterior leaves of the broad ligament were then opened. The same procedure was done to the left. The infundibulopelvic ligament on the right was then identified. The ureter was found to be well out of the way, and a curved Heaney clamp × 2 was placed across the infundibulopelvic ligament and this ligament excised. A 0-Vicryl free tie, as well as a 0-Vicryl suture ligation, was performed with good hemostasis. Next, the same procedure was done on the left, obtaining the left round ligament and infundibulopelvic ligament in the same manner. Next, the bladder flap was dissected off the low uterine segment and cervix. Once this was done appropriately, the uterine artery on the left side was skeletonized, and curved Heaney clamps were used to obtain this Suture ligation was performed with 0-Vicryl. The uterine artery was then obtained on the right. Straight Heaney used in succession to obtain the cardinal ligaments. The patient was noted to have endometriosis on her ovaries, as well as a lot oozing with aberrant blood vessels at this time, and it was decided to go ahead with a supracervical hysterectomy due to the nature of the patient's tissue and difficulty of going any deeper into the pelvis. A Bovie was used to cauterize and remove the fundal portion of the uterus and lower uterine segment, and a portion of the cervix as well. The remaining cervical stump was cauterized en mill, and 0-Chromic was first used to reapproximate the inside edges of the cervix, then 0-Vicryl was used on the outside

Continued

through the cervix in a running locking manner for hemostasis. Once this was done, all areas were inspected for any further bleeding. Bovie cautery or figure-of-eight sutures were placed as necessary. The bladder flap was placed over the cervical stump in the midportion. A 2-0 Chromic was used to anchor this. The right ureter was identified and found to be peristalsing normally. The left ureter could not be seen but was palpated low in the pelvis. Irrigation was performed. No further bleeding was noted, so all the instruments were removed, counts were correct; the rectus muscles were reapproximated with 0-Chromic in an interrupted manner. The fascia was closed with 0-Vicryl in the running manner. The subcutaneous tissue was thoroughly irrigated and the skin was closed with staples. This ended the procedure. The patient tolerated it well and went to recovery room in good condition.

09/09/11 09:24:26

You Code It!

What are the best, most accurate codes?

Diagnosis Codes: _____

Procedure Codes: _____

Anesthesia Codes (when applicable): _____

HCPCS Level II codes (when applicable): _____

PATIENT NAME: LEFFERTY, LORETTA
MRN: LEFLO01
Admission Date: 15 September 2011
Discharge Date: 16 September 2011

Operative Report
Date: 15 September 2011

Preoperative Dx: Pelvic mass
Postoperative Dx: Peritoneal inclusion cyst with involvement of the left fallopian tube and a portion of the left ovary
Operation: Laparoscopy, exploratory laparotomy, removal of mass

Surgeon: Rodney L. Cohen, MD
Assistant: None
Anesthesia: General
Complications: None
Findings: See body of dictation
Specimens: Adnexal mass and Fallopian tube

INDICATIONS: The patient is a 47-year-old Latin-American female status post total abdominal hysterectomy with pelvic mass on ultrasound, mildly symptomatic.

PROCEDURE: The patient was taken to the OR after the induction of adequate general anesthesia and prepped and draped in the dorsolithotomy position. A catheter was introduced into her bladder. Bimanual exam revealed a fullness near the vaginal cuff.

Small subumbilical incision was made to the skin, and the Veress needle was inserted. Peritoneal cavity was insufflated with 2 L of carbon dioxide. 10-mm trocar sleeves were placed in through this, and it was noted that the omentum, which was adherent to the anterior abdominal wall, had been perforated with the trocar and sleeve. There was no evidence of bleeding during the course of the initial scope; however, later, as the scope was removed, there was noted to be a small amount of bleeding where the omentum and the abdominal wall fused.

Examination with laparoscopy revealed a 5- to 6-cm multiloculated pelvic mass that was encapsulated with bowel and that was plastered against the vaginal cuff. There was no evidence of any pedicles, and it was not felt that this would be amenable to laparoscopic therapy.

The trocar sleeves were removed. The incision was closed with a single fascial 0-Chromic suture and 4-0 skin sutures.

Attention was then turned. A Pfannenstiel incision was made and extended to the subcutaneous tissue and fascia. The muscle and fascia were bluntly separated, and the peritoneal cavity was entered atraumatically. The mass was seen to be arising from the left adnexal area. The right ovary was identified and was plastered against the sidewall; it was normal in size and without evidence of visible abnormalities other than being plastered against the sidewall. The mass had bladder adherent over the anterior portion and bowel adherent over the posterior portion. Tedious and careful dissection was accomplished to separate the mass from all of these. The mass appeared to have clear fluid within it and seemed to be in at least three different loculations. The infundibulopelvic ligament was identified running into the mass. Thus it was felt to be ovarian and tubular in complex nature. The left ureter was dissected away from the mass and just as the mass was beginning to be almost completely isolated, it ruptured and poured forth clear fluid, but this allowed access to the inside portion of the mass. The mass was then removed along with what appeared to be the entire portion of the tube. There was a

Continued

portion of the left ovary which was still plastered against the superior portion of the vagina and this was left intact in light of there being no pathology at that point. The pelvic sidewall had been opened, and there were multiple small bleeding points that were coagulated. The infundibulopelvic ligament that had been isolated, clamped, and cut was provided with complete hemostasis. There was a small rent in the ligamentous tissue that was adherent to the mass, and multiple small figure-of-eight sutures using 2-0 Chromic or coagulation were used to provide hemostasis. Tedious examination of all cut surfaces revealed no evidence of bleeding at this point. Irrigation was accomplished and reexamination revealed the area to be dry. Examination of the omentum where the initial laparoscopy had been performed revealed a small amount of bleeding, and coagulation was used to provide hemostasis, and a single figure-of-eight suture was used to secure the fascia from the underneath portion to prevent any future hernia formation. The self-retaining retractor that had previously been placed was then removed. The laps were removed. The bowel was allowed to return to the peritoneal cavity, but prior to this a single sheet was placed over all of the cut surfaces on the left adnexal and superior bladder area to attempt to provide further reduction of adhesion formation. Having removed all the instruments, the muscles were reapproximated across the midline with
a 0-Chromic suture, and subfascia hemostasis were achieved. The fascia was closed with 0-Vicryl. Subcutaneous irrigation and hemostasis were achieved, and the skin was closed with skin staples.

The urine was clear throughout the procedure. The sponge, needle, and instrument counts were correct. The mass was sent to pathology and felt to be involving apportion of the infundibulopelvic ligament, fallopian tube, some peritoneal reflection, and possibly a small portion of the ovary.

The patient is being awakened and prepared for transfer to the recovery room.

09/15/11 07:58:10

You Code It!

What are the best, most accurate codes?

Diagnosis Codes: _____

Procedure Codes: _____

Anesthesia Codes (when applicable): _____

HCPCS Level II codes (when applicable): _____

THE WOMEN'S HEALTH CENTER
671 SENORA LANE • LOVELAND, FL 32772 • 407-555-8541

PATIENT NAME:	TAYLOR, THOMASINA
MRN:	TAYTH01
Admission Date:	5 September 2011
Discharge Date:	6 September 2011

Operative Report Date:	5 September 2011
Preoperative Dx:	1. First trimester missed abortion; 2. Undesired fertility
Postoperative Dx:	Same
Operation:	1. Dilation and curettage with suction; 2. Laparoscopic bilateral tubal ligation using Kleppinger bipolar cautery
Surgeon:	Rodney L. Cohen, MD
Assistant:	None
Anesthesia:	General endotracheal anesthesia
Complications:	None
Findings:	The patient had products of conception at the time of dilatation and curettage. She also had normal-appearing uterus, ovaries, fallopian tubes, and liver edge.
Specimens:	Products of conception to pathology
Disposition:	To PACU in stable condition

PROCEDURE: The patient was taken to the OR and placed in the dorsal supine position. General endotracheal anesthesia was administered without difficulty. The patient was placed in dorsal lithotomy position. She was prepped and draped in the normal sterile fashion. A red rubber tip catheter was placed gently to drain the patient's bladder. A weighted speculum was placed in the posterior vagina, and a Deaver retractor was placed anteriorly. A single-tooth tenaculum was placed in the anterior cervix for retraction. The uterus sounded to 9 cm. The cervix was dilated with Hanks dilators to 25 French. This sufficiently passed a #7 suction curet. The suction curet was inserted without incident, and the products of conception were gently suctioned out. Good uterine cry was noted with a serrated curet. No further products were noted on suctioning. At this point, a Hulka tenaculum was placed in the cervix for retraction. The other instruments were removed.

Attention was then turned to the patient's abdomen. A small vertical infraumbilical incision was made with the knife. A Veress needle was placed through that incision. Confirmation of placement into the abdominal cavity was made with instillation of normal saline without return and a positive handing drop test. The abdomen was then insufflated with sufficient carbon dioxide gas to cause abdominal tympany. The Veress needle was removed, and a 5-mm trocar was placed in the same incision. Confirmation of placement into the abdominal cavity was made with placement of the laparoscopic camera. Another trocar site was placed two fingerbreadths above the pubic symphysis in the midline under direct visualization. The above noted intrapelvic and intraabdominal findings were seen. The patient was placed in steep Trendelenburg. The fallopian tubes were identified and followed out to the fimbriated ends. They were then cauterized four times on either side. At this point, all instruments were removed from the patient's abdomen. This was done under direct visualization during the insufflation. The skin incisions were reapproximated with 4-0 Vicryl suture. The Hulka tenaculum was removed without incident.

Continued

The patient was placed back in the dorsal supine position. Anesthesia was withdrawn without difficulty. The patient was taken to the PACU in stable condition. All sponge, instrument, and needle counts were correct in the OR.

09/05/11 10:40:36

You Code It!

What are the best, most accurate codes?

Diagnosis Codes: _____

Procedure Codes: _____

Anesthesia Codes (when applicable): _____

HCPCS Level II codes (when applicable): _____

THE WOMEN'S HEALTH CENTER
671 SENORA LANE • LOVELAND, FL 32772 • 407-555-8541

PATIENT NAME:	GAULT, IONA
MRN:	GAUIO01
Admission Date:	5 September 2011
Discharge Date:	6 September 2011

Operative Report	
Date:	5 September 2011
Preoperative DX:	Multiparity, desiring permanent sterilization
Postoperative Dx:	Same
Operation:	Postpartum bilateral tubal ligation
Surgeon:	Gary Rothman, MD
Assistant:	None
Anesthesia:	General endotracheal anesthesia
Complications:	None
Specimens:	Fallopian tube
Findings:	Normal postpartum anatomy

PROCEDURE: After appropriate consents were signed, the risks and alternatives of the surgery were explained to the patient, and the patient agreed to the operation. The patient was taken to the OR, was given general endotracheal anesthesia, and was prepped and draped in the usual fashion. Through a transverse infraumbilical incision, the peritoneal cavity was entered. Army-Navy retractors were placed. The right fallopian tube was picked up with Babcock, followed all the way to the fimbria for identification. Then, in the midampullary portion two times of 0 chromic were placed and tube was cut and sent to pathology for identification. A similar thing was done on the left side. Then, fascia was closed with 0 Vicryl in a running locking fashion. The skin was closed with 4-0 Vicryl in a subcuticular fashion and was infiltrated with Marcaine 0.5%. The patient was extubated in the operating room and taken to the recovery room in stable condition.

D: 09/05/11 12:51:41   T: 09/07/11 01:16:18

You Code It!

What are the best, most accurate codes?

Diagnosis Codes: _____

Procedure Codes: _____

Anesthesia Codes (when applicable): _____

HCPCS Level II codes (when applicable): _____

PATIENT NAME: PHELPS, MAXINE
ACCOUNT #: PHEMA01
Date: 13 December 2011

Attending Physician: Yamira E. Newadha, MD
Location: Office

HISTORY OF PRESENT ILLNESS: This is a 40-year-old female who a month ago noted a lump in her right breast (8 o'clock position of the right breast just outside the areola). This prompted bilateral screening mammography. The mammo demonstrated a linear area of increased density and architectural distortion at the 12 o'clock position in the right periareolar region.

This was suspicious mammographically, and a biopsy of this was recommended. The patient had follow-up ultrasound as well. The ultrasound demonstrated a lobulated cyst of 6 mm at the 8 o'clock position corresponding to the patient's area of palpable abnormality. No other lesions were noted.

Due to the mammogram, the patient has an incidental finding of an area of increased density at the 12 o'clock position and requires biopsy. This is not appreciable on examination and requires needle localization and excisional biopsy for which she is here today.

The patient has no family history of breast cancer. Age of menarche: 13. She was pregnant three times with one child, first child born at age 20.

PAST MEDICAL HISTORY: No coronary disease, hypertension, or diabetes

PAST SURGICAL HISTORY: None

MEDICATIONS: None

ALLERGIES: None

SOCIAL HISTORY: The patient does not smoke, does not drink. No history of drug use.

PHYSICAL EXAMINATION:

BREASTS: The patient examined in erect and supine. Both breasts are symmetric. There is no skin dimpling. There is no nipple inversion. There is no mass appreciated in either breast, with careful attention paid to the right breast overlying the 8 o'clock region as well as the 12 o'clock region. Again, no mass was appreciated. She has no axillary, cervical, supraclavicular, or infraclavicular adenopathy notes.

LUNGS: Clear

HEART: Regular rhythm

IMPRESSION: Right breast mass

Continued

This is a 40-year-old who has an incidental finding of an area of increased density at the 12 o'clock position of the right breast. This cannot be appreciated on physical examination. She will require needle loc/excisional biopsy. The indication, alternatives, and complications of the procedure have been discussed with this patient. She understands and wishes to proceed.

Yamira E. Newadha, MD

YEM/mg   D: 12/13/11 12:51:41   T: 12/15/11 01:16:18

You Code It!

What are the best, most accurate codes?

Diagnosis Codes: _____

Procedure Codes: _____

Anesthesia Codes (when applicable): _____

HCPCS Level II codes (when applicable): _____

THE WOMEN'S HEALTH CENTER - AMBULATORY SURGICAL CENTER
671 SENORA LANE • LOVELAND, FL 32772 • 407-555-8541

PATIENT NAME: TOMLINSON, THERESA
ACCOUNT #:   TOMTH01
Date: 15 December 2011

Preoperative Diagnosis: Right breast mass
Postoperative Diagnosis: Same (pending pathology)
Operation: Excision of right breast mass, intermediate wound closure—4 cm

Surgeon: Roweena L. Macomba, MD
Assistant: None
Anesthesiologist: Terence Abnernathy, MD
Anesthesia: MAC/1% lidocaine diluted 50% with Bicarbonate (10cc)
Specimens: Breast tissue

HISTORY: This is a 51-year-old female admitted to the minor surgery suite for excision of a 1-cm palpable nodule in the superficial aspect of the right breast in the 12 o'clock axis near the periphery. The indications, alternatives, and possible complications were reviewed and consent was obtained.

PROCEDURE: With the patient in the supine position, the area in question was prepped and draped in the usual sterile fashion using Betadine. After adequate IV sedation, 1% lidocaine without epinephrine was used to infiltrate the soft tissues at that level to create a field block.

An elliptical incision was made about the lesion itself, considering its intimate association with the overlying skin. The 4-cm incision was deepened into the subcutaneous space. The mass was excised in its entirety with a rim of normal appearing breast, fat, and surrounding skin. Adequate hemostasis was secured within the depths of the wound. The wound was closed in layers. The deeper breast tissue was approximated using interrupted 3-0 chromic sutures. The subcuticular layer was approximated using interrupted 4-0 Biosyn sutures. The skin edges were closed using 4-0 Vicryl in the subcuticular space in a continuous fashion. Mastisol and Steri-Strips were applied. A dressing was applied. The procedure was terminated. Needle, sponge and instrument counts were correct. Estimated blood loss was minimal.

DISPOSITION: The patient tolerated the procedure and was discharged from the minor operating department in satisfactory condition.

_____

Roweena L. Macomba, MD

RLM/mg   D: 12/15/11 12:55:01   T: 12/18/11 09:50:16

You Code It!

What are the best, most accurate codes?

Diagnosis Codes: _____

Procedure Codes: _____

Anesthesia Codes (when applicable): _____

HCPCS Level II codes (when applicable): _____

PATIENT NAME: HARRIS, ROSEANNE
ACCOUNT #:   HARRO01
Date: 01 October 2011

In the 41st week of her first pregnancy, a 37-year-old woman arrived at Labor and Delivery at 6:30 a.m. for a planned induction of labor due to mild, pregnancy-induced hypertension.

After intravaginal placement of misoprostol, the nurse observed her briefly and, at 11:00 a.m., discharged her from the unit. She went for a walk with her husband in a park next to the hospital.

Patient's membranes spontaneously ruptured, and she returned to the labor and delivery unit. A recently hired new graduate nurse admitted the patient, took her vital signs, and checked the fetal heart rate. The mother's blood pressure was 176/95, but the nurse thought this was related to nausea, vomiting, and discomfort from the contractions.

The resident examined the mother, determined that her cervix was 5-6 cm, 90 percent effaced and the vertex was at 0 station. An internal fetal heart monitor was placed because the mother's vomiting and discomfort caused her to move around too much in the bed, making it hard to record the fetal heart rate with an external monitor. The internal monitor revealed a steady fetal heart rate of 120 and no decelerations.

The mother continued to complain of painful contractions and requested an epidural. Shortly after placement of the epidural, the monitor recorded a prolonged fetal heart rate deceleration. The heart rate returned slowly to the baseline rate of 120 as the nurse repositioned the mother, increased her intravenous fluids and administered oxygen by mask.

An epidural analgesia infusion pump was started. The fetal heart rate strip indicated another deceleration that recovered to baseline. The nurse informed the resident who checked the tracing and told her to "keep an eye on things."

The primary nurse noted in the labor record that the baseline fetal heart rate was "unstable, between 100-120," but she did not report this to the resident.

The nurse recorded that the fetal heart rate was "flat, no variability." As the nurse was documenting this as a nonreassuring fetal heart rate pattern, the patient expressed a strong urge to push and the nurse called for an exam.

A resident came to the bedside, examined the mother, and noted that she was fully dilated with the caput at +1. A brief update was written in the chart, but the clinician who had performed the exam was not noted.

The mother was repositioned and began pushing.

The fetal heart rate suddenly dropped and remained profoundly bradycardic for 11 minutes. The resident was called and attempted a vacuum delivery since the fetal head was at +2 station. The attending then entered and attempted forceps delivery.

An emergency cesarean delivery was performed; the baby was stillborn. The physician identified a uterine rupture that required significant blood replacement.

Roland F. LaScala, MD

RFL/mg   D: 10/01/11   T: 10/03/11

You Code It!

What are the best, most accurate codes?

Diagnosis Codes: _____

Procedure Codes: _____

Anesthesia Codes (when applicable): _____

HCPCS Level II codes (when applicable): _____

THE WOMEN'S HEALTH CENTER
671 SENORA LANE • LOVELAND, FL 32772 • 407-555-8541

PATIENT NAME: JOCQUIN, YASMINE
ACCOUNT #: JOCYA01
DATE: 1 October 2011

This is a 26-year-old, G1P0, O+, VDRL NR, rubella immune, HBsAg negative female at 27 weeks gestation presenting to labor and delivery with a 2-day history of headache and facial swelling. Maternal history is remarkable for a single prenatal visit in the first trimester.

EXAM: VS T 37, P 75, RR 14, BP 170/100. Her exam is remarkable for facial and pretibial edema and hyperreflexia.

LABS: Urine dipstick positive for 3+ protein. Ultrasound demonstrates decreased amniotic fluid. The fetus is in the breech position, and no fetal abnormalities are noted. Estimated fetal weight is 650 grams.
    A decision is made to deliver the infant by cesarean section following maternal treatment with betamethasone sodium phosphate 0.5 mg/d.
    Labor and delivery occurs without incident.
    Infant taken to NICU. Neonatologist paged.
    Mother taken to recovery in good condition.

Roland F. LaScala, MD

RFL/mg   D: 10/01/11   T: 10/03/11

You Code It!

What are the best, most accurate codes?

Diagnosis Codes: _____

Procedure Codes: _____

Anesthesia Codes (when applicable): _____

HCPCS Level II codes (when applicable): _____

Oncology Cases and Patient Records

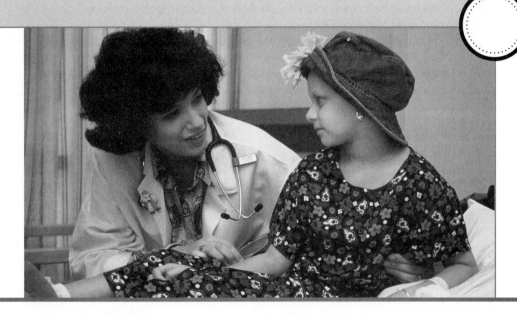

INTRODUCTION

The following case studies are from an oncology practice. In a physician's office of this type, a professional coding specialist is likely to see patients with different kinds of malignant tumors.

Oncologists are physicians who specialize in the diagnosis and treatment of malignancies, the second greatest cause of mortality (death) in the United States. They may be involved in determining the type and extent of cancer and providing such treatments as surgery, radiation, or chemotherapy.

These health care professionals may be board-certified in medical oncology through the Board of Internal Medicine, which is recognized by the American Board of Medical Specialties.

You can use these cases to practice coding diagnoses, E/M, procedures, DME, or other HCPCS Level II items, as applicable; code for the physician or the facility; code inpatient and outpatient services, as applicable:

1. Code for the physician.
2. Code for the anesthesiologist, when applicable.
3. Code for the hospital, when applicable.
4. Code for the pathology and laboratory, when applicable.
5. Code HCPCS Level II codes, when applicable.

SWANSON ONCOLOGY
969 TURNABOUT LANE • REMISSION, FL 32811 • 407-555-9573

PATIENT:	BACHELDER, JEFFREY
MRN:	BACJE001
Admission Date:	13 October 2011
Discharge Date:	13 October 2011
Date:	13 October 2011
Preoperative Dx:	Malignant neoplasm, scrotum, CA in situ
Postoperative Dx:	Same
Procedure:	Resection of scrotum, needle biopsy of testis, laparoscopy with a ligation of spermatic veins
Surgeon:	Daniel Macintosh, MD
Assistant:	None
Anesthesia:	General

INDICATIONS: The patient is a 59-year-old male with a recent diagnosis of malignancy of the scrotum.

PROCEDURE: The patient was placed on the table in supine position. General anesthesia was administered by Dr. Cattan. He was placed in proper position. A needle biopsy was taken of the testis, and then a surgical resection of the scrotum was performed. Before closing, a surgical laparoscopy with a ligation of the spermatic veins was performed, as well.

10/13/11 11:47:39

You Code It!

What are the best, most accurate codes?

Diagnosis Codes: _____

Procedure Codes: _____

Anesthesia Codes (when applicable): _____

HCPCS Level II codes (when applicable): _____

SWANSON ONCOLOGY
969 TURNABOUT LANE • REMISSION, FL 32811 • 407-555-9573

PATIENT: MARSHALL, BARRY
ACCOUNT/EHR #:   MARBA001
Date: 11/09/11

Attending Physician: Willard B. Reader, MD

S: Pt is a 51-year-old male who comes in concerned about a sore he noticed on his left temple, directly at the hairline. He states that his mother died 6 years ago from melanoma and that his brother was diagnosed with precancerous cells of the epidermis. Pt states he is the captain of a beach volleyball team and volunteers at the local YMCA as a water aerobics instructor. He says that he tries to be diligent about sunscreen, but sometimes he forgets.

O: Ht 5'11" Wt. 189 lb. R 20. T 98.6. BP 120/95 Cultures of lesion were taken and sent to our in-house lab. The pathology report confirms the lesion is malignant. I discussed options with the patient and recommended surgical removal of the lesion as soon as possible.

A: Malignant melanoma of skin of scalp

P: Pt to call to make appointment for surgical procedure

_____

Willard B. Reader, MD

WBR/pw   D: 11/09/11 09:50:16   T: 11/13/11 12:55:01

You Code It!

What are the best, most accurate codes?

Diagnosis Codes: _____

Procedure Codes: _____

Anesthesia Codes (when applicable): _____

HCPCS Level II codes (when applicable): _____

SWANSON ONCOLOGY
969 TURNABOUT LANE • REMISSION, FL 32811 • 407-555-9573

PATIENT: UNDERWOOD, PRICILLA
MRN: UNDPR001
Date: 25 September 2011

DX Medulloblastoma
Procedure: Central venous access device (CVAD) insertion
Physician: Frank Vincent, MD
Anesthesia: Conscious sedation

PROCEDURE: Patient is a 4-year-old female with a recent diagnosis of malignancy. Due to an upcoming course of chemotherapy, the CVAD is being inserted to ease administration of the drugs. The patient was placed on the table in supine position. The patient is given Versed to achieve conscious sedation. The incision was made to insert a central venous catheter centrally. During the placement of the catheter, a short tract (nontunneled) is made as the catheter is advanced from the skin entry site to the point of venous cannulation. The catheter tip is set to reside in the subclavian vein. The patient was gently aroused from the sedation and was awake when transported to the recovery room.

Frank Vincent, MD

FV/mg   D: 09/25/11 09:50:16   T: 09/25/11 12:55:01

You Code It!

What are the best, most accurate codes?

Diagnosis Codes: _____

Procedure Codes: _____

Anesthesia Codes (when applicable): _____

HCPCS Level II codes (when applicable): _____

SWANSON ONCOLOGY
969 TURNABOUT LANE • REMISSION, FL 32811 • 407-555-9573

PATIENT: TRANSIL, BRENDA
ACCOUNT/EHR #:   TRABR001
Date: 09/29/11

Attending Physician: Benjamin L. Johnston, MD

Referring Physician: James I. Cipher, MD

HPI: The patient is well known to me from her earlier hospitalization. This is a 71-year-old female with a past history of metastatic follicular carcinoma of the thyroid who had been recently retreated at this medical center for superior vena cava syndrome and obstruction with anticoagulation. At that time, she developed a febrile illness, for which infectious disease was consulted.

It turned out that an infectious disease workup was negative, and it was felt that she had an underlying autoimmune type basis for her fever and was put on prednisone. On the prednisone, her fever resolved and all the other symptoms resolved, and she had been doing quite well.

In the interim, it was determined that she did have metastatic thyroid carcinoma disease, and so she was admitted today for radioactive iodine therapy. However, during the physical examination at the clinic yesterday, Dr. Radner discovered an abdominal mass. She denied any history of trauma and denied fevers, chills, sweats, or other systemic symptoms. She had been doing quite well actually since going home on low-dose maintenance prednisone therapy.

A CT was done that showed a retroperitoneal mass, and a CT-guided biopsy was done this morning that revealed frank pus. She subsequently underwent drainage of 500 cc of grossly purulent material, described as pea-green soup. We are now asked to consult to help with the antibiotic management. The fluid did not apparently appear to be foul smelling but did look green and thick.

The patient, again, continues to deny any fevers, chills, sweats, or systemic symptoms. At the time the subsequent drainage was done today, two drainage catheters were placed into the abscess. She experienced hypotension, nausea, and diaphoresis, which resolved with some fluid boluses. She is now in the IMC for further management because of the episode of hypotension and a concern of sepsis.

Again, on talking to the patient, she denies any history of trauma to the area. She denies any history of abdominal pain, fevers, chills, sweats, nausea, vomiting, diarrhea, or systemic symptoms. She has no past history of diverticulitis or diverticular diseases. She has not had any diarrhea or abdominal pain.

The preliminary Gram stain results shows a few white blood cells; no organisms. Cultures are pending.

Her white count at this time was 12,800, with a left shift but she is on oral prednisone. The sedimentation rate was 42. The PT was 12.4 and the PTT is 25. The chemistries are remarkable for a glucose of 115, albumin of 3.6, and cholesterol of 235, and the liver function tests were normal.

PAST MEDICAL HISTORY: As stated, the past medical history is significant for follicular cell carcinoma of the thyroid, status post subtotal thyroidectomy, 03/07/96; status post right internal jugular repair from tumor invasion into the jugular; and biopsy of mediastinal metastatic disease. The patient is also status post carcinoma. She is status post mastectomy for breast carcinoma in 07/05. She had post-thoracotomy syndrome in 03/07, with fever and effusion, which resolved. She has a history of a small clot at the site of the venogram entry of the left leg. She had been on Coumadin and may possibly have had a retroperitoneal bleed. She also has a history of hypocalcemia secondary to her thyroidectomy and is on calcium maintenance.

MEDICATIONS: Her medications at this time include Nolvadex 10 mg po bid; Os-Cal 1000 mg po tid; Rocaltrol 0.25 mcg po bid; and prednisone 10 mg po qam.

ALLERGIES: She is ALLERGIC TO PENICILLIN and SULFA.

Continued

REVIEW OF SYSTEMS: As stated, the review of systems is essentially unremarkable. She denies fevers, chills, sweats, abdominal pain, nausea, vomiting, and diarrhea. The fevers had resolved on the prednisone.

PHYSICAL EXAM: BP 100/60; P 90; T 98.4

APPEARANCE: Alert, oriented, in no acute distress.

HEAD: Normocephalic, atraumatic.

EYES: Pupils are equal, round, and reactive to light and accommodation. Extraocular movements full.

MOUTH/TONGUE/PHARYNX: Throat clear. No thrush or exudates.

NECK: Supple. No stiffness.

LUNGS: Few crackles at both bases. Scattered rhonchi bilaterally. Good air exchange.

CARDIVASC: Regular rhythm. Normal S1 and S2. No murmurs.

ABDOMEN: Soft. Some tenderness in the right middle quadrant, with drainage catheters in place and no definite mass appreciated at this time.

EXTREMITIES: No joint effusions or deformities. Trace edema of the ankles.

SKIN: Some scattered ecchymoses. No significant rashes or lesions noted.

NEURO: Grossly normal. No focal deficits.

IMPRESSION:
1. Retroperitoneal mass appears to be an abscess; may possibly have been secondary to a possible bleed that secondarily got infected. She has had no preceding systemic signs of infection or trauma to the area. Other etiologies would be some type of relationship to possible abdominal disease, but she has no history of diverticular disease and this would be less likely. The most likely organisms to consider, again, would be *Staphylococcus, Streptococcus,* anaerobes, and gut flora.
2. Metastatic thyroid follicular carcinoma; to receive radiation therapy.

PLAN/RECOMMENDATIONS:
1. Will start her empirically on intravenous antibiotic therapy with clindamycin and Cipro, which should cover *Staphylococcus, Streptococcus,* anaerobes, and gram-negatives, until more culture results are known.
2. Monitor vital signs carefully and provide supportive care if she becomes hypotensive again.
3. Will check blood cultures as well as urine culture.
4. Would not give radioactive iodine at this time until we have cleared up her infection.

Thanks for the consultation. Will follow.

Benjamin L. Johnston, MD

BLJ/mg   D: 09/29/11 09:50:16   T: 10/01/11 12:55:01

You Code It!

What are the best, most accurate codes?

Diagnosis Codes: _____

Procedure Codes: _____

Anesthesia Codes (when applicable): _____

HCPCS Level II codes (when applicable): _____

SWANSON ONCOLOGY
969 TURNABOUT LANE • REMISSION, FL 32811 • 407-555-9573

PATIENT: ABERNATHY, CARTER

ACCOUNT/EHR #:   ABECA001

Date: 10/15/11

Attending Physician: Valerie R. Victors, MD

S: Pt is a 45-year-old male diagnosed with carcinoma of the inner cheek three months ago. He has chewed tobacco for the last 20 years. Pt states he quit chewing six weeks ago. He presents today for his therapeutic injection.

O: Pt is brought into the examining room, and given an injection of Interferon Alfa-2a, 3 million units, IM.

A: Malignant carcinoma, cheek, internal

P: Series of injections to continue on daily basis

_____

Valerie R. Victors, MD

VRV/mg   D: 10/15/11 09:50:16 T: 10/17/11 12:55:01

You Code It!

What are the best, most accurate codes?

Diagnosis Codes: _____

Procedure Codes: _____

Anesthesia Codes (when applicable): _____

HCPCS Level II codes (when applicable): _____

SWANSON ONCOLOGY
969 TURNABOUT LANE • REMISSION, FL 32811 • 407-555-9573

PATIENT: LANGER, DENNY
ACCOUNT/EHR #: LANDE001
Date: 10/15/11

Attending Physician: Valerie R. Victors, MD

Diagnosis on Admission: History of Ewing's sarcoma with recurrent chemotherapy for progressive disease

Final Diagnosis: Known Ewing's sarcoma with pulmonary metastases, with apparent resolution of thoracic and vertebral involvement

Consultations and Procedures during Course of Hospital Stay: Routine imaging studies, including 1. Chest x-ray; 2. CT scan of the thorax; 3. Nucleotide bone scan

HISTORY OF PRESENT ILLNESS AND BRIEF HOSPITAL COURSE BY SYSTEM: Briefly, the patient is a 32-year-old male with a known history of Ewing's sarcoma of the left lower extremity, first diagnosed in 1998. The patient was subsequently found to have pulmonary metastases. He has been seen previously in the hematology/oncology clinic for routine chemotherapy consisting of vincristine, cyclophosphamide, doxorubicin, and routine bone marrow rescue with GCSF therapy. Current therapy includes a regime of Cytoxan, cyclophosphamide and topotecan which corresponds to pediatric oncology group protocol #9354.

In current admission at presentation, patient was well appearing with no significant medical problems, except for his known Ewing's. He was hydrated as per protocol and tolerated the chemotherapy routine well. Serum chemistries remained stable during the course of the hospital stay. Significant findings during the course of the hospital stay included the results of the imaging studies alluded to previously. 1. Routine chest x-ray obtained 07/28/11 showed the presence of a port-a-cath well positioned in the superior vena cava. In addition, there appeared to be an improving pattern of pulmonary metastases from the known Ewing's sarcoma when compared to films from 06/11/00. 2. Computerized spiral tomography of the thorax, obtained 07/28/11, when compared to similar films from 5/9/00, showed significant interval improvement of metastatic disease, involving both the pulmonary parenchyma and the mediastinum of known Ewing's sarcoma. There were persistent small numerous pulmonary nodules which appeared to be in resolution when compared to earlier films. 3. Nucleotide-99 HTP bone scan obtained 07/28/11, compared with a previous study of 06/12/00, showed (a) a persistent left posterior skull and possible left side of the L2 vertebra to have activity, which, however, was less intense than on the previous study; (b) an expansile lesion present in the distal left femur that was a similar distribution of activity but again seemed to be less intense; and c) resolution of activity that had previously been noted on the right side of the T8 vertebra and the sixth costal rib posteriorly.

Patient is admitted to begin a chemotherapeutic regime.

Valerie R. Victors, MD
VRV/mg   D: 10/15/11 09:50:16   T: 10/17/11 12:55:01

You Code It!

What are the best, most accurate codes?

Diagnosis Codes: _____

Procedure Codes: _____

Anesthesia Codes (when applicable): _____

HCPCS Level II codes (when applicable): _____

SWANSON ONCOLOGY
969 TURNABOUT LANE • REMISSION, FL 32811 • 407-555-9573

PATIENT: ALLMAN, SERITA
ACCOUNT/EHR #:   ALLSE001
Date: 10/15/11

Attending Physician: Matthew Saunders, MD

CC: Patient with Ewing's sarcoma, routine chemotherapy

HPI: This is a 10-year-old female with Ewing's sarcoma of the left lower extremity diagnosed in 2005. The patient was scheduled for radiation in 2006 when significant pulmonary metastases were found. Last admission was July 6, 2006, for chemotherapy consisting of vincristine, cyclophosphamide, doxorubicin, mesna and G-CSF. Previous admission was June 11, 2006, for ifosfamide, cyclophosphamide, and etoposide chemotherapy. Previous sick hospital admission was May 8, 2006 for a pleural effusion. The patient has had no intercurrent illnesses, no nausea, vomiting, diarrhea, or constipation since the last admission. No fevers. The patient has noted some mucositis following the past chemotherapy, which resolved with Miles Magic mouthwash eight days ago.

PAST MEDICAL HISTORY: Is as above for Ewing's sarcoma of left lower extremity; the patient has received chemotherapy. Last chemotherapy consisting of pediatric oncology group #9354, regime A with ICE.

BIRTH HISTORY: The patient was born at 34 weeks gestation, birth weight of six pounds, no complications following delivery.

DEVELOPMENTAL HISTORY: The patient had normal milestones. Immunizations are up to date to 3 years of age.

PAST SURGICAL HISTORY: The patient had multiple catheter replacements and a bone marrow biopsy.

ALLERGIES: Phenergan

MEDICATIONS: None

SOCIAL HISTORY: The patient lives with her mother, father, two brothers, and one sister. They have no pets. There are no smokers in the home.

FAMILY HISTORY: Paternal grandmother with breast cancer.

PE: VITAL SIGNS: Temperature 98.1, pulse 115, respirations 20, blood pressure 110/61, height 143.5 cm, weight 28.1 kilos.

GENERAL: The patient is a female with alopecia in no acute distress.

HEENT: Complete alopecia, normocephalic, atraumatic. Pupils are equal and reactive to light, fundi are visualized without lesions. TMs are gray bilaterally with good landmarks. Pharynx is clear, mucous membranes are without lesions.

NECK: No lymphadenopathy is noted.

LUNGS: Clear to auscultation bilaterally.

CHEST: There is a PermCath in the right chest which is intact without tenderness.

HEART: Cardiac exam is with regular rate and rhythm without murmurs or rubs.

ABDOMEN: Positive bowel sounds, nontender, nondistended with no hepatosplenomegaly noted, the patient's abdomen is soft.

PELVIC/RECTAL: GU deferred.

Continued

EXTREMITIES: No clubbing, cyanosis, or edema. Pulses are 2+ femorals, distal posterior tibial pulses, dorsalis pedis and radial pulses. Capillary refill is less than two seconds.

NEURO: The patient was alert and oriented and responds to questions appropriately. Cranial nerves II-XII are grossly intact. Sensation is intact bilaterally. The patient's muscle strength is 5/5 bilaterally. Deep tendon reflexes are 2+ in all groups.

ASSESSMENT: This is a 10-year-old patient with metastatic Ewing's sarcoma here for routine chemotherapy: Pediatric Oncology Group #9464 consisting of cyclophosphamide, topotecan chemotherapy.

1. Oncology. The patient will have lab-drawn CBC with diff, retic count, complete metabolic profile, LDH, and UA prior to starting chemotherapy. Other labs: The patient will have chest x-ray, AP and lateral, CT scan, bone scan during hospital stay. The patient will be prehydrated with 550 cc of D5 1/4 normal saline over 30 minutes q.d. times 5 days. The patient will receive Zofran 4 mg IV q8h times 5 days. The patient will receive cyclophosphamide 275 mg. in 55 cc of normal saline IV over 30 minutes q.d. times 5 days. The patient will received topotecan 0.8 mg in 50 cc D5W IV over 30 minutes q.d. times 5 days. The patient will continue hydration post chemotherapy D5 1/4 normal saline at 75 cc/hour until next day of chemo, q.d. times 5 days. On day 6, the patient will be on G-CSF 140 mcg subcu q.d. times 10-14 days post nadir of absolute neutrophil count greater than or equal to 5,000.
2. Hematologic. The patient will have type and cross on parents' blood for direct donated white blood cells if needed; the patient will be sent to the Blood Bank for type and donation.
3. ID. The patient will be observed for fever.
4. Social. Patient plan discussed with parents with me present. The parents agree to chemotherapy.
5. The patient will have a regular diet, routine vital signs, and activity as tolerated.

Matthew Saunders, MD

MS/mg   D: 10/15/11 09:50:16   T: 10/17/11 12:55:01

You Code It!

What are the best, most accurate codes?

Diagnosis Codes: _____

Procedure Codes: _____

Anesthesia Codes (when applicable): _____

HCPCS Level II codes (when applicable): _____

SWANSON ONCOLOGY
969 TURNABOUT LANE • REMISSION, FL 32811 • 407-555-9573

PATIENT: GARRISON, THEODORE
ACCOUNT/EHR #:   GARTH001
Date: 10/13/11

Attending Physician: Matthew Saunders, MD

1. Metastatic colon carcinoma, on palliative systemic chemotherapy with second line chemotherapy combination at this time.
2. Obstructive uropathy, status postreplacement of internal ureteral stent.

COMPLICATIONS: None

SPECIAL PROCEDURES: Replacement of ureteral stent by Dr. Surikian on 06/30/08; port placement by Dr. Madison on 06/26/11.

DISCHARGE MEDICATIONS: OxyContin 40 mg p.o. q12 hours, Neurontin 300 mg p.o. t.i.d., Vicodin one or two every four hours as needed for breakthrough pain, Zantac 150 mg p.o. b.i.d., Magic mouth wash one or two teaspoons for symptomatic sore mouth and sore throat.

DISPOSITION: The patient will be followed by the MD Anderson Cancer Center in t2 weeks' time, at which time restaging studies will be scheduled.

HOSPITAL COURSE: Patient is a pleasant 38-year-old unfortunate black male with progressive metastatic colon carcinoma, having failed first line chemotherapy with Camptosar, 5FU, and Leucovorin and currently on 5FU infusion therapy at monthly intervals with Mitomycin added to every odd numbered cycle of same. He was admitted on 06/26/11 for cycle #3 of 5 FU with Mitomycin this time. He tolerated the chemotherapy quite well. To facilitate ongoing therapy, a port was placed at my request on the day of admission by Dr. Madison, and also at the patient's request, a urology consultation with Dr. Surikian was requested for replacement of the internal ureteral stent, which was accomplished on 06/30/11.

     The patient remained stable with good performance status at 70% or better on a Karnofsky scale throughout the hospital course.

     Vital signs have remained stable, and he is being discharged in stable condition with the above follow-up instructions.

Matthew Saunders, MD

MS/mg   D: 10/13/11 09:50:16   T: 10/17/11 12:55:01

You Code It!

What are the best, most accurate codes?

Diagnosis Codes: _____

Procedure Codes: _____

Anesthesia Codes (when applicable): _____

HCPCS Level II codes (when applicable): _____

SWANSON ONCOLOGY
969 TURNABOUT LANE • REMISSION, FL 32811 • 407-555-9573

PATIENT: HAWAN, MARILYN
ACCOUNT/EHR #:   HAWMA001
Date: 10/15/11

Preop DX: Right ureteral obstruction secondary to colon cancer
Postop DX: Same
Operation: 1. Cystoscopy
                        2. Right retrograde pyelogram
                        3. Removal and replacement of double-J stent

Surgeon   Michael Surikian, MD
Anesthesia: General

HISTORY/INDICATIONS: This is a 28-year-old black female with a history of colon cancer and secondary right ureteral obstruction who had a stent inserted a number of months ago. At this time, she is in the hospital and it is time for a stent change. Consequently, the patient presents for the procedure.

PROCEDURE: The patient was taken to the operating room, and there she was given general anesthetic and positioned in the dorsal lithotomy position, the genitalia scrubbed and prepped with Betadine. Sterile towels and sheets were utilized to drape the patient in the usual fashion. A cystoscope was introduced into the bladder. The ureteral catheter was identified. It was grabbed and removed without any difficulty. Subsequently, the cystoscope was reinserted into the bladder and the right ureteral orifice was identified over a Pollack catheter. A glide wire was inserted into the right collecting system. Some contrast was injected, and a hydronephrotic right side was noted. Then, the wire was placed through the Pollack catheter. With the wire in position, over the wire a 7 French 26 cm double-J stent was inserted. Excellent coiling was noted fluoroscopically in the kidney and distally with a cystoscope. The bladder was then drained, and again it was inspected prior to stent removal. There was no evidence of any tumors or lesions in the bladder. The stent was in good position. The cystoscope was removed and the patient was taken to the recovery room awake and in stable condition.

Michael Surikian, MD

MS/mg   D: 10/15/11 09:50:16 T: 10/17/11 12:55:01

You Code It!

What are the best, most accurate codes?

Diagnosis Codes: _____

Procedure Codes: _____

Anesthesia Codes (when applicable): _____

HCPCS Level II codes (when applicable): _____

SWANSON ONCOLOGY
969 TURNABOUT LANE • REMISSION, FL 32811 • 407-555-9573

PATIENT: YANNI, HASAN
ACCOUNT/EHR #:   YANHA001
Date: 10/15/11

Surgeon: Lawrence Lafferty, MD

Preop DX: Malignant pleural effusion
Postop DX: Same
Procedure: Tubular thoracostomy

DESCRIPTION OF PROCEDURE: The procedure was done at the bedside with sterile technique. A #24 French chest tube was inserted, and 1200 cc of serosanguineous fluid was aspirated into the suction control apparatus without any problems. The fluid was tidalling well.

The patient tolerated the procedure well, and 1200 cc was aspirated initially.

A chest x-ray was pending at the time of this dictation.

10/15/11 11:47:39

You Code It!

What are the best, most accurate codes?

Diagnosis Codes: _____

Procedure Codes: _____

Anesthesia Codes (when applicable): _____

HCPCS Level II codes (when applicable): _____

SWANSON ONCOLOGY
969 TURNABOUT LANE • REMISSION, FL 32811 • 407-555-9573

PATIENT: PEPPER, SCOTT
ACCOUNT/EHR #:   PEPSC001
Date: 10/15/11

Diagnosis on Admission:
1. Malignant effusion
2. Dyspnea
3. History of metastatic bone disease
4. Small cell carcinoma of the lung
5. Hepatic metastases

CHIEF COMPLAINT: This 71-year-old white man was admitted for evaluation and management of his rather large, right-sided pleural effusion and dyspnea. He has had somewhat of a dry cough. He has had somewhat of a scattered bone pain syndrome. He denies fevers, chills, or sweats.

PAST MEDICAL/SURGICAL HISTORY: See the progress notes of Dr. Hammond, now part of this record, 10/23/95.

MEDICATIONS: At home, he was on Prilosec, Tenormin, Hytrin, digoxin, and Megace (see orders for doses).

ALLERGIES: Iodine dye

SOCIAL HISTORY: Noncontributory

FAMILY HISTORY: Noncontributory

REVIEW OF SYSTEMS: Noncontributory PE: BP: 140/70 Pulse: 80 regular Resp: 20, slightly labored T: 98.6

HEAD: Negative

EYES: Negative

EARS: Negative

NOSE: Negative

MOUTH/TONGUE/PHARYNX: Negative

NECK: No jugular venous distention or bruits. Supple.

LYMPH NODES: Negative in all groups examined at this time

CHEST: Dullness on the right side three-fourths of the way up. Clear on the left.

CARDIVASC: Distant S1 and S2. No murmurs, gallops, or rubs.

ABDOMEN: Slightly obese. No masses or organomegaly.

GENITALIA: Not done

RECTAL: Not done

EXTREMITIES: No clubbing or cyanosis, but he did have 21 pedal edema to the knee, slightly pitting. There were some superficial varicosities.

SKIN: Dry. No rashes.

Continued

NEURO: Central nervous system intact. Anxious.

CHEST X-RAY: Large right-sided plural effusion

BONE SCAN OF 10/95: Diffuse skeletal metastases

LABORATORY DATA: ProTime and PTT — normal. Platelet count — normal. Chemistries — unremarkable except for total protein of 5.8, albumin 2.6, total CO_2 content 33, calcium 7.9, and alkaline phosphatase of 210.

Note: Thoracentesis fluid from 04/03/96—positive for malignant cells, consistent with non-small-cell carcinoma (report now in this chart, part of the record). Hemoglobin 10.6, with a white count of 10.1

ASSESSMENT: Diagnoses as above.

PLAN/RECOMMENDATIONS:
1. Tube thoracostomy
2. After fluid is drained adequately, pleurodesis.

Robyn Bennito, MD

10/15/11 11:47:39

You Code It!

What are the best, most accurate codes?

Diagnosis Codes: _____

Procedure Codes: _____

Anesthesia Codes (when applicable): _____

HCPCS Level II codes (when applicable): _____

PATIENT: PRESSLER, GAYLE
ACCOUNT/EHR #:   PRESGA001
DATE: 10/15/11
H&P:

CHIEF COMPLAINT/HISTORY OF PRESENT ILLNESS: Patient is a female with cervical cancer. The patient is undergoing radiation therapy and chemotherapy. The patient admitted with nausea, vomiting, and dehydration. The patient was just discharged from the hospital with the same problem. She is readmitted with progressive nausea and vomiting, and she has become weak and is dehydrated. She has poorly described lower abdominal pain. There have been no fevers.

PAST MEDICAL HISTORY:

MEDICAL: Hypertension, cervical cancer, undergoing chemotherapy radiation. Apparent recent diagnosis of Hodgkin's disease via excision of a groin lymph node.

ALLERGIES: Negative

MEDICATIONS: Vasotec, Ativan p.r.n, Duragesic patch 75 mcg q.3 days

SOCIAL HISTORY: Unchanged

FAMILY HISTORY: Unchanged

REVIEW OF SYSTEMS: As above

PHYSICAL EXAMINATION:

GENERAL: She is a female in modest distress due to malaise and nausea.

VITAL SIGNS: She is afebrile. Vitals are stable. Blood pressure 130/70.

HEENT: Remarkable for dry mucous membranes. There is no thrush.

NECK: Supple

LUNGS: Clear with decrease breath sounds generally

CARDIAC: Regular rate and rhythm without murmur, gallop or rub

ABDOMEN: Exam reveals soft abdomen. There is tenderness in the lower quadrants without rebound. There is no palpable mass or hepatosplenomegaly.

EXTREMITIES: Reveal no edema

SKIN: Poor turgor

LABORATORY DATA: Pending

Continued

IMPRESSION/PLAN: Female with locally advanced cervical cancer undergoing chemotherapy radiation. The patient admitted with nausea, vomiting, weakness, and dehydration.

　　The patient will be admitted to a regular medical floor and will be given fluids and antiemetics. We will check routine labs. Her nausea and vomiting are probably due to radiation enteritis, although we may have GI see her to see if they have any other suggestions with reference to her nausea and vomiting, which are fairly intractable and persistent. There may be a functional component. We will review the pathology of lymph node biopsy showing what I understand is Hodgkin's. Dr. Buckman will continue on radiation therapy for now, and until the nausea resolves, we will hold chemotherapy.

Robyn Bennito, MD

10/15/11 11:47:39

You Code It!

What are the best, most accurate codes?

Diagnosis Codes: _____

Procedure Codes: _____

Anesthesia Codes (when applicable): _____

HCPCS Level II codes (when applicable): _____

PATIENT: DEIGHTON, SAMANTHA
ACCOUNT/EHR #:   DEISA001
Date: 10/15/11
H&P

Reason for Admission: Placement of afterload in tandem and ovoid for cervix cancer.

CC/HPI: Patient is a 49-year-old female who was recently diagnosed with a locally advanced cervix cancer. Shortly after diagnosis she was also found to have a left inguinal lymph node biopsy — which returned Hodgkin's disease. She received external beam radiotherapy to her pelvis and groin and now presents for her first afterload in tandem and ovoid.

PMH: History of migraine headaches. No other significant medical or surgical illnesses.

ALLERGIES: None

MEDICATIONS: OxyContin, Lomotil

SOCIAL HISTORY: Patient has a long smoking/drinking history.

FAMILY HISTORY: No significant family history of cancer

REVIEW OF SYSTEMS: Noncontributory

PHYSICAL EXAMINATION:

GENERAL APPEARANCE: Well-developed, well-nourished female in no distress

SKIN: No palpable cervical or supraclavicular adenopathy

LUNGS: Clear to auscultation

ABDOMEN: Soft, nontender without palpable mass or organomegaly. She has desquamation from previous external beam radiotherapy in the groins bilaterally.

EXTREMITIES: Without edema

PELVIC/RECTAL:

IMPRESSION: Squamous cell carcinoma of the cervix

DISPOSITION: The patient will be brought to the operating room for placement of tandem and ovoid. She will be hospitalized for approximately two days. This is her first out of two planned treatments.

10/15/11 11:47:39

You Code It!

What are the best, most accurate codes?

Diagnosis Codes: _____

Procedure Codes: _____

Anesthesia Codes (when applicable): _____

HCPCS Level II codes (when applicable): _____

SWANSON ONCOLOGY
969 TURNABOUT LANE • REMISSION, FL 32811 • 407-555-9573

PATIENT: LIGHTFOOT, WANITA
ACCOUNT/EHR #:   LIGWA001
Date: 10/15/11

Preop DX: Cervical cancer
Post op DX: Same
Operation: Examination under anesthesia and placement of tandem for
                        afterloading radiation

Surgeon: Jacob Sapperstein, MD/David Buckman, MD
Assistant: Caroline Blythe, MD
Anesthesia: General anesthesia

PROCEDURE: After adequate induction of general anesthesia, the patient was placed in the dorsal lithotomy position and she was prepped and draped in the usual sterile manner for vaginal surgery. An exam under anesthesia was performed. The patient has had a significant response to her external beam radiation and chemotherapy. Initially, she had a large 3B lesion with tumor extending from side wall to side wall. Today she has fibrosis in both parametria. The right parametrium is free from the sidewall and there is some movement allowed there. The left side is not as free, but again it mostly feels like smooth fibrosis as opposed to nodular tumor. The upper vagina is very small due to the radiation changes, and there is no viable-appearing tumor on the cervix. We could not identify cervix today. There was an os uterus. After exam under anesthesia, she was prepped and draped and a weighted speculum was placed in the vagina. A Deaver retractor was utilized to identify the upper vagina. A sound was used, the os was identified, and the uterus sounded to 7 cm. We dilated the cervix then and allowed placement of a tandem. The vaginal walls were too small and too close together to allow placement of even the smallest ovoid we had available, and so Dr. Buckman decided to just place the tandem in, so the tandem was packed. Foley catheter was placed. Five cc of radiopaque dye were placed in the Foley bulb. After packing the tandem in place, we then sutured the labia to the tandem so that it would not move during treatment. The patient tolerated the procedure well. Blood loss was minimal, and she was taken to recovery in stable condition.

10/15/11 11:47:39

You Code It!

What are the best, most accurate codes?

Diagnosis Codes: _____

Procedure Codes: _____

Anesthesia Codes (when applicable): _____

HCPCS Level II codes (when applicable): _____

PATIENT: SOUTTER, ANDREA
ACCOUNT/EHR #: SOUTAN001
Date: 10/15/11

CC: The patient is a 31-year-old woman admitted from the outpatient department with a chief complaint of bloating and gas for 1 week.

HPI: The patient had been on a cruise with her husband and had about a one-week history of bloating, gas per rectum, as well as burping, early satiety, and indigestion. These symptoms were similar to what she had prior to her cholecystectomy, as well as when she first diagnosed with gastroparesis. The symptoms are worse after eating meat. The patient also has been noticing increased swelling or bloating of her abdomen. She denies cough, paroxysmal nocturnal dyspnea, palpitations, chest pain, or diaphoresis.

In the outpatient department, she had an electrocardiogram done, which was unremarkable. Abdominal and pelvic ultrasound showed tumors in left ovary and what appears to be a large cyst in the right ovary.

PAST MEDICAL HISTORY: Hypercholesterolemia; hypertension; diabetes, insulin requiring; gastroparesis; stress test two years ago, which was normal; endoscopy three years ago

PAST SURGICAL HISTORY: Cholecystectomy

MEDICATIONS: At home, Dyazide 1 tablet a day; Vasotec 5.0 mg a day; Mevacor 20 mg a day; Prilosec 20 mg a day; Reglan 20 mg twice a day; insulin 70/30, 35 Iu in the morning, and 20 Iu in the evening

ALLERGIES: No known drug allergies

SOCIAL HISTORY: The patient does not smoke and drinks about one to two shots of vodka every night to help her sleep. She is recently started a new job as an elementary school teacher and lives with her husband and is active.

REVIEW OF SYSTEMS: The review of systems is also positive for weight gain, occasional loose stool without blood or diarrhea, and chronic sleeplessness. Her diabetes is well controlled.

PHYSICAL EXAMINATION

BP: 127/70; Pulse 88; Resp 16; T: afebrile

APPEARANCE: The patient looked well, is obese, and has good skin.

HEAD: Clear

EYES: Clear

EARS: Clear

NOSE: Clear

MOUTH/TONGUE/PHARYNX: Clear

NECK: She has a mild goiter.

LUNGS: Good bilateral air entry, resonant, with a few bibasilar crackles

CARDIOVASC: Regular rate and rhythm, with a normal jugular venous pressure. Heart sounds 1 and 2, with no rubs, murmurs, or gallops, and no carotid bruits.

Continued

ABDOMEN: Obese but soft, non-tender, with a large cholecystectomy scar. Bowel sounds were very active.

EXTREMITIES: The lower extremity examination was remarkable for 2+ pitting edema and 3+ pulses, with no evidence of deep venous thrombosis.

NEUROLOGIC: Grossly normal

ELECTROCARDIOGRAM: The electrocardiogram showed sinus rhythm with right bundle branch block but no acute or old myocardial infarction and no ischemic changes.

DIAGNOSES:
1. This is a 31-year-old female with abdominal symptoms. Possible ovarian cancer unlikely, although this needs to be ruled out. Patient is still of childbearing age and wants to have children in the future.
2. Probable diabetic gastroparesis worsening but also exacerbated by excesses on the cruise.
3. Fluid retention due to increased sodium/water intake.
4. Pulmonary embolus is very unlikely.

PLAN/RECOMMENDATIONS:
1. Admit for exploratory surgery of abdomen for ovarian cancer
2. Check SMA-20, CBC, urinalysis, TSH, and serial cardiac enzymes and electrocardiograms.
3. Also, check chest x-ray and KUB.
4. Call in gynecology for consult
5. She will be started on Propulsid 10 mg t.i.d. and gastroesophageal reflux disease precautions.
6. She will also be seen by the dietician for weight reduction.
7. We will continue to control her diabetes.

Robyn Bennito, MD

10/15/11 11:47:39

You Code It!

What are the best, most accurate codes?

Diagnosis Codes: _____

Procedure Codes: _____

Anesthesia Codes (when applicable): _____

HCPCS Level II codes (when applicable): _____

SWANSON ONCOLOGY
969 TURNABOUT LANE • REMISSION, FL 32811 • 407-555-9573

PATIENT: GREEN, SHAWNNA
ACCOUNT/EHR #:   GREESH001
Date: 10/15/11

HPI: The patient is a 45-year-old woman who was readmitted from the outpatient department. She came in complaining of chronic hoarseness, dyspnea, and occasional dysphagia. Upon palpation, patient stated there was pain in her neck. A hard nodule is evident on a thyroid that appears to be enlarged. The patient was admitted for further workup.

    The patient's alcohol consumption is one to two drinks every night to help her sleep. Occasionally, she has none for a week, but usually no more than two.

PMH: The patient's past medical history includes hypercholesterolemia, hypertension, diabetes type II insulin requiring, gastroparesis, cholecystectomy and obesity. Father died of thyroid cancer five years ago.

MEDICATIONS: Lasix 20 mg a day, Potassium chloride, Vasotec 5 mg a day, Mevacor 20 mg a day, Prilosec 50 mg a day, Propulsid 10 mg t.i.d., Insulin 70/30, 20 in the morning and 10 in the evening

PHYSICAL EXAMINATION

VITAL SIGNS: Stable

HEAD: Clear

EYES: Clear

EARS: Clear

NOSE: Clear

MOUTH/TONGUE/PHARYNX: Clear

CHEST: Clear

CARDIOVASC: Regular rate and rhythm. Heart sounds S1, S2. Jugular venous pressure was normal. No S3.

ABDOMEN: The abdomen is obese and very distended. It was difficult to ascertain splenomegaly, and there was ascites on percussion.

EXTREMITIES: The lower extremities showed 2+ edema and good pulses.

ELECTROCARDIOGRAM: The electrocardiogram showed a sinus rhythm with no changes to previous one.

LABORATORY: Serum alkaline phosphatase, and serum calcitonin assay indicate silent medullary carcinoma.

Outpatient department performed needle biopsy three days ago. Pathology report confirms node on thyroid is hypofunctional.

Continued

DX: Medullary malignancy

PLAN/RECOMMENDATIONS:
1. The plan is to admit.
2. The patient will undergo staging of tumor with possible total thyroidectomy.
3. Once staging has been completed, a treatment plan can be developed.

Robyn Bennito, MD

10/15/11 11:47:39

You Code It!

What are the best, most accurate codes?

Diagnosis Codes: _____

Procedure Codes: _____

Anesthesia Codes (when applicable): _____

HCPCS Level II codes (when applicable): _____

SWANSON ONCOLOGY
969 TURNABOUT LANE • REMISSION, FL 32811 • 407-555-9573

PATIENT: REESE, REBECCA
ACCOUNT/EHR #: REERE001
Date: 10/05/11

Rebecca is an 18-month-old female brought by her parents to the office on referral from Dr. Herrin, her pediatrician. He noted something during the ophthalmoscopy exam during her last well-baby exam.

PAST MEDICAL HISTORY: There is no history of weight loss, anorexia, crossed eyes, fever, or irritability.

EXAM: VS T 37.0, P 110, R 26, BP 92/42. Height, weight, head circumference are all at the 40th percentile. She is alert and active. On a routine ophthalmoscopy exam, Dr. Herrin noted that the child does not have a red reflex in the right eye. Leukocoria is present in the right eye. A normal red reflex observed in the left eye. The ophthalmoscopy exam performed today reveals a tumor in the posterior pole of the right eye. An orbital CT demonstrates that the tumor is confined to the globe (i.e., no spread outside the eye). Pupils are equal and reactive. The eyes are conjugate. Facial function is good. The remainder of the physical examination is negative.

DX: Tumor, posterior pole, right eye

CLINICAL COURSE: Since the tumor is small, it is treated with laser photoablation. Careful follow-ups are scheduled to monitor for recurrences or development of secondary tumors.

Robyn Bennito, MD

10/05/11 11:47:39

You Code It!

What are the best, most accurate codes?

Diagnosis Codes: _____

Procedure Codes: _____

Anesthesia Codes (when applicable): _____

HCPCS Level II codes (when applicable): _____

SWANSON ONCOLOGY
969 TURNABOUT LANE • REMISSION, FL 32811 • 407-555-9573

PATIENT: LUCAS, MORGAN
ACCOUNT/EHR #:   LUCMO001
Date: 12/15/11

Morgan is a 10-year-old boy, brought into the ED by his parents, with epistaxis for two hours and hematemesis. He complains of nausea, constipation, severe hip pain, and headache. He has a history of recurrent Stage IV neuroblastoma, initially diagnosed two years ago, treated with chemotherapy and a bone marrow transplant. He received chemotherapy again when his cancer recurred six months ago. Initially his tumor responded, but eventually it progressed and includes bone marrow involvement. He has started experimental chemotherapy at the request of his parents, with his assent. He has multiple metastatic bone lesions, most pronounced on his head and right hip. He has required increasing doses of pain medications. He has been attending school a few hours a day, but this week he has been increasingly tired with increased pallor. This morning, he woke up with epistaxis that would not stop with pressure. About one hour later he started vomiting bright red blood. He is currently taking 8 mg of hydromorphone (Dilaudid) orally every six hours around the clock for pain. He rates his current pain level as a 6 on a scale of 1-to-10.

EXAM: VS T 37, P 120, RR 18, BP 100/50. His skin is pale and dry with multiple bruises. He has multiple lumps on his scalp. Dried blood, blood clots, and some oozing blood is noted in both nares. Subconjunctival hemorrhages and pallor are noted. His neck is supple with no lymphadenopathy. Heart regular rate without murmurs. Lungs are clear. A central venous catheter is present in his left anterior chest. His abdomen is soft with no hepatosplenomegaly. There is mild tenderness. Exam of his extremities is significant for bruising and pallor. He has moderate tenderness over his back, hips, and pelvis.

LAB: WBC 2.4, 70% neutrophils, Hgb 6.2, Hct 19.6, platelet count 3,000.

HOSPITAL COURSE: He receives packed RBC transfusions to correct his anemia (which may also improve his stamina) and platelet transfusions, which stop his epistaxis. He is started on MS Contin (slow release morphine) 60 mg PO q12 hr with morphine 15 mg PO for breakthrough pain as needed, which controls his pain well. His physician discusses the future use of IV morphine on a patient-controlled analgesia (PCA) pump. He is started on Senokot (senna) to prevent constipation. Since he seems to improve, or at least remain stable, with the experimental chemotherapy, this is continued.

Linda F. Rasmussen, MD

12/15/11 11:47:39

You Code It!

What are the best, most accurate codes?

Diagnosis Codes: _____

Procedure Codes: _____

Anesthesia Codes (when applicable): _____

HCPCS Level II codes (when applicable): _____

Ophthalmology Cases and Patient Records

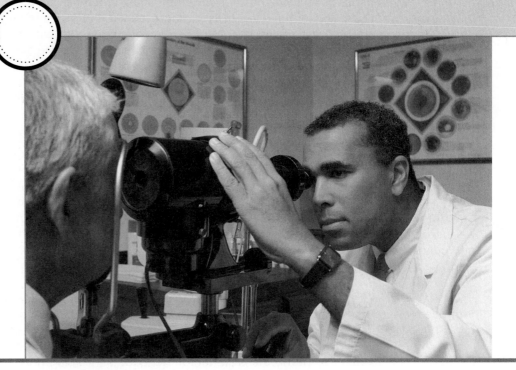

INTRODUCTION

The following case studies are from an ophthalmology practice. In an ophthalmology office, a professional coding specialist is likely to see many different types of health conditions, including preventive health care services. When it comes to caring for the eyes of a patient, there may be three different types of eye care specialists involved.

Ophthalmologists are trained to diagnose and treat eye diseases, such as macular degeneration, conjunctivitis, and ophthalmia neonatorum. In addition, they care for patients with injuries to the eye, such as a foreign objects lodged in the eye or a detached retina, and perform surgery, such as cataract removal, glaucoma correction, or LASIK surgery.

An optometrist is a health care professional who is trained and licensed to perform eye examinations and to prescribe eyeglasses and contact lenses. While an ophthalmologist may also prescribe eyeglasses or contact lenses in addition to other services, an optometrist is limited to this work.

The eye care specialist who will typically provide those glasses or lenses is called an optician. Opticians are not permitted to examine the eyes or prescribe glasses or lenses. They are professionals trained in grinding and forming lenses.

Ophthalmologists may decide to maintain a subspecialty, such as a retina specialist or a pediatric ophthalmologist.

Ophthalmologists are board-certified by the Board of Ophthalmology, which is recognized by the American Board of Medical Specialties.

You can use these cases to practice coding diagnoses, E/M, procedures, DME, or other HCPCS Level II items, as applicable; code for the physician or the facility; code inpatient and outpatient services, as applicable:

1. Code for the physician.
2. Code for the anesthesiologist, when applicable.
3. Code for the hospital, when applicable.
4. Code for the pathology and laboratory, when applicable.
5. Code HCPCS Level II codes, when applicable.

OPHTHALMOLOGY CARE CENTER
6481 SIGHT BOULEVARD • ANYTOWN, FL 32719 • 407-555-5137

PATIENT: PORTLAND, BROOKE
ACCOUNT/EHR #: PORTBR002
Date of Operation: 06/17/11

Preoperative Diagnosis: Nuclear sclerosis 2+ with a 2+ posterior subcapsular cataract, right eye
Postoperative Diagnosis: Same
Operation: Phacoemulsification of cataract with posterior chamber intraocular lens implantation, right eye

Surgeon: Julian Gallagher, MD
Assistant: Cindy Morse, MD
Anesthesia: Local

DESCRIPTION OF OPERATIVE PROCEDURE: Local anesthesia was obtained with retrobulbar and modified Van Lint injection using a 50-50 mixture of 4 percent Lidocaine and 0.75 percent Marcaine with Wydase. A Honan balloon was placed for approximately 15 minutes. The patient was positioned, prepped, and draped in the usual sterile fashion. A wire lid speculum was inserted, and the operating microscope was brought into position. A temporal limbal corneal incision was made with a 2.75-mm keratome, and Viscoat was injected into the anterior chamber. Using a cystotome and Utrata forceps, a continuous tear capsulorrhexis was performed. A limbal paracentesis stab incision was made at 6 o'clock with a diamond blade. Hydrodissection and hydrodelineation of the lens was accomplished with balanced salt solution via cannular injection. Phacoemulsification of the lens proceeded as the lens was sectioned into quadrants with each quadrant removed. Residual lens cortex was removed with irrigation and aspiration. The posterior capsule was polished with an irrigating Graether collar button. Viscoat was injected into the capsular bag, and the cataract incision was opened with the keratome. Using lens-folding forceps, an Alcon, Model MA60VM, 6.0 mm optic, 21.5 diopter posterior chamber intraocular lens was inserted into the capsular bag. A Sinskey hook was used to facilitate rotation and centration of the lens. Residual anterior chamber Viscoat was removed with irrigation and aspiration. Balanced salt solution was injected into the anterior chamber, and the wound was observed to be watertight. Subconjunctival Celestone and Cefazolin were injected. Topical Iopidine solution and Maxitrol ophthalmic ointment were instilled. Dressing included eye pad and Fox shield. The patient tolerated the procedure well without complications.

Julian Gallagher, M.D.

JG/mg   D: 06/17/11 09:50:16   T: 06/19/11 12:55:01

You Code It!

What are the best, most accurate codes?

Diagnosis Codes: _____

Procedure Codes: _____

Anesthesia Codes (when applicable): _____

HCPCS Level II codes (when applicable): _____

OPHTHALMOLOGY CARE CENTER
6481 SIGHT BOULEVARD • ANYTOWN, FL 32719 • 407-555-5137

PATIENT: WESTERBY, ELMO
ACCOUNT/EHR #: WESTEL001
Date: 09/16/11

Attending Physician: Suzanne R. Taylor, MD

Preoperative DX: Orbital mass, OD
Postoperative DX: Herniated orbital fat pad, OD
Procedure: Excision of mass and repair, right superior orbit

Surgeon: Raul Sanchez, MD
Anesthesia: Local

PROCEDURE: After proparacaine was instilled in the eye, it was prepped and draped in the usual sterile manner and 2.0 % Lidocaine with 1:200,000 epinephrine was injected into the superior aspect of the right orbit. A corneal protective shield was placed in the eye. The eye was placed in down-gaze.

The upper lid was everted and the fornix examined. The herniating mass was viewed and measured at 0.75 cm in diameter. Westcott scissors were used to incise the fornicele conjunctiva. The herniating mass was then clamped, excised, and cauterized. It appeared to contain mostly fat tissue, which was sent to pathology.

The superior fornix was repaired by using running suture of 6-0 plain gut. Bacitracin ointment was applied to the eye followed by an eye pad. The patient tolerated the procedure well and left the operating room in good condition.

Suzanne R. Taylor, MD

SRT/pw   D: 09/16/11 09:50:16   T: 09/18/11 12:55:01

You Code It!

What are the best, most accurate codes?

Diagnosis Codes: _____

Procedure Codes: _____

Anesthesia Codes (when applicable): _____

HCPCS Level II codes (when applicable): _____

OPHTHALMOLOGY CARE CENTER
6481 SIGHT BOULEVARD • ANYTOWN, FL 32719 • 407-555-5137

PATIENT: GROENENDAL, PETER
ACCOUNT/EHR #:   GROEPE001
Date: 09/16/11

The patient is a 61-year-old male who came into the office due to progressive right eye swelling and loss of vision. He was diagnosed with Type 2 diabetes approximately five years ago. Patient complained about severe headaches on the right side of his head, which began about one week ago. He also has had a fever and blurred vision during that time period. There is a personal history of frequent nasal congestion and sinus tenderness for which he took over-the-counter decongestants and blew his nose forcibly. During this same week he had been admitted to the hospital for erythema and swelling over the right eye and received IV antibiotics for five days. WBC 18,600 with 72% PMN and 11% band forms, glucose 364, lumbar puncture 8 WBC, protein 90 mg% and glucose 130 mg%. CT scan suggested right retrobulbar density and maxillary sinusitis.

On PE, severe proptosis of the right eye with conjunctival and scleral edema and minimal eye movement. No vision or light perception. Bilateral frontal and ethmoid sinus tenderness (RT>LT): otherwise PE within normal limits. Patient placed on nafcillin, ceftazidime, and Flagyl for orbital cellulites versus cavernous sinus thrombosis. Mucormycosis entertained, but amphotericin B not administered. Multiple cultures (blood, superficial, operative) negative. Surgery included orbitotomy, ethmoidotomy, and sphenoidotomy.

CT with contrast revealed marked proptosis of the right orbit and thrombosis and enlargement of the right superior ophthalmic vein, as well as increased density and prominence of the right cavernous sinus. There was opacification of the sphenoid and ethmoid sinuses and the left maxillary sinus. Changes suggesting chronic sinusitis also observed in the right maxillary sinus and both frontal sinuses.

_____

Suzanne R. Taylor, MD

SRT/pw   D: 09/16/11 09:50:16   T: 09/18/11 12:55:01

You Code It!

What are the best, most accurate codes?

Diagnosis Codes: _____

Procedure Codes: _____

Anesthesia Codes (when applicable): _____

HCPCS Level II codes (when applicable): _____

OPHTHALMOLOGY CARE CENTER
6481 SIGHT BOULEVARD • ANYTOWN, FL 32719 • 407-555-5137

PATIENT: ROBINET, RENAY
ACCOUNT/EHR #:   ROBIRE001
Date: 10/07/11

Attending Physician: Walter P. Henricks, MD
Referring Physician: Valerie Victors, MD

This new Pt is a 36-year-old female who lost her right eye in a skiing accident. She presents today for the prescription, fitting, and placement of her ocular prosthesis (artificial eye).

P: Follow-up in one month.

_____

Walter P. Henricks, MD

WPH/mg   D: 10/07/11 09:50:16   T: 10/09/11 12:55:01

You Code It!

What are the best, most accurate codes?

Diagnosis Codes: _____

Procedure Codes: _____

Anesthesia Codes (when applicable): _____

HCPCS Level II codes (when applicable): _____

OPHTHALMOLOGY CARE CENTER
6481 SIGHT BOULEVARD • ANYTOWN, FL 32719 • 407-555-5137

PATIENT: DENTMER, BARNEY
ACCOUNT/EHR #:   DENTBAR001
Date: 10/07/11

Attending Physician: Walter P. Henricks, MD

This is a 4-week-old male infant born to a 26-year-old G2P2 O+, rubella immune, group B strep-negative, HBsAg-negative, VDRL-negative, GC- and Chlamydia-negative married female at 40 weeks gestation via spontaneous vaginal delivery with Apgar scores of 8 and 9 at 1 and 5 minutes. Pregnancy, delivery, and postpartum hospital course were uncomplicated. He presents with his mother to our office with a 2-day history of bilateral eye drainage. He had been in good health until 2 days ago when he developed yellow drainage and mild periorbital swelling.

Review of systems is negative except for the recent development of a cough that he "probably caught from his older brother."

EXAM: VS T 37.5, P 120, RR 60, BP 60/40, oxygen saturation 94% in room air, weight 4.0 kg (50 %ile). He is a well developed, well nourished, nontoxic male infant with mild tachypnea and staccato cough, but in no acute distress. His upper and lower eyelids are edematous. There is mild conjunctival infection with moderate amounts of mucopurulent drainage bilaterally. Pseudomembranes are seen with eversion of the upper eyelids. Coarse breath sounds are appreciated bilaterally with occasional rales and fine expiratory wheezes. The remainder of his exam is unremarkable.

The conjunctiva is swabbed for gram stain, culture, and chlamydia direct fluorescence antibody staining. Complete blood count is remarkable for eosinophilia. Chest radiograph reveals bilateral patchy infiltrates with hyperinflation. After receiving positive chlamydia DFA results, I informed the mother of the diagnosis. Initially shocked, she admits that 6 months ago, she and her husband had separated briefly, but are now back together.

DX: Ophthalmia neonatorum, due to *Chlamydia trachomatis*

PLAN: Order written for testing for other STDs in the infant. In addition, both parents are urged to be tested for STDs by their own physicians. Parents are counseled regarding a reported association between oral erythromycin and infantile hypertrophic pyloric stenosis. Retesting for *C. trachomatis* is not indicated once treatment has been completed unless symptoms persist. The mother is informed that, if left untreated, chlamydia conjunctivitis will subside within 2–3 weeks, but chronic infection is common.

RX: Oral erythromycin (50 mg/kg/day in 4 divided doses) for 14 days

---

Walter P. Henricks, MD

WPH/mg   D: 10/07/11 09:50:16   T: 10/09/11 12:55:01

You Code It!

What are the best, most accurate codes?

Diagnosis Codes: _____

Procedure Codes: _____

Anesthesia Codes (when applicable): _____

HCPCS Level II codes (when applicable): _____

OPHTHALMOLOGY CARE CENTER
6481 SIGHT BOULEVARD • ANYTOWN, FL 32719 • 407-555-5137

PATIENT: ULTON, SOPHIA
ACCOUNT/EHR #:   ULTOSO001
Date: 10/07/11

Attending Physician: Walter P. Henricks, MD

This is a 6-month-old female who is brought to my office by her parents for a well-child examination. She has had no problems in the past with her eyes and, according to her parents, she tracks well and reaches for objects. Her parents deny any crossing of the eyes when she looks at objects from a distance; however, her mother mentions that she had a lazy eye when she was a child and needed to be operated on.

EXAM: Vital signs are normal for age. Her red reflex and corneal light reflex tests are normal. Cover test is negative for strabismus. Her extraocular movements appear intact, and she is able to follow objects 180 degrees.

DX: Normal eye examination

PLAN: Next appointment at 9 months old or earlier prn

_____

Walter P. Henricks, MD

WPH/mg   D: 10/07/11 09:50:16   T: 10/09/11 12:55:01

You Code It!

What are the best, most accurate codes?

Diagnosis Codes: _____

Procedure Codes: _____

Anesthesia Codes (when applicable): _____

HCPCS Level II codes (when applicable): _____

OPHTHALMOLOGY CARE CENTER
6481 SIGHT BOULEVARD • ANYTOWN, FL 32719 • 407-555-5137

PATIENT: AMBRO, MEGAN
ACCOUNT/EHR #:   AMBRME001
Date: 10/11/11

Attending Physician: Walter P. Henricks, MD

A 6-month-old female infant is brought to our office, referred by her pediatrician, Dr. Houseman, due to a concern regarding her crossed eyes. Her parents say her eyes have been crossed since birth, and the left eye seems to cross more than the right. They deny any problem with her vision. They report that she plays with toys and recognizes people across the room. She was a full-term infant without perinatal complications and has no known medical problems.

EXAM: She is alert and playful.

EXTERNAL: Her left eye is clearly esotropic (crossed inward). There is no facial hemiparesis.

VISION: She tracks toys well using both eyes. With the left eye covered, she fixes and follows easily. However, she fusses when the right eye is covered and has more trouble following with the left eye (i.e., she is fussing when the right eye is covered because she can't see as well with her left eye).

MOTILITY: Full extraocular movements. There does not seem to be any retraction of the globe on adduction. No nystagmus.

PUPILS: Equally round and reactive to light; no afferent pupil defect. No leukocoria. Corneal reflection test (Hirschberg test): A penlight is directed toward the cornea, and the reflected image is located temporal to the center of the left pupil.

COVER-UNCOVER TEST: On covering the right eye, there is an outward shift of the left eye. When the eye is uncovered, the left eye shifts back inward.

ALTERNATE-COVER TEST: On switching the cover to the left eye, there is an outward shift of the right eye. When the cover is alternated from one eye to the other, there is always an outward shift of the opposite eye.
    No structural ocular abnormalities are found, and there is no significant refractive error.

DX: Infantile esotropia; amblyopia, left eye

PLAN: Parents are told to have her wear a patch 6 hours a day over the right eye for a month, to effect improvement of vision in her left eye.
    Once this has been accomplished, we will schedule surgery to correct her strabismus.

Walter P. Henricks, MD
WPH/mg   D: 10/11/11 09:50:16 T: 10/13/11 12:55:01

You Code It!

What are the best, most accurate codes?

Diagnosis Codes: _____

Procedure Codes: _____

Anesthesia Codes (when applicable): _____

HCPCS Level II codes (when applicable): _____

OPHTHALMOLOGY CARE CENTER
6481 SIGHT BOULEVARD • ANYTOWN, FL 32719 • 407-555-5137

PATIENT: BROOKSTONE, FREDERICK
ACCOUNT/EHR #:   BROOFR001
Date: 10/17/11

Attending Physician: Walter P. Henricks, MD

A 28-month-old male is referred to our office by his pediatrician, Dr. Katzman, with a swollen right upper eyelid for one day. His mother states that the eyelid had a small red lump two days prior, but the eyelid became progressively swollen. The patient has a low-grade fever, but he is otherwise still playful.

    The pediatrician had diagnosed the patient with right upper eyelid cellulitis and prescribed oral antibiotics and warm compresses. After two days of antibiotics, the eyelid is still swollen and red. At this point, the patient is referred here.

EXAM: T 102F. Edema, erythema, warmth, and pain of the eyelid are observed at the right upper eyelid. Visual acuity, eye motility, and pupillary reaction are all normal. There appears to be very little pain on eye movement.

DX: Preseptal eyelid cellulitis (periorbital cellulitis), caused by *Haemophilus influenzae* type B

PLAN: Admit into the hospital pediatrics ward for intravenous antibiotics

---

Walter P. Henricks, MD

WPH/mg   D: 10/17/11 09:50:16 T: 10/19/11 12:55:01

You Code It!

What are the best, most accurate codes?

Diagnosis Codes: _____

Procedure Codes: _____

Anesthesia Codes (when applicable): _____

HCPCS Level II codes (when applicable): _____

OPHTHALMOLOGY CARE CENTER
6481 SIGHT BOULEVARD • ANYTOWN, FL 32719 • 407-555-5137

PATIENT: SWANKLEE, CLAUDIA
ACCOUNT/EHR #:   SWANCL001
Date: 12/07/11

Attending Physician: Walter P. Henricks, MD

An 8-year-old female is brought in to the emergency department by her parents with moderately severe right eye pain six hours after riding her bicycle through some low hanging leaves from a tree. She didn't notice the tree branches until a few leaves hit her in the face. She has no bleeding wounds. I was called in for the ophthalmologic consultation by the attending physician, Dr. Morgan.

EXAM: VS are normal. She does not want to open her right eye because of discomfort. Some anesthetic eye drops are instilled into her right eye. She complains that this burns a lot and she begins to cry. After 10 minutes (topical anesthetic usually works within minutes), she is able to open her eye. Her visual acuity was 20/20 in the left eye and 20/30 in the right eye. Her pupils are equal and reactive. Her conjunctiva is slightly infected. No hyphema is visible. A drop of saline is placed on a fluorescein paper strip. This drop is then touched to her lower eyelid so fluorescein dye flows over the surface of her eye. With an ultraviolet light, a 0.5 cm linear abrasion is seen in the lateral aspect of her right cornea.

DX: Corneal abrasion

PLAN: Her eye is rinsed with saline to remove excess fluorescein. A single drop of homatropine (a cycloplegic agent) is instilled into her right eye. Antibiotic ointment is instilled into her eye, and a pressure eye patch is applied. She is instructed to take over-the-counter analgesics for pain.

_____

Walter P. Henricks, MD

WPH/mg   D: 12/07/11 09:50:16 T: 12/09/11 12:55:01

You Code It!

What are the best, most accurate codes?

Diagnosis Codes: _____

Procedure Codes: _____

Anesthesia Codes (when applicable): _____

HCPCS Level II codes (when applicable): _____

OPHTHALMOLOGY CARE CENTER
6481 SIGHT BOULEVARD • ANYTOWN, FL 32719 • 407-555-5137

PATIENT: BRUCE, LLOYD
ACCOUNT/EHR #:   BRUCLL001
Date: 10/21/11

Attending Physician: Walter P. Henricks, MD

This is an 80-year-old male who was referred by Dr. Tellmon due to recurrent episodes of blurry vision and hyphema in his left eye. Each episode was associated with high intraocular pressures.

PAST MEDICAL HISTORY: Significant for bilateral cataract extraction and lens implantation 19 years ago.

EXAM: His BCVA was 20/20 OU, and pressures were 20 OU. In the left eye, he had 2+ cells (mostly RBCs), a patent PI, a sulcus PCIOL in the vertical position, an intact posterior capsule, and an area of blood staining between optic and capsule. In the right eye, there was no cell or flare, two patent PIs, an ACIOL in the vertical position, and an open posterior capsule. There was no rubeosis, transillumination defects OU, pseudophakodonesis or pseudoexfoliation OU. Gonioscopy revealed open structures 360 degrees OU with no PAS. A UBM revealed the inferior haptic of the left eye sulcus IOL pressing on the ciliary body/iris junction. The superior haptic was OK.

DX: Uveitis-glaucoma-hyphema (UGH) syndrome OS

PLAN: Treatment of UGH syndrome is discussed with patient. He requests time to discuss this with his daughter who lives in another state. He will return in one week.

_____

Walter P. Henricks, MD

WPH/mg   D: 10/21/11 09:50:16   T: 10/23/11 12:55:01

You Code It!

What are the best, most accurate codes?

Diagnosis Codes: _____

Procedure Codes: _____

Anesthesia Codes (when applicable): _____

HCPCS Level II codes (when applicable): _____

OPHTHALMOLOGY CARE CENTER
6481 SIGHT BOULEVARD • ANYTOWN, FL 32719 • 407-555-5137

PATIENT: ROTHSTEIN, PHIL
ACCOUNT/EHR #: ROTHPH001
Date: 10/07/11

Attending Physician: Walter P. Henricks, MD

This is a 32–year-old male being evaluated for repair of LUL ptosis.

HPI: Patient noted progressive ptosis of the LUL for three years, which now blocks his vision. He has no other complaints or problems.

POH/PMH: Healthy, no history of eye problems.

EXAM: Vision 20/20 OU without correction. Extraocular motility with −2 elevation defect OU. VF full OD, VF with ~20% superior VF cut OS.
   Pupils: 5.0 mm in the dark, 3 mm in the light, no RAPD, equally reactive IOP 18 mmHg OU Anterior segment normal. DFE normal.
   Pt is able to maintain chin-up position. RUL retraction and marked ptosis OS is evident. Palpebral fissures are 10 mm OD and 5 mm OS with palpebral function of 15 mm OD and 10 mm OS. There is a twitching of the LUL when the patient looks up after looking down.

DX: Myasthenia gravis

TREATMENT
   1. Refer patient for neurology consultation.
   2. Rx pyridostigmine bromide 60 mg PO qid with dosage adjustment according to response.
   3. Monitoring with consideration for surgery to remove the thymoma.

_____

Walter P. Henricks, MD

WPH/mg   D: 10/07/11 09:50:16   T: 10/09/11 12:55:01

You Code It!

What are the best, most accurate codes?

Diagnosis Codes: _____

Procedure Codes: _____

Anesthesia Codes (when applicable): _____

HCPCS Level II codes (when applicable): _____

PATIENT: BERRY, PAIGE
ACCOUNT/EHR #:   BERRPA001
Date: 10/07/11

Attending Physician: Walter P. Henricks, MD

This patient is an 11-year-old female being seen for evaluation of an open globe and traumatic cataract.

HPI: Patient was referred to me by Dr. Timmons for evaluation of a possible open globe. One day prior, while hammering on a stained glass project for her Girl Scout troop, a glass shard flew into her right eye. She complained of pain and a foreign body sensation and was taken to the local emergency treatment center for evaluation. A slit lamp examination failed to reveal a foreign body. Early the next morning, she awoke with worsening pain and decreased vision. Her pediatrician referred her to us.
       Upon arrival, she continued to complain of pain and decreased vision in her right eye.

PAST OCULAR HISTORY: No prior ocular injury, surgery, or illness

PAST MEDICAL HISTORY: Noncontributory

MEDICATIONS: Gatifloxacin (Zymar) ophthalmic drops, 4 times a day, in the right eye, prescribed by the emergency room physician

FAMILY AND SOCIAL HISTORY: Noncontributory

OCULAR EXAM:
- Visual acuity, without correction: right eye (OD)—20/70; left eye (OS)—20/20
- Motility: Normal; no restrictions
- Confrontation visual fields: Full, both eyes (OU)
- Intraocular pressure: OD—15; OS not attempted due to risk of open globe
- Pupils: No relative afferent pupillary defect (RAPD)
- Slit lamp examination, OD:
- 2.5-mm diameter full-thickness stellate corneal laceration (Seidel negative)
- Anterior chamber—deep with 1+ cell and flare
- Anterior capsular tear—from 11:00 to 4:00 position and extending to the zonules
- Cortical lens material protruding through the tear
- Dilated fundus exam (DFE): No foreign body. No vitreous hemorrhage or vitreitis. Normal macula, vessels, and periphery, OU.

Maxillofacial CT: No IOFB detected

Ocular echography: No IOFB detected

b-scan echography: The posterior lens capsule appeared to be intact

Continued

DX: Self-sealing corneal laceration with traumatic cataract and anterior capsular rupture

PLAN: Cataract extraction scheduled for tomorrow.

Walter P. Henricks, MD

WPH/mg   D: 10/07/11 09:50:16   T: 10/09/11 12:55:01

You Code It!

What are the best, most accurate codes?

Diagnosis Codes: _____

Procedure Codes: _____

Anesthesia Codes (when applicable): _____

HCPCS Level II codes (when applicable): _____

OPHTHALMOLOGY CARE CENTER
6481 SIGHT BOULEVARD • ANYTOWN, FL 32719 • 407-555-5137

PATIENT: GRAYSON, WALLACE
ACCOUNT/EHR #:   GRAYWA001
Date: 10/07/11

Attending Physician: Walter P. Henricks, MD

This is a 49-year-old male who has been on amiodarone therapy. At this time, the patient denies visual problems. He present to our office today for a routine ophthalmologic examination.

HPI: Patient has a history of atrial fibrillation and hypertension. He has been on amiodarone therapy for several years. Patient reports that, six weeks ago, his primary care doctor, Dr. LaBelle, made a change in his cardiac medications that included the removal of amiodarone from his medication regimen.

PMH: Atrial fibrillation and hypertension. No other ocular or health problems.

OCULAR EXAM:
- VA 20/20 OD and OS
- Intraocular Pressures and Confrontation Visual Fields normal
- DFE normal OU
- EOM Full OU
- SLE notable for corneal deposits in the cornea at the level of the basal epithelium, inferiorly OU. Deposits form a faint golden-brown whorl pattern evident in both corneas.

DX: Corneal Verticillata

TREATMENT:
Depositing drugs are stopped with the expectation that the condition will eventually self-correct.

_____
Walter P. Henricks, MD

WPH/mg   D: 10/07/11 09:50:16   T: 10/09/11 12:55:01

You Code It!

What are the best, most accurate codes?

Diagnosis Codes: _____

Procedure Codes: _____

Anesthesia Codes (when applicable): _____

HCPCS Level II codes (when applicable): _____

OPHTHALMOLOGY CARE CENTER
6481 SIGHT BOULEVARD • ANYTOWN, FL 32719 • 407-555-5137

PATIENT: WARREN, BONITA
ACCOUNT/EHR #:   WARRBO001
Date: 10/08/11

Attending Physician: Walter P. Henricks, MD

This new patient is a 44-year-old female with a lesion on her left lower lid.

HPI: The patient noted that the lesion has been present for the last 18 months. She states that it occasionally becomes inflamed and then heals, but it always comes back. She has not noted any change in the size of the lesion over the course of this time frame.

PAST EYE HISTORY: No previous ocular history. No eye surgery nor eye trauma.

PAST MEDICAL HISTORY: Hypothyroidism

CURRENT MEDICATIONS: Levothyroxine

FAMILY AND SOCIAL HISTORY: Noncontributory. Patient is a nonsmoker and occasionally consumes alcohol.

OCULAR EXAM:
- Visual acuity, with correction: OD, OS—20/20
- Pupils, motility, and intraocular pressure: normal, OU
- External and anterior segment examination:
- OD: normal; OS: normal but for the eyelid lesion on the left lower lid, as noted. The lesion is 3 × 5 mm in size, with central ulceration and rolled, pearly borders with telangiectatic vessels. There are lashes missing (madarosis) in the area of the lesion.

DX: Nodular Basal Cell Carcinoma (BCC)

TREATMENT: An excisional biopsy is performed and demonstrates skin with central ulceration of the epidermis and multiple islands of basophilic neoplastic cells in the superficial dermis. The neoplastic cells appear to arise from surface epidermis. The diagnosis is consistent with basal cell carcinoma.
    Mohs surgery with oculoplastic reconstruction is planned.

Walter P. Henricks, MD

WPH/mg   D: 10/08/11 09:50:16 T: 10/09/11 12:55:01

You Code It!

What are the best, most accurate codes?

Diagnosis Codes: _____

Procedure Codes: _____

Anesthesia Codes (when applicable): _____

HCPCS Level II codes (when applicable): _____

OPHTHALMOLOGY CARE CENTER
6481 SIGHT BOULEVARD • ANYTOWN, FL 32719 • 407-555-5137

PATIENT: RODRIQUEZ, IMANI
ACCOUNT/EHR #: RODRIM001
Date: 10/27/11

Attending Physician: Walter P. Henricks, MD

This patient is a 4-year-old female who presents with a dog bite to left side of face.

HPI: Approximately three hours ago, patient was playing with a pit bull, the pet of a neighbor. Family witnessed the dog make a single lunge at the girl's face. Due to the adults' attempts to intervene, only the top jaw made contact. The dog did not attack further, and the incomplete bite to the left face was the only injury sustained.

POH/PMH/SH: No past ocular history. No past medical history. No current medications or allergies. Well- adjusted preschool child lives at home with both parents. Childhood immunizations are up-to-date, according to the mother.

OCULAR EXAM:
- VA 20/25 OD and OS without correction
- Extraocular motility and IOP were normal, OU
- CVF: Full OD, OS
- Lids: Right side—Normal
- Lids: Left side—2 lacerations on the left upper lid; the larger and deeper of the laceration passes just medial to the upper punctum. Initial exploration of laceration raises concerns for probable canalicular involvement, but further detailed examination in this anxious pediatric patient was unable to be accomplished.
- Continuation of the examination in the operating suite revealed that the remainder of the anterior segment examination and DFE were normal.

TREATMENT: Primary surgical repair of the lacerated or avulsed canaliculus using pigtail probes is performed immediately. The patient was taken to the operating suite for examination under anesthesia (EUA) and laceration repair, likely to include canalicular repair.

DX: Superior canalicular laceration

Walter P. Henricks, MD

WPH/mg   D: 10/27/11 09:50:16   T: 10/29/11 12:55:01

You Code It!

What are the best, most accurate codes?

Diagnosis Codes: _____

Procedure Codes: _____

Anesthesia Codes (when applicable): _____

HCPCS Level II codes (when applicable): _____

OPHTHALMOLOGY CARE CENTER
6481 SIGHT BOULEVARD • ANYTOWN, FL 32719 • 407-555-5137

PATIENT: HARDY, DERRICK
ACCOUNT/EHR #:   HARDDE001
Date: 11/27/11

Attending Physician: Walter P. Henricks, MD

This 25-year-old male comes into the office complaining of watery, red, irritated eyes; left more than right. I have not seen this patient since last year.

HPI: Patient states that his eyes began to feel watery and irritated about five days ago. He noted that his left eye was tearing, slightly blurry, and starting to get red throughout. The eye gradually became increasingly red and irritated over the ensuing days, and the patient noted increased crusting in the mornings. There was a mild "scratchy" sensation noted then as well. Symptoms did not remit with antibiotic drops, and eye continued to worsen, with early redness and watery sensation in the contralateral eye. Patient states he had an upper respiratory infection about two months prior to any ocular symptoms. He denies any medical treatment for this URI and states that it resolved on its own.

PMH/FH/POH: No previous ocular or health problems. No eye surgery, trauma, nor contact lens use.

EXAM OCULAR:
- Anterior segment: Evident crusting on lashes and watery d/c, OU. The bulbar conjunctiva is injected OS>OD. A follicular reaction is evident on the palpebral conjunctiva, especially inferiorly, OU. There is mild chemosis and palpebral edema, again L>R.
- Palpable pre-auricular lymphadenopathy (LAD), L>R

DX: Adenoviral conjunctivitis

TREATMENT:
- Patient advised to apply cool compresses and OTC artificial tears for comfort several times a day.
- To prevent contagious spread, patient is given an instruction sheet on washing sheets and pillowcases and handwashing.

_____

Walter P. Henricks, MD

WPH/mg   D: 11/27/11 09:50:16   T: 11/29/11 12:55:01

You Code It!

What are the best, most accurate codes?

Diagnosis Codes: _____

Procedure Codes: _____

Anesthesia Codes (when applicable): _____

HCPCS Level II codes (when applicable): _____

OPHTHALMOLOGY CARE CENTER
6481 SIGHT BOULEVARD • ANYTOWN, FL 32719 • 407-555-5137

PATIENT: HAMMOND, DARLENE
ACCOUNT/EHR #: HAMMDA001
Date: 10/17/11

Attending Physician: Walter P. Henricks, MD

CHIEF COMPLAINT: Chronic, stable, mildly diminished vision

HISTORY OF PRESENT ILLNESS: 47-year-old female with the presumptive diagnosis of cone dystrophy was referred to us for further evaluation of chronic, mildly diminished visual acuity and dyschromatopsia by her optometrist, Dr. Wassau. The patient reported that her vision has never been correctable to 20/20. The best visual acuity she remembers having is 20/30 in the left eye.

PAST EYE HISTORY: She was diagnosed with amblyopia in the right eye as a child and underwent a trial of patching at age 10. She is anisometropic, and her vision has always been worse in the right eye, presumably due to amblyopia.

PAST MEDICAL HISTORY: None.

MEDICATIONS: She takes no medications on a regular basis. She has never taken hydroxychloroquine or antipsychotic medications.

FAMILY HISTORY: She has several family members with mildly subnormal vision. Her mother, brother, sister, and son all have mildly reduced vision, in the range of 20/30 to 20/50. All of the affected family members are able to drive.

SOCIAL HISTORY: She works as a clerk. Her social history is otherwise unremarkable.

OCULAR EXAM:
- Visual acuity (with corrective lenses): Right eye—20/70; Left eye—20/40
- Current spectacle correction: Right eye: $-0.75 +2.50 \times 037$; Left eye: -3.00 sphere
- Manifest Refraction (MRx) improves the acuity of the right eye to 20/60 while the left eye remains unchanged
- Motility: Orthophoric (normally aligned) in primary gaze; Versions full.
- Intraocular pressure: Right eye—12 mmHg; Left eye—14 mmHg
- Pupils: Normal in both eyes. No relative afferent pupillary defect.
- External and anterior segment examination: Normal in both eyes
- Dilated fundus exam: There was optic disc pallor, predominantly temporal, in both eyes. Peripapillary atrophy and grey temporal crescent were noted in the left eye. The macula, vessels, and periphery were normal in both eyes.
- Ishihara plates: 2/14 OD, 3/14 OS
- Nagel anomaloscope: Protanomalous match
- Goldmann Visual Field testing: Right eye—baring of blind spot with mildly constricted I2e isopter; Left eye—constricted I2e isopter
- Electroretinogram (ERG): Scotopic bright flash 589 microvolts in the right eye, 572 microvolts left eye; scotopic dim flash 405 microvolts right eye, 340 microvolts left eye; photopic bright flash 180 microvolts right eye, 185 microvolts left eye

Continued

DX: Autosomal dominant optic atrophy, or dominant optic atrophy (DOA)

TREATMENT: A blood sample for molecular studies was obtained. The clinical and genetic features of autosomal dominant optic atrophy were discussed. More information will follow when results of the genetic testing are complete. The patient returned to the care of her local eye doctor.

Walter P. Henricks, MD

WPH/mg   D: 10/17/11 09:50:16   T: 10/19/11 12:55:01

You Code It!

What are the best, most accurate codes?

Diagnosis Codes: _____

Procedure Codes: _____

Anesthesia Codes (when applicable): _____

HCPCS Level II codes (when applicable): _____

OPHTHALMOLOGY CARE CENTER
6481 SIGHT BOULEVARD • ANYTOWN, FL 32719 • 407-555-5137

PATIENT: ERICSON, FRANK
ACCOUNT/EHR #:   ERICFR001
Date: 01/07/12

Attending Physician: Walter P. Henricks, MD

CC: 30-year-old male referred for bilateral macular lesions

HPI: Patient was found to have bilateral macular lesions on routine examination. He has no visual complaints and denies any history of "night blindness." His family history is negative for eye diseases.

PMH: Healthy. FH: Noncontributory.

EXAM:
- Best corrected visual acuities: 20/25 OD & OS
- Color Vision: normal
- Pupils: normal, no RAPD
- VF: full to CF OU
- EOM: normal
- IOP: normal OU
- SLE: normal

DX: Best Vitelliform macular dystrophy

TREATMENT:
- Treat associated choroidal neovascular membrane (CNVM).
- Genetic testing available via Dr. McCoy's lab.
- Visual potential is usually very good.
- Avoid subfoveal surgery because outcomes can be poor.

Walter P. Henricks, MD

WPH/mg   D: 01/07/12 09:50:16   T: 01/09/12 12:55:01

You Code It!

What are the best, most accurate codes?

Diagnosis Codes: _____

Procedure Codes: _____

Anesthesia Codes (when applicable): _____

HCPCS Level II codes (when applicable): _____

Orthopedics Cases and Patient Records

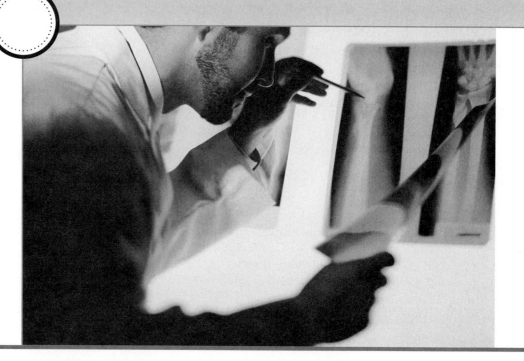

INTRODUCTION

The following case studies are from an orthopedic practice. In an orthopedic office, a professional coding specialist is likely to see many different types of health situations relating to musculoskeletal concerns.

Physicians who specialize in conditions of the musculoskeletal system are called orthopedic specialists. These health care professionals care for patients with seemingly ordinary conditions, such as a fractured leg or a case of carpal tunnel syndrome. They also work with patients suffering with congenital disorders like clubfoot or muscular dystrophy, conditions such as osteomyelitis, or deformities such as kyphosis or scoliosis.

Those orthopedists trained in surgical procedures are called upon to perform corrective procedures, such as a laminectomy or spinal fusion for a patient with a herniated disk, or joint replacement, often performed on patients with a bad knee or hip.

Some orthopedic surgeons specialize in specific areas, such as knee surgery, hand surgery, or joint replacement. Others may specialize in types of injuries, such as sports medicine.

Orthopedic surgeons are board-certified through the Board of Orthopedic Surgery, which is recognized by the American Board of Medical Specialties.

You can use these cases to practice coding diagnoses, E/M, procedures, DME, or other HCPCS Level II items, as applicable; code for the physician or the facility; code inpatient and outpatient services, as applicable:

1. Code for the physician.

2. Code for the anesthesiologist, when applicable.

3. Code for the hospital, when applicable.

4. Code for the pathology and laboratory, when applicable.

5. Code HCPCS Level II codes, when applicable.

HALVERSON ORTHOPEDIC CENTER
1212 DOG LEG ROAD • ANYTOWN, FL 32722 • 407-555-8523

PATIENT: HICKS, LOTTIE
ACCOUNT/EHR #:   HICKLO010
Date of Operation: 11/09/2011

Preoperative Diagnosis: Hallux limites, right foot
Postoperative Diagnosis: Same
Operation: Shortening, osteotomy, first metatarsal, right foot, with screw fixation
                              and cheilectomy, first metatarsal head, right foot

Surgeon: Allen Roberston, DPM
Assistant: None
Anesthesia: IV sedation with local anesthesia

DESCRIPTION OF OPERATIVE PROCEDURE: Following the customary sterile preparation and draping, the right limb was elevated approximately five minutes in order to facilitate circulatory drainage, at which time the pneumatic cuff, which had previously been placed on her right ankle, was inflated to a pressure of 250 mmHg. The right limb was then placed in the operative position. The operative site was injected with 2% Xylocaine mixed with 0.5% Marcaine. Upon having achieved anesthesia, a curvilinear incision was created on the plantar medial aspect of the first metatarsophalangeal joint of the right foot. The incision was deepened with sharp dissection; traversing veins were cauterized. Capsule was identified on the medial and dorsomedial aspect. Capsule was longitudinally incised on the dorsomedial aspect and meticulously dissected to expose the head of the first metatarsal into the operative site. At this point, it was noted that the cartilage of the first metatarsal head was healthy; however, there was distinct irritation to the dorsal portion of the metatarsal head with an apparent flattening of the metatarsal head secondary to the hallux limites. Using a rongeur, the hypertrophic exuberant portion of the first metatarsal head was resected, and the remaining surface was rasped smooth in order to recreate a ball joint. Using an oscillating saw, an osteotomy was performed from medial to lateral in a V-shaped fashion with the apex centrally located and the dorsal arm longer than the plantar arm. A segment of bone was removed from the dorsal arm in order to shorten and plantar flex the metatarsal head. Upon having done so, two 2.0-mm screws were obliquely driven into the osteotomy site; following range of motion was noted that the osteotomy remained stable. At this point, the hallux had approximately 90 degrees of motion to the metatarsal shaft. The area was copiously irrigated with sterile saline. The capsular tissue was repaired using 4-0 Vicryl; subcutaneous tissue was repaired using 5-0 Vicryl. Operative site was injected with dexamethasone, Betadine-soaked Adaptic was applied to the incision site, then sterile gauze and Kling. The pneumatic cuff was deflated. Normal color, circulation, was noted to return to all digits immediately. The patient tolerated the surgery well. Vital signs remained stable throughout the entire procedure. The patient returned to the recovery room in good condition.

Allen Roberston, DPM

AR/mg   D: 11/09/11 09:50:16 T: 11/12/11 12:55:01

You Code It!

What are the best, most accurate codes?

Diagnosis Codes: _____

Procedure Codes: _____

Anesthesia Codes (when applicable): _____

HCPCS Level II codes (when applicable): _____

HALVERSON ORTHOPEDIC CENTER
1212 DOG LEG ROAD • ANYTOWN, FL 32722 • 407-555-8523

PATIENT: PETRY, MASON
ACCOUNT/EHR #:   PETRMA001
Date: 09/25/11

Attending Physician: Sandford Lockard, MD

S: Patient is a 45-year-old male seen by his regular physician after his car was struck from behind on the street near his home. Patient is complaining of severe neck pain and difficulty turning his head.

O: PE reveals tightness upon palpitation of ligaments neck and shoulders, most pronounced C3 to C5. X-rays are taken of head and neck including the cervical vertebrae. Radiologic review denies any fracture.

A: Anterior longitudinal cervical sprain.

P: 1. Cervical collar to be worn during all waking hours
     2. Rx Vicodin (hydrocodone) 500 mg po prn
     3. 1,000 mg aspirin q.i.d.
     4. Pt to return in 2 weeks for follow-up

_____

Sandford Lockard, MD

SL/mg   D: 09/25/11 09:50:16   T: 09/30/11 12:55:01

You Code It!

What are the best, most accurate codes?

Diagnosis Codes: _____

Procedure Codes: _____

Anesthesia Codes (when applicable): _____

HCPCS Level II codes (when applicable): _____

HALVERSON ORTHOPEDIC CENTER
1212 DOG LEG ROAD • ANYTOWN, FL 32722 • 407-555-8523

PATIENT: WHITE, SASHA
ACCOUNT/EHR #:   WHITSA001
Date: 09/16/11

Attending Physician: Sandford Lockard, MD

S: This new Pt is a 25-year-old female who was involved in a two-car MVA while driving on the job. She is complaining about some neck pain. She has tingling into her hand and her feet. She states that her arm hurts when she tries to pull it overhead. She apparently was told by a friend that she should likely need to see a spine doctor, but somehow she came to see me first. PMH is remarkable for kidney trouble. Past bronchoscopy, laparoscopy, and kidney stone surgery, otherwise noncontributory as per the medical history form completed by the patient and reviewed at this visit.

O: Ht 5'5" Wt. 179 lb. R 16. Pt presented in a sling. She was told to use it by the same friend. She states if she does not use it, her arm does not feel any different, so I had her remove it. On exam, the left shoulder demonstrates full passive motion. She has normal strength testing. She has no deformity. She has some tenderness over the trapezial area. The reflexes are brisk and symmetric. X-rays of her chest two views and C spine AP/LAT are relatively benign, as are complete x-rays of the shoulder.

A: Contusion of upper arm and shoulder

P: 1. MRI to rule/out torn ligament
     2. Rx Naprosyn.
     3. Referral to PT
     4. Referral to orthopedic specialist

Sandford Lockard, MD

SL/mg   D: 09/16/11 09:50:16   T: 09/18/11 12:55:01

You Code It!

What are the best, most accurate codes?

Diagnosis Codes: _____

Procedure Codes: _____

Anesthesia Codes (when applicable): _____

HCPCS Level II codes (when applicable): _____

HALVERSON ORTHOPEDIC CENTER
1212 DOG LEG ROAD • ANYTOWN, FL 32722 • 407-555-8523

PATIENT: BRUTUS, JOHN
ACCOUNT/EHR #:   BRUTJO001
Date: 09/20/11

Attending Physician: Sandford Lockard, MD

S: Pt is a 27-year-old male who was involved in a fist fight at a local bar the previous evening. He complained of an ache in the area of his left eye as well as severe pain around his right ear.

O: Ht 5'10.5" Wt. 209 lb. R 19. Surface hematoma evident in the area surrounding the left eye socket reaching to the upper cheek. Head x-ray of the right side confirmed a closed fracture of the right mandible.

A: Black eye, fracture of the rt mandible, angle (closed)

P: 1. interdental fixation of mandible, closed reduction
      2. NPO except liquids for 3 weeks
      3. Cold wet compresses on eye prn
      4. Return for follow-up in three weeks

Sandford Lockard, MD

SL/mg   D: 09/20/11 09:50:16   T: 09/22/11 12:55:01

You Code It!

What are the best, most accurate codes?

Diagnosis Codes: _____

Procedure Codes: _____

Anesthesia Codes (when applicable): _____

HCPCS Level II codes (when applicable): _____

PATIENT NAME: CONNOR, DENISE
MRN: CONNDE001
Date: 08/20/11

Attending Physician: Gerrard Yahnert, MD

Patient is a 79-year-old female status post MVA. Imaging studies showed a C2 fracture involving the vertebral body. Arrangements were made for placement of halo. The procedure was described in detail to the patient and her husband, and consent was provided by the patient.

The hair was shaved above both ears. The halo ring was placed. Lidocaine was used to numb the tissue. The halo was then placed in the usual manner without difficulty. A lateral cervical spine was obtained, which showed good positioning. The patient tolerated the procedure without difficulty.

Gerrard Yahnert, MD

GY/mgr   D: 08/20/11 12:33:08 PM   T: 08/27/11 3:22:54 PM

You Code It!

What are the best, most accurate codes?

Diagnosis Codes: _____

Procedure Codes: _____

Anesthesia Codes (when applicable): _____

HCPCS Level II codes (when applicable): _____

HALVERSON ORTHOPEDIC CENTER
1212 DOG LEG ROAD • ANYTOWN, FL 32722 • 407-555-8523

NAME: WINGATE, SAMANTHA
PATIENT NUMBER: WINGSA001
Date of Admission: 08/20/2011

Admitting Information

Surgeon: Martin Hande, MD
Primary Care Provider: Sandra Homacker, MD

Financial Class: Workers' Compensation (WC)
Preoperative Diagnosis: Right carpal tunnel syndrome
Postoperative Diagnosis: Same, plus flexor tenosynovitis of the palm and wrist

PROCEDURES: Multiple flexor tenosynovectomies of the palm and wrist. Decompression of the right carpal tunnel with epineurolysis of medial nerve and individual motor branch decompression.

OPERATIVE PROCEDURES AND PATHOLOGIC FINDINGS:
This white female has had bilateral carpal tunnel syndrome, slightly greater on the left than on the right for an undetermined period of time. The patient is deaf. She also had bilateral thumb arthritis. It was elected not to address the latter problem at the present time. She had quite classic symptoms without any history of any rheumatoid type arthritis.

Nerve conduction studies showed significant prolongation of the median nerve conduction times on both sides. She also had bilateral thenar atrophy. Her more symptomatic left side was done in June. At surgery, multiple flexor tenosynovitis was found. She underwent resection of the tenosynovitis along with carpal tunnel decompression. Pathology report did not show a rheumatoid etiology for the tenosynovitis. Plan was to decompress her right side today. She has full extension of her fingers and possibly a slight diminution in flexion related to some degenerative arthritis.

DESCRIPTION OF PROCEDURE: Under satisfactory right IV block, prep and drape were performed. Using 4½ loupe magnification, standard incision was made, which was carried down through the superficial palmar fascia. One proximal crossing branch of the median palmar cutaneous nerve was identified and preserved. Battery-operated cautery was utilized to control some small bleeding points. The superficial palmar fascia and then the transverse carpal ligament were divided in a distal to proximal direction. The distal wrist fascia was decompressed. Inspection of the canal revealed a quite large median nerve with a subligamentous motor branch going into a tight hiatus. This was decompressed.

Further inspection of the canal revealed a picture reminiscent of the left side. Most of the flexor tendons were involved in the tenosynovitis. Systematic flexor tenosynovectomy was then performed down to the level of the lumbrical, removing the tenosynovium. Two of the deep flexors, namely those to the ring and little fingers, had some area of tendon erosions on them. These were excised. This involved the small portion of the tendon and no way weakened it.

The incision was extended 4 to 5 cm to allow some removal of additional tenosynovium in the wrist. After completing this, the median nerve was reinspected. There was a moderate hourglass deformity, and a longitudinal epineurolysis was performed on the ulnar border.

The wound was then thoroughly irrigated with saline. The skin was closed with interrupted 4-0 nylon suture. A Xeroform bulky gauze dressing was applied along with a volar splint out to the PIP joints, putting the wrist in a neutral position.

Continued

The tourniquet was released. Tourniquet time was a little over one hour. There was good color in the fingers. The patient tolerated the procedure quite well and was sent to the ASU for recovery.

Martin Hande, MD

DATE: 08/20/2011

You Code It!

What are the best, most accurate codes?

Diagnosis Codes: _____

Procedure Codes: _____

Anesthesia Codes (when applicable): _____

HCPCS Level II codes (when applicable): _____

HALVERSON ORTHOPEDIC CENTER
1212 DOG LEG ROAD • ANYTOWN, FL 32722 • 407-555-8523

PATIENT NAME: RUMPLE, BETTY
MRN: RUMPBE001
Date: 09/23/11

Attending Physician: Zainab Goupil, MD
Preoperative Diagnosis: C5 compression fracture
Postoperative Diagnosis: Same

PROCEDURE: C5 corpectomy and fusion fixation with fibular strut graft and Atlantis plate

ANESTHESIA: General endotracheal

This is a 25-year-old female status post assault. The patient sustained a C5 compression fracture. MRI scan showed compression with evidence of posterior ligamentous injury. The patient was subsequently set up for the surgical procedure. The procedure was described in detail including the risks. The risks included but not limited to bleeding, infection, stroke, paralysis, death, cerebrospinal fluid (CSF) leak, loss of bladder and bowel control, hoarse voice, paralyzed vocal cord, death, and damage to adjacent nerves and tissues. The patient understood the risks. The patient also understood that bank bone instrumentation would be used and that the bank bone could collapse and the instrumentation could fail or break or the screws could pull out. The patient provided consent.

The patient was taken to the OR. The patient was induced. Endotracheal tube was placed. A Foley was placed. The patient was given preoperative antibiotics. The patient was placed in slight extension. The right neck was prepped and draped in the usual manner. A linear incision was made over the C5 vertebral body. The platysma was divided. Dissection was continued medial to the sternocleidomastoid to the prevertebral fascia. This was cauterized and divided. The longus colli was cauterized and elevated. The fracture was visualized. A spinal needle was used to verify location using fluoroscopy. The C5 vertebral body was drilled out. The bone was saved. The disks above and below were removed. The posterior longitudinal ligament was removed. The bone was quite collapsed and fragmented. Distraction pins were then packed with bone removed from the C5 vertebral body prior to implantation. A plate was then placed with screws in the C4 and C6 vertebral bodies. The locking screws were tightened. The wound was irrigated. Bleeding was helped with the bipolar. The retractors were removed. The incision was approximated with simple interrupted Vicryl. The subcutaneous tissue was approximated and skin edges approximated subcuticularly. Steri-Strips were applied. A dressing was applied. The patient was placed back in an Aspen collar. The patient was extubated and transferred to recovery.

Zainab Goupil, MD

ZG/mgr   D: 09/23/11 12:33:08 PM   T: 09/25/11 3:22:54 PM

You Code It!

What are the best, most accurate codes?

Diagnosis Codes: _____

Procedure Codes: _____

Anesthesia Codes (when applicable): _____

HCPCS Level II codes (when applicable): _____

HALVERSON ORTHOPEDIC CENTER
1212 DOG LEG ROAD • ANYTOWN, FL 32722 • 407-555-8523

PATIENT: STARKER, SHARON
ACCOUNT/EHR #: STARSH001
Date: 08/11/11

Attending Physician: Willard B. Reader, MD

S. Patient is a 41-year-old female, who comes in with a complaint of severe neck pain and difficulty turning her head. She states she was in a car accident two days ago, her car struck from behind when she was driving home from work.

O: PE reveals tightness upon palpitation of ligaments neck and shoulders, most pronounced C3 to C5. X-rays are taken of head and neck including the cervical vertebrae. Radiologic review denies any fracture.

A. Anterior longitudinal cervical sprain

P: 1. Applied cervical collar to be worn during all waking hours
    2. Rx Vicodin (hydrocodone) 500 mg po prn
    3. 1,000 mg aspirin q.i.d.
    4. Pt to return in 2 weeks for follow-up

Willard B. Reader, MD

WBR/pw   D: 08/11/11 09:50:16   T: 08/13/11 12:55:01

You Code It!

What are the best, most accurate codes?

Diagnosis Codes: _____

Procedure Codes: _____

Anesthesia Codes (when applicable): _____

HCPCS Level II codes (when applicable): _____

HALVERSON ORTHOPEDIC CENTER
1212 DOG LEG ROAD • ANYTOWN, FL 32722 • 407-555-8523

PATIENT:	AMATTI, CLIFFORD
MRN:	AMATCL001
Admission Date:	09 October 2011
Discharge Date:	09 October 2011
Date:	09 October 2011
Preoperative DX:	Lacerations of hand, and leg
Postoperative DX:	Same
Procedure:	Simple repair of leg lacerations; layered repair of hand laceration
Surgeon:	Mary Lou Duncan, MD
Assistant:	None
Anesthesia:	General

INDICATIONS: The patient is a 9-year-old male brought to the emergency room by his father. He was helping his father hang a mirror in the bedroom when it fell and shattered. The boy suffered lacerations on his left hand and left leg.

PROCEDURE: The patient was placed on the table in supine position. Satisfactory anesthesia was obtained. The area was prepped, and attention to the deeper laceration of the left palm of the hand was first. A layered repair was performed and the 5.1-cm laceration was closed successfully with sutures. The lacerations on the lower extremity, a 2-cm laceration on the left leg at the base of the patella and a 3-cm laceration on the left shin, were successful closed with 4-0 Vicryl as well. The patient tolerated the procedures well and was transported to the recovery room.

10/09/11 11:47:39

You Code It!

What are the best, most accurate codes?

Diagnosis Codes: _____

Procedure Codes: _____

Anesthesia Codes (when applicable): _____

HCPCS Level II codes (when applicable): _____

HALVERSON ORTHOPEDIC CENTER
1212 DOG LEG ROAD • ANYTOWN, FL 32722 • 407-555-8523

PATIENT: GRANT, AMOS
ACCOUNT/EHR #:   GRANAM001
Date: 11/05/11

Attending Physician: Valerie R. Victors, MD

S: This Pt is a 15-year-old male. I have not seen this patient since last July when he came in for a certificate to play sports in school. Today he is brought in by his father after being tackled during football practice and hurting his left wrist. He is complaining of pain upon flexing and is having difficulty moving his fingers.

O: Tenderness and swelling of the wrist is observed. Pt can move his fingers slightly indicating no fracture; however, AP/lat X-rays are taken to confirm. X-ray does confirm the wrist is sprained. A conforming, nonelastic (nonsterile) bandage, 2 × 35, is applied.

A: Sprain, radiocarpal ligament, wrist

P: Follow-up in one week.

___

Valerie R. Victors, MD

VRV/mg   D: 11/05/11 09:50:16   T: 11/07/11 12:55:01

You Code It!

What are the best, most accurate codes?

Diagnosis Codes: _____

Procedure Codes: _____

Anesthesia Codes (when applicable): _____

HCPCS Level II codes (when applicable): _____

PATIENT: FISCHER, ELVIRA
ACCOUNT/EHR #:   FISCEL001
Date: 12/09/11

Attending Physician: Gena Reynoldo, MD

Technician: Harvey Nickols

Pt is a 37-year-old female hurt during a waterskiing accident. She was performing in a ski show at Water World Adventure Park when she came off the ski jump ramp in the wrong angle and hit the water unevenly, twisting her knee. Her physician, Dr. Cipher, ordered her to use a wheelchair for the next six weeks.

I delivered a standard wheelchair with fixed full-length arms and swing-away, detachable footrests to the patient's home. I spent 20 minutes instructing the patient on the proper way to use the chair, transfer from the chair to standard furniture and back, and transfer to other function furniture, including the toilet and the bed. She was instructed on how to stop and start the chair with the least amount of strain on her upper extremities and how to apply the brakes. Patient stated she clearly understood all instructions.

DX: Torn meniscus, lateral, knee

P: Patient given instruction booklet and technical support number

Harvey Nickols

HN/mg   D: 12/09/11 09:50:16   T: 12/11/11 12:55:01

You Code It!

What are the best, most accurate codes?

Diagnosis Codes: _____

Procedure Codes: _____

Anesthesia Codes (when applicable): _____

HCPCS Level II codes (when applicable): _____

HALVERSON ORTHOPEDIC CENTER
1212 DOG LEG ROAD • ANYTOWN, FL 32722 • 407-555-8523

PATIENT: MELMANN, MICHAEL
ACCOUNT/EHR #:   MELMMI001
Date: 12/09/11

Attending Physician: Gena Reynoldo, MD

This is a 13-year-old male who presents with a chief complaint of right forearm pain. While playing soccer earlier that day, the patient fell onto his right hand and heard a snapping sound. He reports that the pain in his forearm increases with movement. It is visibly swollen and deformed.

EXAM: VS are normal except for a resting tachycardia secondary to pain. He is alert and cooperative but subdued, in moderate pain. His head, neck and torso show no signs of external trauma. Heart, lungs and abdomen are normal. Upper extremities: Swelling and deformity is observed at the right midforearm, corresponding to his area of greatest pain. Radial pulses and sensation are intact.

    An IV is started, and he is given 3 mg of IV morphine. AP and lateral radiographs of his right forearm demonstrate displaced, angulated fractures of the radius and ulna with overriding (overlapping) ends.

    The patient is sedated and given additional analgesia. A closed reduction is performed with good alignment of the radius and ulna. Immobilization is accomplished with a fiberglass cast extending from the hand to the proximal humerus.

Gena Reynoldo, MD

GR/mg   D: 12/09/11 09:50:16 T: 12/11/11 12:55:01

You Code It!

What are the best, most accurate codes?

Diagnosis Codes: _____

Procedure Codes: _____

Anesthesia Codes (when applicable): _____

HCPCS Level II codes (when applicable): _____

HALVERSON ORTHOPEDIC CENTER
1212 DOG LEG ROAD • ANYTOWN, FL 32722 • 407-555-8523

PATIENT: O'DAY, SHANNON
ACCOUNT/EHR #:   ODAYSH001
Date: 12/09/11

Attending Physician: Gena Reynoldo, MD

This is a 7-year-old female who presents with a chief complaint of left wrist pain. She was rollerblading with several friends and was accidentally pushed from behind. She fell forward with outstretched, pronated arms. She denies hitting her head, loss of consciousness, vomiting, and abdominal pain.

EXAM: VS T37.0, P105, R20, BP 117/75. She is comfortable, alert and appears to be in no distress. Mild abrasions are noted on her left knee and palmar surfaces of both hands. No obvious puncture wounds are present. She has mild discomfort upon palpation of her left knee, but she is able walk, stand, and jump without difficulty or discomfort. Her right wrist is normal, but tenderness is elicited upon palpation of her left distal radius. Slight wrist swelling is noted, but no angular deformity is present. The remainder of her exam is unremarkable.

Radiographs reveal a nondisplaced distal radius fracture of the left wrist without angulation. She is placed in a forearm sugar tong splint, and her mother is given instructions to follow-up in three weeks.

Gena Reynoldo, MD

GR/mg   D: 12/09/11 09:50:16   T: 12/11/11 12:55:01

You Code It!

What are the best, most accurate codes?

Diagnosis Codes: _____

Procedure Codes: _____

Anesthesia Codes (when applicable): _____

HCPCS Level II codes (when applicable): _____

HALVERSON ORTHOPEDIC CENTER
1212 DOG LEG ROAD • ANYTOWN, FL 32722 • 407-555-8523

PATIENT:	YAEGER, DAVID
ACCOUNT/EHR #:	YAEGDA001
Date:	12/09/11
Surgeon:	Brice McArdle, MD
Anesthesiologist:	Nancy Ferguson, MD
Preop Diagnosis:	Osteoarthritis, right knee
Postop Diagnosis:	Same
Procedure:	Right total knee replacement

PATHOLOGY: The patient is a 57-year-old male with severe osteoarthritis of both knees, which has been refractory to long-term conservative treatment. He now presents for a total knee placement.

OPERATIVE FINDINGS: The patient's right knee had advanced tricompartmental osteoarthritis.

DESCRIPTION OF PROCEDURE: General anesthesia, supine position, right above-knee tourniquet, routine sterile prep and drape of the right lower extremity, intravenous antibiotics, laminar air flow room.

   The right lower extremity was wrapped with an Esmarch and a tourniquet inflated to 300 mmHg. An anterior incision was made over the right knee with dissection to the superficial retinaculum, which was then sharply split and mobilized medially. A medial parapatellar arthrotomy was performed.

   The patella was dislocated laterally. Sharp dissection was performed along the mediolateral proximal tibial plateau. The knee was flexed to expose the anterior joint. The meniscal remnants of the anterior cruciate were debrided. Osteophytes were removed from the distal femur and proximal femur using a rongeur.

   Intramedullary cutting jigs were subsequently applied to the distal femur and cuts made with an oscillating saw. The trial femur was noted to fit perfectly. The patella was then measured with the caliper and the articular surface removed with an oscillating saw. A drill-hole guide was applied and drill holes created. The patella trial was noted to fit well. A lateral retinacular release was required to obtain good tracking.

   An external alignment guide was then applied to the proximal tibia and the proximal tibia transected with an oscillating saw. Trial reductions were then performed to determine the size of the tibial plate and also confirmed soft tissue balance and axial alignment. The proximal tibial was then further broached with a cruciate driver.

   All trial components were then removed and the wound thoroughly pulse lavaged. The components were then cemented in place, beginning with the tibia and patella, followed by the femur. All extraneous cement was removed. A polyethylene liner was then applied to the tibia, and the knee was completed. The knee had excellent range of motion from 0–125 degrees with good tracking and no instability.

Continued

The tourniquet was then deflated and hemostasis performed. A Sauvage drain was placed within the knee, existing over the anterolateral thigh. The capsule was then closed with multiple interrupted sutures of #1-0 Vicryl. The superficial retinaculum was closed with interrupted vertical mattress sutures of #3-0 nylon. A sterile compressive dressing and a knee immobilizer and PAS stockings were applied.

Estimated blood loss was 200 cc. The final sponge, instrument counts were correct. Tourniquet time was 50 minutes.

The patient was transported to recovery in stable condition. Immediate neurovascular examination of the right leg showed intact pulsation, sensation and motor. There were no complications.

Brice McArdle, MD

BM/mg   D: 12/09/11 09:50:16   T: 12/11/11 12:55:01

You Code It!

What are the best, most accurate codes?

Diagnosis Codes: _____

Procedure Codes: _____

Anesthesia Codes (when applicable): _____

HCPCS Level II codes (when applicable): _____

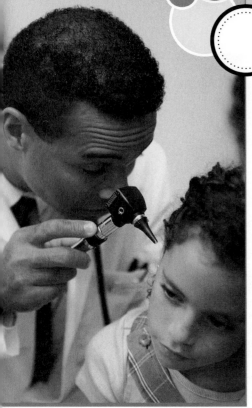

CHAPTER

17

Otolaryngology Cases and Patient Records

INTRODUCTION

The following case studies are from an ear-nose-throat (ENT) practice. In a physician's office of this type, a professional coding specialist is likely to see many different kinds of health situations, including preventive health care services.

The medical term used to identify a physician who specializes in conditions of the ears, nose, and throat (ENT) is otolaryngologist or oto-rhinolaryngologist.

Otolaryngologists diagnose and treat conditions and diseases that range from allergies to sleep apnea to laryngeal malignancies. These specialists care for patients with diseases such as myringitis, Ménière's disease, or suffering from nasal polyps. Allergy/immunology is a subspecialty because of the vast number of signs and symptoms that patients suffer and that affect the upper portion of the respiratory system. An additional subspecialty focuses on hearing and deafness. These otolaryngologists are the surgeons who perform cochlear implants or excise tumors in the ear canal.

Otolaryngologists are board-certified through the Board of Otolaryngology, which is recognized by the American Board of Medical Specialties.

You can use these cases to practice coding diagnoses, E/M, procedures, DME, or other HCPCS Level II items, as applicable; code for the physician or the facility; code inpatient and outpatient services, as applicable:

1. Code for the physician.
2. Code for the anesthesiologist, when applicable.
3. Code for the hospital, when applicable.
4. Code for the pathology and laboratory, when applicable.
5. Code HCPCS Level II codes, when applicable.

THE E.N.T. MEDICAL CENTER
Otolaryngology
321 HATCH STREET • ANYTOWN, FL 32711 • 407-555-9876

PATIENT: CAMMEN, JAN
ACCOUNT/EHR #:   CAMMJA001
Date: 10/13/11

Attending Physician: James I. Cipher, MD

This patient is a 25-year-old male with a history of recurrent sinus infections. He denies any health problems until five days before he went to his family physician's office about a year ago. He presented with fever, severe frontal headache, facial pain, and runny nose. He was treated for acute sinusitis with antibiotics and pseudoephedrine (OTC) with resolution of his symptoms. Over the next 6 months, he had recurrent bouts of frontal and left-sided headache, fever, and nasal congestion, which always improved on oral antibiotics. Over the recent 6 months, he received three courses of oral antibiotics. The last course finished 10 days before this encounter. The family physician, Dr. Blanchard, referred this patient to me.

HISTORY: No known allergies. Because of recent difficulty in concentrating, he asked the physician for an evaluation. Nonfocal neurologic examination was performed. Tenderness over frontal and left maxillary sinuses. Afebrile.

    CT scan, taken this morning in our facility, shows opacification of both frontal and left maxillary and sphenoid sinuses and a possible large nonenhanced lesion in the brain.

    Parasagittal MRI and axial MRI show a large (7-cm) well-circumscribed epidural collection compressing the left frontal lobe.

DX: Epidural abscess with frontal lobe lesions caused by significant compression on frontal lobe.

PLAN: Recommend surgery to evacuate the large epidural abscess.

James I. Cipher, MD

JIC/mg   D: 10/13/11 09:50:16   T: 10/15/11 12:55:01

You Code It!

What are the best, most accurate codes?

Diagnosis Codes: _____

Procedure Codes: _____

Anesthesia Codes (when applicable): _____

HCPCS Level II codes (when applicable): _____

THE E.N.T. MEDICAL CENTER
Otolaryngology
321 HATCH STREET • ANYTOWN, FL 32711 • 407-555-9876

PATIENT: KRAUS, MAYNARD
ACCOUNT/EHR #:   KRAUMA001
Date: 10/13/11

Attending Physician: James I. Cipher, MD

S: This new Pt is a 35-year-old male who works in a mattress factory. He states that he has had a piercing ringing sound in his left ear that began six months ago. He noticed the ringing sound in his ear upon awakening one morning, and it remains a considerable annoyance all day long, interfering with his ability to enjoy television, movies, and even conversation. Pt states he has trouble sleeping, as well.

O: Pt taken to testing suite for a bilateral tinnitus assessment: pitch (frequency) matching, loudness matching, and masking procedures are included. Findings of the testing indicate a positive determination of tinnitus. Patient is informed of the outcome, along with the recommendations for remediation therapy.

A: Acute tinnitus

P: Follow-up with masking therapy treatment plan

_____

James I. Cipher, MD

JIC/mg   D: 10/13/11 09:50:16   T: 10/15/11 12:55:01

You Code It!

What are the best, most accurate codes?

Diagnosis Codes: _____

Procedure Codes: _____

Anesthesia Codes (when applicable): _____

HCPCS Level II codes (when applicable): _____

THE E.N.T. MEDICAL CENTER
Otolaryngology
321 HATCH STREET • ANYTOWN, FL 32711 • 407-555-9876

PATIENT: ALBANNO, LOUISE
ACCOUNT/EHR #:   ALBALO001
Date: 10/13/11

Attending Physician: James I. Cipher, MD

This patient is an 81-year-old Caucasian woman referred by Dr. Stevenson due to complaints of dysphagia and dyspnea exacerbated by swallowing. She reports a 3-week history of progressive dysphagia, initially for solids and subsequently for fluids, leading to total dysphagia. She also reports regurgitation, cough, and hoarseness of voice.

HISTORY: The patient has a history of progressive dysphagia and the accumulation of food debris lead to megaesophagus.

FAMILY HISTORY: There was no significant medical, family or social history.

PHYSICAL EXAMINATION: Pulse is rapid and irregular; no other cardiovascular-respiratory abnormalities are identified. Abdominal examination: unremarkable; indirect laryngoscopy shows pooling of saliva in the hypopharynx.

IMAGING: Lateral soft tissue radiograph reveals widening of the upper mediastinum, and subsequent barium swallow shows achalasia with food debris filling the cervical esophagus. An electrocardiogram (ECG) showed evidence of ischemia and atrial fibrillation with a ventricular response rate of 120–150.

LAB: Hematologic and biochemical laboratory investigations were within the normal limits.

DX: Atrial fibrillation secondary to a megaesophagus

PLAN: Patient to be admitted to hospital for resuscitation with intravenous fluids, followed by nasoesophageal lavage and removal of 300 mL of retained food debris from the cervical esophagus. A follow-up ECG is to be performed 8 hours afterward.

James I. Cipher, MD

JIC/mg   D: 10/13/11 09:50:16   T: 10/15/11 12:55:01

You Code It!

What are the best, most accurate codes?

Diagnosis Codes: _____

Procedure Codes: _____

Anesthesia Codes (when applicable): _____

HCPCS Level II codes (when applicable): _____

THE E.N.T. MEDICAL CENTER
Otolaryngology
321 HATCH STREET • ANYTOWN, FL 32711 • 407-555-9876

PATIENT: PARMER, DIETRA
ACCOUNT/EHR #: PARMDI001
Date: 10/17/11

Attending Physician: James I. Cipher, MD

This is a 41-year-old female who underwent routine FESS and was not packed nasally after the procedure for recurrent sinusitis.

HPI: Preoperatively she was noted to have bilateral concha bullous on CT scan with subsequent obstruction of both osteomeatal complexes. Attempts to control the symptoms with medication, using both steroid sprays and antibiotics, provided no relief. FESS was discussed with the patient, and she opted to have the procedure.

FESS was scheduled for early this morning. The operation was performed at the Hilltown Ambulatory Surgical Center, which has no facilities for inpatient care. Nasal preparation used was Otrivin 30 minutes beforehand, followed by injection of 2% lidocaine in a solution of 1:80000 adrenaline into both uncinate processes and middle turbinates. Bilateral uncinectomy with middle meatal antrostomies were performed prior to reduction of both middle turbinates. There was little bleeding noted during the procedure and also after completion of the surgery. Insertion of nasal packs was therefore not deemed to be necessary. She was transferred to the recovery room in good condition. Immediate postoperative recovery was routine.

Six hours after the procedure she started bleeding, and nasal packs were inserted. She soon developed unilateral periorbital bruising and within hours her condition had worsened so much that the viability of the left eye became questionable. The patient was then transported and admitted into the hospital. She was taken in for immediate medial and lateral canthotomies. The hematomas were evacuated surgically, particularly laterally, and the tenseness of the orbit was markedly reduced. A specific bleeding point was not identifiable. She made an uneventful postoperative recovery. Postoperative CT scan revealed normal ocular anatomy, with no evidence of re-collection of hematoma. Ophthalmologic opinion stated no abnormality and orthoptics were normal.

DX: Orbital complications following functional endoscopic sinus surgery (FESS)

James I. Cipher, MD

JIC/mg   D: 10/17/11 09:50:16   T: 10/19/11 12:55:01

You Code It!

What are the best, most accurate codes?

Diagnosis Codes: _____

Procedure Codes: _____

Anesthesia Codes (when applicable): _____

HCPCS Level II codes (when applicable): _____

THE E.N.T. MEDICAL CENTER
Otolaryngology
321 HATCH STREET • ANYTOWN, FL 32711 • 407-555-9876

PATIENT: PAPPIETTE, JUANITA

ACCOUNT/EHR #:   PAPPJA001

Date: 10/13/11

Attending Physician: James I. Cipher, MD

The patient is a 61-year-old female with a chief complaint of involuntary movements of jaw-opening triggered mainly by talking and/or eating. She states that she has been symptomatic for the preceding three years. Her symptoms made eating difficult, requiring her to bite down with effort in order to keep her mouth from opening. She wore out her regular dentures, and special dentures had to be manufactured for her. Yelling would ameliorate the involuntary movements.

PERSONAL/FAMILY HISTORY: Unremarkable for other neurologic disorders. The patient denies any exposure to dopamine-blocking drugs. She denies any weight loss but admitted to eating difficulty and social embarrassment due to the jaw-opening OMD. Her neurologic examination was otherwise unremarkable.

DX: Oromandibular dystonia (OMD)

PLAN: BTX-A injections to her lateral pterygoids (75 units/side)

James I. Cipher, MD

JIC/mg   D: 10/13/11 09:50:16   T: 10/15/11 12:55:01

You Code It!

What are the best, most accurate codes?

Diagnosis Codes: _____

Procedure Codes: _____

Anesthesia Codes (when applicable): _____

HCPCS Level II codes (when applicable): _____

THE E.N.T. MEDICAL CENTER
Otolaryngology
321 HATCH STREET • ANYTOWN, FL 32711 • 407-555-9876

PATIENT: PAPPACCI, JUNE
ACCOUNT/EHR #:   PAPPJU002
Date: 10/13/11

Attending Physician: James I. Cipher, MD

DX: Foreign body in maxillary sinus

PROCEDURE: Endoscopically-assisted procedure for removal of a foreign body from the maxillary sinus

The patient is a 37-year-old female seen for chronic pain in the region of the upper first molar/right side.

HISTORY: Patient states that she had a root canal of her right upper first molar three years ago. She states that she has had previous symptoms in the last two years of maxillary sinusitis, including tenderness in the left infraorbital region and nasal stuffiness.

PHYSICAL EXAM: The left upper first molar region is painful upon light pressure. Orthopantomography shows a radiopacity of the left maxillary sinus. CT scan shows the presence of a foreign body located in the superomedial aspect of the maxillary sinus, near the natural maxillary ostium. The FB appears to be a partially formed calcium deposit. A partial mucosal thickening of the sinus upon the roots of the upper first molar was also present. Video-rhinoscopy shows hypertrophy of the inferior turbinates bilaterally.

PROCEDURE: Once patient is successfully under anesthesia, and draped in the usual, sterile fashion, standard surgical technique is used to create a small osteotomy in the lateral antral wall upon the roots of the upper first left molar. The antrum is examined through the endoscope and the foreign body is easily identified and gently removed. A contemporary endodontic surgical treatment of the upper first left molar roots and an endoscopic reduction of inferior turbinates is also performed.

   Patient is brought out of the anesthesia and taken to recovery. Her postoperative course was satisfactory, with no evidence of sinus infection.

James I. Cipher, MD

JIC/mg   D: 10/13/11 09:50:16   T: 10/15/11 12:55:01

You Code It!

What are the best, most accurate codes?

Diagnosis Codes: _____

Procedure Codes: _____

Anesthesia Codes (when applicable): _____

HCPCS Level II codes (when applicable): _____

THE E.N.T. MEDICAL CENTER
Otolaryngology
321 HATCH STREET • ANYTOWN, FL 32711 • 407-555-9876

PATIENT: APPLEMANN, DERRICK
ACCOUNT/EHR #:   APPLDE001
Date: 10/13/11

Attending Physician: James I. Cipher, MD

The patient is a 15-month-old male who presents with a mass lesion in the left postauricle region.

HISTORY: The mass was present at birth and has gradually increased in size.

EXAM: The measurement of the mass is currently 9-5-5 cm. The skin covering it is unremarkable. The balance of ROS examination is unremarkable. A noncontrast CT of the head and neck revealed the mass in the left postauricular region. There is no intracranial involvement.

DX: Congenital alveolar rhabdomyosarcoma (RMS)

PROCEDURE: Complete excision of the mass

SURGICAL PATHOLOGY:

Gross Exam: The mass is fairly well circumscribed, multinodular with a glistening, gelatinous gray-white surface. Neither hemorrhage nor necrosis is present.

Microscopic Exam: It revealed a varying degree of cellularity with densely packed cellular areas separated by a framework of hyalinized fibrous septa. The tumor cells are noncohesive in the center. The individual cells are large and round with darkly staining hyperchromatic nuclei, inconspicuous nucleoli, and scant indistinct cytoplasm. High mitotic rate is noticed. The tumor cells ($\approx$40%) are positive for desmin and myogenin immunostains. The other panels of immunostains used are CD45, CD20, MIC-2, CK, neuron-specific enolase, and myeloperoxidase, all of which are negative.

    Ultrastructurally, the tumor cells show few cytoplasmic organelles and occasional bundles of thin myofilaments measuring 4–6 mm in diameter. Bone marrow examination didn't reveal any metastatic deposit. A cytogenetic analysis was not performed because of technical reasons.

James I. Cipher, MD

JIC/mg   D: 10/13/11 09:50:16 T: 10/15/11 12:55:01

You Code It!

What are the best, most accurate codes?

Diagnosis Codes: _____

Procedure Codes: _____

Anesthesia Codes (when applicable): _____

HCPCS Level II codes (when applicable): _____

THE E.N.T. MEDICAL CENTER
Otolaryngology
321 HATCH STREET • ANYTOWN, FL 32711 • 407-555-9876

PATIENT: DONALDSON, KEIANNA
ACCOUNT/EHR #:   DONAKE001
Date: 10/23/11

Attending Physician: James I. Cipher, MD

The patient is a 27-year-old female who complains of right-sided hemicrania and difficult nasal breathing associated with recurrent right-sided maxillary sinusitis.

Nasal endoscopy revealed a substantial nasal obstruction on the right side that was caused by a marked hypertrophy of the turbinates and a deviated nasal septum. After shrinkage of the turbinate with a nasal decongestant, examination revealed a long septal ridge along the middle portion of the septum on the right side, which extended from anterior to posterior. The ridge was projecting into the right inferior turbinate, displacing it laterally. There was no significant obstruction on the left side of the nasal passage.

The patient was administered local anesthesia, and a longitudinal posterior-to-anterior incision was made over the ridge with a sickle knife. The superior and inferior mucosal flaps were elevated with the sharp end of a Cottle elevator. When the entire ridge was fully exposed, it was easily removed with a powered endoscopic excision. The mucosal flaps were repositioned, and a piece of Gelfoam was placed over the incision.

Patient got through the procedure well.

_____

James I. Cipher, MD

JIC/mg   D: 10/23/11 09:50:16   T: 10/25/11 12:55:01

You Code It!

What are the best, most accurate codes?

Diagnosis Codes: _____

Procedure Codes: _____

Anesthesia Codes (when applicable): _____

HCPCS Level II codes (when applicable): _____

THE E.N.T. MEDICAL CENTER
Otolaryngology
321 HATCH STREET • ANYTOWN, FL 32711 • 407-555-9876

PATIENT: BANKS, ARTHUR
ACCOUNT/EHR #: BANKAR001
Date: 11/13/11

Attending Physician: James I. Cipher, MD

This patient is a 39-year-old male who noted an increasing difficulty speaking audibly in noisy situations. He states that approximately five months ago he began to experience persistent vocal fatigue after he gave a 25-minute speech. He had also experienced persistent hoarseness during the same period prior to this evaluation. The patient reported no antecedent illness or other vocal abuse. He has had several examinations by his family physician, Dr. Dominguez, and was started on a proton-pump inhibitor for laryngopharyngeal reflux. Dr. Dominguez referred this to me.

EXAMINATION: Strobovideolaryngoscopy revealed mild supraglottic hyperfunction, normal motion of the vocal folds, and a large vascular mass that was centered on the anterior third of the right vocal fold. A large varicose vessel was observed leading to the mass, and the entire right side of the vocal fold was discolored yellow and red. It was also observed that there is some thickening on the left vocal fold along the contact area as well as the presence of an anterior web. On stroboscopic examination, the right vocal fold exhibited a severely decreased amplitude and wave form.

   The patient was prescribed a brief course of voice therapy to decrease his hyperfunction and to prepare him for safe phonation following surgery.

PROCEDURE: Patient was taken for microlaryngoscopy and excision of the right vocal fold mass. After the laryngoscope was suspended, the right vocal fold was infused with saline-and-epinephrine solution. The vascular mass could not be elevated from the vocal ligament, indicating a deep fibrotic reaction attaching the mass to the vocal ligament. An incision was made along the superior surface of the mass, and the mass was carefully dissected from its deep attachments. During dissection, the vocal ligament was identified anteriorly and preserved. The remaining mucosal attachments were then incised, and the mass was sent for pathologic examination. A steroid was injected underneath the yellowish mucosa and into the region of the vocal ligament in an attempt to reduce the amount of scarring. The small anterior web was left undisturbed. Pathologic examination of the mass revealed an organized hematoma without evidence of hemangioma.

PLAN: The patient should be kept on voice rest for 10 days postoperatively. He will then be allowed to slowly increase his voice use under the close observation of a laryngologist and a speech-language pathologist.

_____

James I. Cipher, MD

JIC/mg   D: 11/13/11 09:50:16   T: 11/15/11 12:55:01

You Code It!

What are the best, most accurate codes?

Diagnosis Codes: _____

Procedure Codes: _____

Anesthesia Codes (when applicable): _____

HCPCS Level II codes (when applicable): _____

THE E.N.T. MEDICAL CENTER
Otolaryngology
321 HATCH STREET • ANYTOWN, FL 32711 • 407-555-9876

PATIENT: HOLMES, RHODA
ACCOUNT/EHR #:   HOLMRH001
Date: 11/23/11

Attending Physician: James I. Cipher, MD

This patient is a 3-year-old female who presents with a history of congestion, runny nose, occasional cough, and fever. Her mother is concerned the cough is worsening. She states that the discharge from the child's nose is mostly clear; however, she has observed it cloudy on occasion. The child has not been wheezing per the mother. She has little exposure to ill children since her aunt takes care of her during the day. Her cousins, with ages ranging from 2 to 9 years, are rarely ill.

When asked about her ear, the child states, "My ear hurts, Mommy." Upon further questioning, her mother reveals no other symptoms. She states that her boyfriend and maternal grandmother, who both have similar symptoms, have been around the child recently.

The mother mentions that her grandmother had suggested some homemade remedies. She stated that she applied an OTC rub to the child's chest. She made some nose drops with salt and water and a bulb syringe, and that seemed to help the congestion much better than the OTC cough medicine, or the OTC infant's drops. She states that she has been giving the child plenty of fluids. She states that the girl has been in good health and all of her immunizations are current. She denies any previous ear infection.

FAMILY/SOCIAL HISTORY: Positive for asthma in the maternal uncle and first cousin. The mother denies any pets or smoking at home.

PHYSICAL EXAM:

GENERAL: Alert, smiling, awake, female in no acute distress

VITAL SIGNS: Wt. 18kg Pulse 90 Temp 36.3C R 36

HEENT: Normocephalic/atraumatic, eyes normal, ears—tympanic membranes pearly white and mobile bilaterally, mouth is moist, no erythema of throat

NODES: Posterior cervical shotty nodes, nontender

LUNGS: Normal respiratory rate, symmetrical breath sounds, some upper airway noises with no wheezes, clear

BREAST: Normal

CARDIOVASCULAR: RRR, no audible heart murmur, normal pulses

ABDOMINAL: Soft nondistended, positive bowel sounds and no palpable masses

NEUROLOGIC: Grossly normal and moves all extremities, no evidence of seizures, no focal findings

DX: Viral upper respiratory infection

Continued

PLAN:
1. Continue home remedy with saline nose drops.
2. Avoid over-the-counter medications, as well as herbs and vitamin supplements.
3. Nutritional supplement could include chicken broth—the heat, the liquid, and the antibiotic activity of garlic, a common ingredient, can ease symptoms and support the immune system.
4. Humidifier-cool mist would be preferable since bacteria can grow in a constant warm environment. May use the periodic steamy shower. Also remember whether the humidifier is cold or warm to change its filter since mold and bacteria love moist environments.
5. Given that this is a viral upper respiratory infection, there is no need for antibiotic treatment at this time. If she (the patient) does not improve after 2–3 days, she should be rechecked by her pediatrician to make certain that she has not developed an illness requiring antibiotics, such as otitis media or pneumonia.

James I. Cipher, MD

JIC/mg   D: 11/23/11 09:50:16   T: 11/25/11 12:55:01

You Code It!

What are the best, most accurate codes?

Diagnosis Codes: _____

Procedure Codes: _____

Anesthesia Codes (when applicable): _____

HCPCS Level II codes (when applicable): _____

THE E.N.T. MEDICAL CENTER
Otolaryngology
321 HATCH STREET • ANYTOWN, FL 32711 • 407-555-9876

PATIENT: MONTESETTO, OSCAR
ACCOUNT/EHR #:   MONTOS001
Date: 10/19/11

Attending Physician: James I. Cipher, MD

The patient is a 68-year-old right-handed man was brought in by his wife who reported, "All of a sudden he dropped the coffee, his face sagged and now he can't talk." I last saw this patient two years ago.

ROS: Wife states that problem occurred about 2 hours ago when they were having breakfast. The patient suddenly dropped a cup of coffee from his right hand, and the wife noticed a right facial droop. More strikingly, he, normally quite a chatterbox, completely ceased speaking. He could grunt and say "hello," but that was all. The wife was understandably alarmed by his state and said, "We need to go see the doctor." The patient not only could follow the commands given by his wife but, unlike his usual self, walked to the car without further coercion.

      Since the onset of the problem, patient's condition neither worsened nor remitted. There were no other symptoms around this time such as repetitive movements or complaints of H/A, CP, or palpitations before the onset of symptoms.

FH: Parents died of old age, has two sons and one daughter, all three in good health.

SH: Lives with wife of 30 years, who encourages patient to take meds and not take cigarettes. Unfortunately, he remains quite compliant on his pack per day habit of 50 years. He drinks two beers per day and does not take illicit drugs. He is a retired steel worker.

PMH: Significant for hypertension, hypercholesteremia, and type II DM. He is noncompliant on medication. Patient stated in the past, "I don't like drugs and I don't like doctors; you can give 'em to me, but I don't have to take 'em." The patient's wife recalls an episodic "mini-stroke" one year ago; the patient presented with loss of vision in one eye lasting 15 minutes. Subsequently, he was convinced to undergo a carotid endarterectomy for symptomatic carotid stenosis of 98%. Since that time, he has been lost to F/U.

ALLERGIES: NKDA

MEDS: HCTZ 25 mg PO qd, Captopril 50 mg PO bid, Glyburide 6 mg PO qAM, Zocor 20 mg qd and baby aspirin qd, but patient admits to taking it only when he feels his blood pressure or blood sugar is high.

EXAM: VITAL SIGNS: Temp: 37.0, BP: 170/100, Pulse: 88, Resp: 20.

GENERAL APPEARANCE: Obese patient, appears stated age, NAD.

HEENT: PERRL, EOMI, left fundi with cholesterol (Hollenhorst) plaques, mucus membranes moist.

NECK: No bruit bilaterally. No jugular venous distension.

HEART: RRR without murmur, rub, or gallop.

LUNGS: Clear to auscultation B.

ABD: Obese, nontender, nondistended, + B.S.

EXT: No cyanosis, clubbing, or edema.

Continued

NEURO:

MENTAL STATUS: Alert. Patient cannot repeat, cannot name, speech is restricted to word "hello." Follows commands appropriately. Patient cannot write sentence, writes "Hello." Can copy figures.

CRANIAL NERVES:
II: right homonymous inferior quadrantanopia.
III, IV, VI: EOMI
V: facial sensation intact.
VII: Right lower facial droop, flattened nasolabial fold. Wrinkles brow symmetrically.
VIII: Hearing grossly intact.
IX, X: gag intact, palate rises symmetrically.
XI: shrugs symmetrically.
XII: tongue midline.

MOTOR: RUE 0/5 proximally and distally. RLE 4/5 proximally, 5/5 distally.
    All left extremities are 5/5 proximally and distally.

REFLEXES: No reflexes, RUE in all muscle groups. Otherwise 2/4 and symmetric with downgoing toes.

SENSORY: Pin, vibration, position tested. All slightly decreased in RUE. Otherwise preserved.

CEREBELLAR FUNCTION: nl. Finger to nose on L. Nl. Heel shin B.

GAIT: nl. Romberg: nl.

LABS: CT: wnl. Some evidence of cortical atrophy.

DX: Dysphasia, probable stroke.

PLAN: Admit to hospital immediately.

James I. Cipher, MD

JIC/mg   D: 10/19/11 09:50:16   T: 10/21/11 12:55:01

You Code It!

What are the best, most accurate codes?

Diagnosis Codes: _____

Procedure Codes: _____

Anesthesia Codes (when applicable): _____

HCPCS Level II codes (when applicable): _____

PATIENT:	WATERS, SELENE
ACCOUNT/EHR #:	WATESE001
Date:	09/13/11

Attending Physician: James I. Cipher, MD

This patient is a 27-year-old female who presents for the first time to our office because she has recently had difficulty keeping up with her friends in her biweekly volleyball game. She had a "cold" five weeks ago (stuffy nose, cough, sore throat), which has gotten better except for the persistent cough. The cough is productive of green phlegm, and she gets short of breath with exertion. She states that she thinks she's got "bronchitis," because she got bronchitis frequently as a child. She is here requesting antibiotics because that's what her doctor "always" gave her for the bronchitis. She has recently tried over-the-counter inhalers, but finds they offer little relief of her symptoms. She does not smoke. She coughs daily and is awakened from sleep at least 1 or 2 nights a week with cough. Her cough is worsened by cold weather and she is noticing decreased exercise tolerance over the past several months. She volunteers, "I do NOT have asthma."

Review of systems is otherwise negative. There is no personal history of asthma. She thinks her mom had asthma and her brother has "allergies." She has never been hospitalized. She denies any allergies to medication or environmental allergens. The patient denies symptoms of GERD.

EXAM:

GENERAL: She is a neatly dressed white female appearing her stated age and in no respiratory distress.

VITALS: BP 110/70 RR 12 HR 68 T 97.5 Ht: 6'1" Wt: 190 lb

HEENT: PERRL, EOMI, anicteric sclera, tympanic membranes visualized bilaterally, clear nasal discharge noted, nasal mucosa pink and without inflammation. No frontal or maxillary sinus tenderness. Pharynx without erythema, tonsils without exudate. Neck is supple, without adenopathy; no thyromegaly.

CV: Heart rate regular without m/r/g

LUNGS: Clear to auscultation in all fields bilaterally

ABD: Soft, positive bowel sounds, nontender, nondistended, no masses, guarding, organomegaly

GU/RECTAL: Deferred

EXTREMITIES: Without clubbing, cyanosis, edema

CHEST X-RAY: Showed no infiltrate, no mass, no cardiomegaly or increased vascular markings. The patient's peak flow is 350 (expected is 630).

The patient read about the recent outbreak of pertussis and wondered if she has the disease. However, she then remembered that she is fully vaccinated against pertussis.

Continued

DX: Asthma symptoms (cough, decrease exercise tolerance) and has likely had asthma since childhood.

PLAN: A low dose inhaled steroid two puffs QID and albuterol two puffs q4hours prn. Patient is given a peak flow meter and taught how to use it and to record her daily readings.

James I. Cipher, MD

JIC/mg   D: 09/13/11 09:50:16   T: 09/15/11 12:55:01

You Code It!

What are the best, most accurate codes?

Diagnosis Codes: _____

Procedure Codes: _____

Anesthesia Codes (when applicable): _____

HCPCS Level II codes (when applicable): _____

Pathology and Laboratory Cases and Patient Records

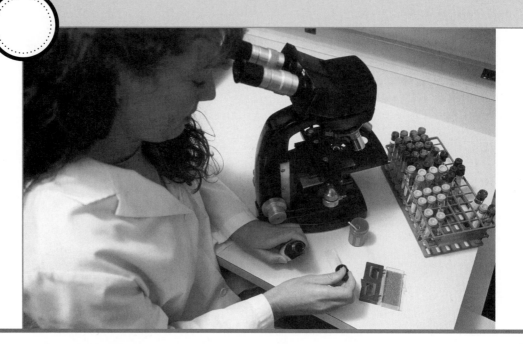

INTRODUCTION

The following case studies are from a pathology laboratory. Labs may be located within a hospital or other health care facility or a freestanding independent facility.

Pathologists are physicians who specialize in the examination of anatomical tissue and body fluid samples in order to identify disease.

Pathologists analyze and evaluate many different types of specimens. They may receive tissues (such as a swab, excised lesion, mole, or polyp) removed from a patient during surgery or a biopsy. They also analyze blood, urine, sperm, saliva, and other bodily fluid samples. Very often, it is the results of a pathology report (test results interpreted by a pathologist) that confirm or deny a suspected diagnosis or the progress of a disease or therapeutic procedure.

A medical examiner or coroner, a clinical professional who performs autopsies, is a subspecialty of pathology.

Pathologists are board-certified in a number of subspecialties through the American Board of Pathology, which is recognized by the American Board of Medical Specialties.

You can use these cases to practice coding diagnoses, E/M, procedures, DME, or other HCPCS Level II items, as applicable; code for the physician or the facility; code inpatient and outpatient services, as applicable:

1. Code for the physician.
2. Code for the anesthesiologist, when applicable.
3. Code for the hospital, when applicable.
4. Code for the pathology and laboratory, when applicable.
5. Code HCPCS Level II codes, when applicable.

AMERICAN TESTING & DIAGNOSTICS
792 TREMONT DRIVE • HAMLIN, FL 32744 • 407-555-9764

PATIENT: FRANKLIN, FRANCES
MRN: FRANFR001
Date: 17 October 2011

Procedure Performed: Comprehensive metabolic panel

Pathologist: Caryn Simonson, MD

Referring Physician: Valerie R. Victors, MD

Indications: Routine physical exam

IMPRESSIONS:

Albumin	3.9
Bilirubin	Small*
Calcium	8.9
Carbon dioxide (CO_2)	28
Chloride	96 L
Creatinine	1.2
Glucose	102
Phosphatase, alkaline	90
Potassium	3.9
Protein, total	30*
Sodium	138
Transferase, alanine amino (ALT)(SGPT)	30
Transferase, aspartate amino (AST)(SGOT)	29
Urea nitrogen (BUN)	18

* = Abnormal, L = Low, H = High

Caryn Simonson, MD

CS/mg   D: 10/17/11 09:50:16   T: 10/20/11 12:55:01

You Code It!

What are the best, most accurate codes?

Diagnosis Codes: _____

Procedure Codes: _____

Anesthesia Codes (when applicable): _____

HCPCS Level II codes (when applicable): _____

AMERICAN TESTING & DIAGNOSTICS
792 TREMONT DRIVE • HAMLIN, FL 32744 • 407-555-9764

PATIENT: TRANSIL, BRENT

MRN: TRANBRO01

Date: 29 September 2011

Procedure Performed: Tissue, skin, head, mutation identification

Pathologist: Caryn Simonson, MD

Referring Physician: James I. Cipher, MD

INDICATIONS: Suspected melanoma

IMPRESSIONS: Abnormal cells present

MOLECULAR DIAGNOSTICS; mutation identification by sequencing, single segment

---

Caryn Simonson, MD

CS/mg   D: 09/29/11 09:50:16   T: 09/30/11 12:55:01

You Code It!

What are the best, most accurate codes?

Diagnosis Codes: _____

Procedure Codes: _____

Anesthesia Codes (when applicable): _____

HCPCS Level II codes (when applicable): _____

PATIENT:	HAVERSTROM, OLIVIA
MRN:	HAVEOL001
Date:	15 November 2011

Procedure Performed: Surgical pathology, gallbladder, gross and microscopic examination

Pathologist: Caryn Simonson, MD

Referring Physician: Valerie R. Victors, MD

INDICATIONS: R/o malignancy

IMPRESSIONS: All tissues unremarkable

Surgical pathology, gross and microscopic examination of gallbladder

---

Caryn Simonson, MD

CS/mg   D: 11/15/11 09:50:16   T: 11/20/11 12:55:01

You Code It!

What are the best, most accurate codes?

Diagnosis Codes: _____

Procedure Codes: _____

Anesthesia Codes (when applicable): _____

HCPCS Level II codes (when applicable): _____

AMERICAN TESTING & DIAGNOSTICS
792 TREMONT DRIVE • HAMLIN, FL 32744 • 407-555-9764

PATIENT: FRIEDMAN, DORIS

MRN: FRIEDO001

Date: 23 September 2011

Procedure Performed: Rectal biopsies, gross and microscopic examination

Pathologist: Caryn Simonson, MD

Referring Physician: Matthew Appellet, MD

INDICATIONS: Inflammatory bowel disease

IMPRESSIONS: All tissues normal

Surgical pathology, gross and microscopic examination, colon biopsy

_____

Caryn Simonson, MD

CS/mg   D: 09/23/11 09:50:16 T: 09/25/11 12:55:01

You Code It!

What are the best, most accurate codes?

Diagnosis Codes: _____

Procedure Codes: _____

Anesthesia Codes (when applicable): _____

HCPCS Level II codes (when applicable): _____

PATIENT: FRANKS, ELMER
MRN: FRANEL001
Date: 17 June 2011

Procedure Performed: Mass (fat tissue), upper eyelid gross and microscopic examination

Pathologist: Caryn Simonson, MD

Referring Physician: Mark C. Welby, MD

INDICATIONS: Herniated orbital fat pad, OD

IMPRESSIONS: Carcinoma in situ

Surgical pathology, gross and microscopic examination, soft tissue tumor, extensive resection

_____

Caryn Simonson, MD

CS/mg   D: 06/17/11 09:50:16   T: 06/20/11 12:55:01

You Code It!

What are the best, most accurate codes?

Diagnosis Codes: _____

Procedure Codes: _____

Anesthesia Codes (when applicable): _____

HCPCS Level II codes (when applicable): _____

AMERICAN TESTING & DIAGNOSTICS
792 TREMONT DRIVE • HAMLIN, FL 32744 • 407-555-9764

PATIENT: BAKER, DORITTA
MRN: BAKEDO001
Date: 19 September 2011

Procedure Performed: Endocervical specimen,

Intraepithelial lesion of the cervix, cytopathology smear

Pathologist: Caryn Simonson, MD

Referring Physician: Rodney L. Cohen, MD

INDICATIONS: Lesion of cervix

IMPRESSIONS: Uncertain behavior neoplasm

Cytopathology, cervical, collected in preservative fluid, automated thin layer preparation; manual screening and rescreening

_____

Caryn Simonson, MD

CS/mg   D: 09/19/11 09:50:16   T: 09/23/11 12:55:01

You Code It!

What are the best, most accurate codes?

Diagnosis Codes: _____

Procedure Codes: _____

Anesthesia Codes (when applicable): _____

HCPCS Level II codes (when applicable): _____

AMERICAN TESTING & DIAGNOSTICS
792 TREMONT DRIVE • HAMLIN, FL 32744 • 407-555-9764

PATIENT: KLOTSKY, STACY

MRN: KLOTST001

Date: 05 October 2011

Procedure Performed: Bladder, biopsy gross and microscopic examination

Pathologist: Caryn Simonson, MD

Referring Physician: Leonard Dupont, MD

INDICATIONS: R/o bladder tumor

IMPRESSIONS: Chronic cystitis with squamous cell metaplasia

Surgical pathology, gross and microscopic examination, urinary bladder, biopsy

Caryn Simonson, MD

CS/mg   D: 10/05/11 09:50:16   T: 10/07/11 12:55:01

You Code It!

What are the best, most accurate codes?

Diagnosis Codes: _____

Procedure Codes: _____

Anesthesia Codes (when applicable): _____

HCPCS Level II codes (when applicable): _____

AMERICAN TESTING & DIAGNOSTICS
792 TREMONT DRIVE • HAMLIN, FL 32744 • 407-555-9764

PATIENT NAME: BIRRSTONE, SHIRLEY

MRN: BIRRSH001

Date: 09/20/2011

Date of Surgery: 02/20/2011

Pathologist: Allan Cantor, MD

Surgeon: Roger Torres, MD

CLINICAL DIAGNOSIS AND HISTORY: Carpal tunnel syndrome. No history of rheumatoid arthritis.

TISSUE(S) SUBMITTED: SYNOVIUM, right hand.

GROSS DESCRIPTION: Specimen is received in fixative and consists of multiple yellow-tan, rubbery, irregular connective tissue fragments, 4 × 2 × 1 cm in aggregate.

MICROSCOPIC DESCRIPTION: 1 microscopic slide examined.

DX: Chronic inflammation and fibrosis, tenosynovium, clinically, right hand.

Allan Cantor, MD

AC:ygc   DD: 09/20/2011   DT: 09/22/2011

You Code It!

What are the best, most accurate codes?

Diagnosis Codes: _____

Procedure Codes: _____

Anesthesia Codes (when applicable): _____

HCPCS Level II codes (when applicable): _____

PATIENT NAME: LARMAR, CARLA
MRN: LARMCA001
Date: 12/04/2011

Date of Surgery: 12/03/2011

Pathologist: Allan Cantor, M.D.

Surgeon: Harriet Fara, M.D.

OPERATION: Bilateral tubal ligation
TISSUE: Left and right tubes
PREOP DX: Undesired fertility
POSTOP DX: Same

HISTOLOGIC DIAGNOSIS: #1 and #2 segments of fallopian tube, right and left: lumen identified

GROSS DESCRIPTION: Received labeled with the patient's name.

Received in formalin, labeled "right and left tubes" are grossly recognizable segment of the right and left fallopian tubes measuring 1.5 × 0.5 × 0.4 cm and 2.0 × 0.6 × 0.4 cm. The serosa is pink-tan, smooth and glistening and the cut surface is grossly unremarkable. Representative section of right and left fallopian tube is submitted in one cassette.

Allan Cantor, MD

AC:ygc   DD: 12/04/2011   DT: 12/09/2011

You Code It!

What are the best, most accurate codes?

Diagnosis Codes: _____

Procedure Codes: _____

Anesthesia Codes (when applicable): _____

HCPCS Level II codes (when applicable): _____

AMERICAN TESTING & DIAGNOSTICS
792 TREMONT DRIVE • HAMLIN, FL 32744 • 407-555-9764

PATIENT NAME: COLUMBO, ENZO
MRN: COLUEN001
Date: 12/15/2011

Date of Surgery: 12/14/2011

Pathologist: Allan Cantor, MD

Surgeon: Harriet Fara, MD

OPERATION: Laparocholecystectomy
TISSUE: Gallbladder
PREOP DX: Cholelithiasis
POSTOP DX: Same

Histologic Diagnosis: Gallbladder: Chronic cholecystitis. Cholelithiasis. T57000, M43000, M30010

GROSS DESCRIPTION: Received labeled with the patient's name.

The specimen is received in formalin in a single container labeled "gallbladder" and consists of one pink-green gallbladder measuring 7 × 2.8 × 2 cm. The serosal surface is smooth and glistening. Surgical staple is removed to reveal a partially obstructed cystic duct due to a thickening of the luminal wall. The specimen is opened to reveal a smooth dark green mucosal surface that is filled with viscous green bile and multiple tan yellow gallstones measuring 1 × 0.6 × 0.8 cm up to 2.2 × 1.5 × 1.2 cm. The gallbladder wall thickness measures 0.4 cm. Representative sections of cystic duct and gallbladder wall are submitted in one cassette.

Allan Cantor, MD

AC:ygc   DD: 12/15/2011   DT: 12/23/2011

You Code It!

What are the best, most accurate codes?

Diagnosis Codes: _____

Procedure Codes: _____

Anesthesia Codes (when applicable): _____

HCPCS Level II codes (when applicable): _____

AMERICAN TESTING & DIAGNOSTICS
792 TREMONT DRIVE • HAMLIN, FL 32744 • 407-555-9764

PATIENT NAME: GONZALEZ, ANITA
MRN: GONZAN001
Date: 09/22/2011

Date of Surgery: 09/21/2011

Pathologist: Allan Cantor, MD

Surgeon: Fredrick Frankel, MD

OPERATION: Laparotomy, appendectomy, right salpingo-oophorectomy
TISSUE: Right tube and ovary and appendix
PREOP DX: Acute abdomen
POSTOP DX: Same

HISTOLOGIC DIAGNOSIS:
1. Fibroconnective tissue with acute and chronic inflammation and microabscess formation consistent with acute peritonitis
2. Right ovary and fallopian tube with congestion, edema, inflammation, fibrous adhesions and serositis.
3. No evidence of malignancy.
Designated right tube and ovary

COMMENT: Despite a meticulous search, no appendiceal tissue is identified grossly or microscopically. Case discussed with Dr. Frankel on 4/23/11.

GROSS DESCRIPTION: The specimen is labeled right tube, ovary, and appendix and consists of a right ovary and fallopian tube which appear adherent to one another via numerous adhesions. The entire specimen weighs 20 grams and measures 6 × 4 × 2.0 cm. The segment of fallopian tube that is present measures 6.0 cm in length. The external surface is pale tan. Sections through the tube reveal a somewhat dilated but patent lumen. The adjacent ovary measures 3.5 × 3.0 × 1.0 cm. Bisection reveals pale tan tissue with areas of hemorrhage. No grossly recognizable appendix is seen. Representative sections in six cassettes.

MICROSCOPIC DESCRIPTION: This specimen has been extensively sampled. Sections of the fallopian tube show areas of vascular congestion and edema. In addition within the serosa are areas of acute and chronic inflammation associated with microabscess formation. Fibrous adhesions are also present.

    Sections of the ovary show surface adhesions, vascular congestion, and corpora albicantia. The serosa of the ovary also shows areas of inflammation.

    Also present are several fragments of fibroconnective tissue with vascular congestion, acute and chronic inflammation, and microabscess formation. No appendiceal tissue is identified. There is no evidence of malignancy.

Allan Cantor, MD

AC:ygc   DD: 09/22/2011   DT: 09/27/2011

You Code It!

What are the best, most accurate codes?

Diagnosis Codes: _____

Procedure Codes: _____

Anesthesia Codes (when applicable): _____

HCPCS Level II codes (when applicable): _____

AMERICAN TESTING & DIAGNOSTICS
792 TREMONT DRIVE • HAMLIN, FL 32744 • 407-555-9764

PATIENT NAME: NATRINU, HERBERT
MRN: NATRHE001
Date: 11/11/2011

Date of Surgery: 11/10/2011

Pathologist: Allan Cantor, MD

Surgeon: Albert Farina, MD

OPERATION: Gastroscopy
TISSUE: Antrum R/O Helicobacter
PREOP DX: GI Bleed
POSTOP DX: Same

PATHOLOGY DIAGNOSIS:
1. Mild chronic active gastritis
2. No intestinal metaplasia identified
3. Few rare *Helicobacter pylori* identified on the Giemsa stain
4. No evidence of malignancy
Designated antrum

GROSS DESCRIPTION: The specimen is labeled antrum r/o *Helicobacter* and consists of a circular fragment of pale tan yellow soft tissue that measures 0.3 cm in greatest dimension. Entirely submitted in one cassette.

Microscopic Description: All of the tissue has been submitted for microscopic examination. Multiple levels have been obtained. Sections show gastric mucosa with vascular congestion and edema. There is a mild increase in the numbers of both acute and chronic inflammatory cells within the lamina propria. No intestinal metaplasia is identified. A few *Helicobacter pylori* are identified on the Giemsa stain. There is no evidence of malignancy.

Allan Cantor, MD

AC:ygc   DD: 10/11/2011   DT: 11/11/2011

You Code It!

What are the best, most accurate codes?

Diagnosis Codes: _____

Procedure Codes: _____

Anesthesia Codes (when applicable): _____

HCPCS Level II codes (when applicable): _____

AMERICAN TESTING & DIAGNOSTICS
792 TREMONT DRIVE • HAMLIN, FL 32744 • 407-555-9764

PATIENT NAME: NATRINU, HERBERT
MRN: NATRHE001
Date: 09/11/2011

Date of Surgery: 09/10/2011

Pathologist: Allan Cantor, MD

Surgeon: Albert Farina, MD

NATURE OF SPECIMEN: Paracentesis fluid

FINAL DX:
Abdominal fluid, aspiration
—positive for malignant cells
—consistent with adenocarcinoma

_____

Allan Cantor, MD

AC:ygc   DD: 09/11/2011   DT: 09/11/2011

You Code It!

What are the best, most accurate codes?

Diagnosis Codes: _____

Procedure Codes: _____

Anesthesia Codes (when applicable): _____

HCPCS Level II codes (when applicable): _____

AMERICAN TESTING & DIAGNOSTICS
792 TREMONT DRIVE • HAMLIN, FL 32744 • 407-555-9764

PATIENT: DENNING, ROSE
ACCOUNT/EHR #:   DENNRO001
Date: 10/15/11

Ordering Dr: Terence Rollin, MD

Clinical Information: Emergency room

TEST	BMP			
(136–144)	SODIUM	L	130	MEQ/L
(3.6–5.1)	POTASSIUM		4.1	MEQ/L
(101–111)	CHLORIDE	L	97	MEQ/L
(22–32)	CO_2 CONTENT		22	MEQ/L
(08–20)	BUN	H	23	MG/DL
(74–118)	GLUCOSE	H	130	MG/DL
(0.9–1.3)	CREATININE		0.9	MG/DL
(7.3–21.7)	BUN/CREAT RATIO	H	25.6	
(280–300)	CALCULATED OSMO	L	275	MOS/KG
(8.9–10.3)	CALCIUM		9.4	MG/DL

Lewis Strumm, MD
Pathologist

LS/fa 10/15/11 11:47:39

You Code It!

What are the best, most accurate codes?

Diagnosis Codes: _____

Procedure Codes: _____

Anesthesia Codes (when applicable): _____

HCPCS Level II codes (when applicable): _____

PATIENT: YAWLIN, LAWRENCE
ACCOUNT/EHR #:   YAWLLA001
Date: 10/15/11

Ordering Dr: Terence Rollin, MD

PATIENT HISTORY: The patient is a 53-year-old male with a 3-year history of an increasing neck mass associated with a choking feeling. The pre-op and post-op diagnoses were "left thyroid mass."

GROSS DESCRIPTION: The specimen is received fresh in one part labeled "left thyroid lobe, superior pole, marked by stitch." It consists of 8.5 × 7.0 × 4.0 cm 125-gram thyroid lobectomy. The specimen is inked and serially sectioned, revealing a single nodule involving most of the specimen, with a 0.5-cm rim of thyroid tissue superiorly. This nodule is encapsulated, revealing a brown, soft, lobulated cut surface with fibrous bands, with focal areas of hemorrhage, cystic degeneration, and necrosis. Sections are frozen in bulk and OCT. A frozen section was performed. Pictures and digital images are taken.

MICROSCOPIC DESCRIPTION: Histologic examination reveals an encapsulated expansile tumor which is seen to compress the normal thyroid tissue around it. The tumor is composed of nests of cells separated by fine fibrous septa. The cells are large and brightly eosinophilic, with a granular cytoplasm and a low nuclear-to-cytoplasmic ratio. In most areas the nuclei are rather monomorphic, with coarse chromatin features and singular prominent eosinophilic nucleoli. Focally, there is nuclear atypia suggesting aneuploidy, but mitotic figures are not easily found. There are focal areas where there seems to be invasion into the capsule, and in one region, frank breaching of the capsule is seen. The tumor appears to track along the blood vessels as they pierce the capsule. Angiolymphatic invasion is identified.

DX: Thyroid, left, lobectomy
A. Well-differentiated Hürthle cell carcinoma (8.5 cm, 125 grams) with angiolymphatic invasion, capsular invasion, and focal areas of degeneration.
B. All margins of resection free of tumor.
C. Stage: T3, Nx, Mx.

Lewis Strumm, MD
Pathologist

LS/fa 10/15/11 11:47:39

You Code It!

What are the best, most accurate codes?

Diagnosis Codes: _____

Procedure Codes: _____

Anesthesia Codes (when applicable): _____

HCPCS Level II codes (when applicable): _____

AMERICAN TESTING & DIAGNOSTICS
792 TREMONT DRIVE • HAMLIN, FL 32744 • 407-555-9764

PATIENT: WALKEN, SERITA
ACCOUNT/EHR #: WALKSE001
Date: 10/15/11

Ordering Dr: Terence Rollin, MD

HISTORY: This patient is a 25-year-old female, referred by her primary care physician, Dr. Kennison, due to complaints of abdominal discomfort and distension, which she has had for about four weeks. The patient reported constipation but denied nausea, vomiting, sharp abdominal pain, and rectal bleeding. Physical examination demonstrated diffuse abdominal tenderness and firmness without guarding. A transvaginal ultrasound revealed a large, complex, cystic and solid soft tissue mass within the pelvis, extending to 2.0 cm above the umbilicus. A CT scan of the abdomen and pelvis showed involvement of the right adnexa. The patient underwent a right salpingo-oophorectomy.

LABORATORY DATA: Alpha-Fetoprotein (AFP) 11023 ng/mL, CA 125 93 U/mL, CA 19-9

GROSS DESCRIPTION: The right salpingo-oophorectomy specimen consisted of an unremarkable fallopian tube and a 19 × 18 × 6 cm solid and cystic ovarian mass. The serosa was intact and smooth. Serial section of the mass demonstrated multiloculated cysts containing yellow, seromucinous fluid. The interior of the cyst wall was red-tan and smooth, with focal edema and intramural hemorrhage. The solid component was fleshy and tan-pink with yellow, rubbery-to-firm stellate areas. Separate from the main solid and cystic mass was a 6.5-cm area containing hair and friable, yellow material.

MICROSCOPIC DESCRIPTION: Histologic sections of the smaller yellow, friable area showed epidermis with adnexal structures.

Sections of the larger cystic and solid mass demonstrated branching papillary structures containing thick basement membrane material and covered with cuboidal to low columnar cells. This arrangement was best seen in a cross-section of an individual papilla. In addition to this pattern, microcystic spaces were prominent in other areas. Eosinophilic globules were present in a few sections and were found to be PAS-positive, diastase-resistant.

IMMUNOHISTOCHEMICAL STAINS: Stains for human chorionic gonadotropin (hCG), placental alkaline phosphatase (PLAP), and epithelial membrane antigen (EMA) were negative.

FINAL DX: Yolk sac tumor arising in association with mature cystic teratoma (dermoid cyst).

Lewis Strumm, MD
Pathologist

LS/fa 10/15/11 11:47:39

You Code It!

What are the best, most accurate codes?

Diagnosis Codes: _____

Procedure Codes: _____

Anesthesia Codes (when applicable): _____

HCPCS Level II codes (when applicable): _____

AMERICAN TESTING & DIAGNOSTICS
792 TREMONT DRIVE • HAMLIN, FL 32744 • 407-555-9764

PATIENT: ABATTI, BRIAN
ACCOUNT/EHR #:   ABATBR001
Date: 10/04/11

Ordering Dr: Terence Rollin, MD

DX:
1. Sepsis. Rule out pneumonitis or urinary tract infection.
2. Acute bronchitis
3. Diabetes mellitus
4. Chronic obstructive pulmonary disease

GRAM STAIN****
  Body Site: Sputum
  Gram Stain   Few epithelial cells, few WBC's, few gram positive cocci and gram positive bacilli

SPUTUM CULTURE****
  Source: Sputum
  Status: Preliminary
  Grade   +1
  Organism   Normal respiratory flora

URINE CULTURE*****
  Source: CATH
  Status: Final
  Organism   No growth 48 hr

THROAT CULTURE*****
  Source: Throat
  Body Site: Throat
  Status: Final
  Organism   Normal upper respiratory flora. No group A Beta Streptococcus isolated.

BLOOD CULTURE #1****
  Source: Blood
  Arm   Right
  Time   1550
  Status   Preliminary
  Organism   No growth 48 hr

Continued

BLOOD CULTURE #2****
    Source: Blood
    Arm   Left
    Time   1600
    Status   Preliminary
    Organism   No growth 48 hr

Lewis Strumm, MD
Pathologist

LS/fa 10/04/11 11:47:39

You Code It!

What are the best, most accurate codes?

Diagnosis Codes: _____

Procedure Codes: _____

Anesthesia Codes (when applicable): _____

HCPCS Level II codes (when applicable): _____

Plastic and Reconstructive Surgery Cases and Patient Records

INTRODUCTION

The following case studies are from a plastic (reconstructive) surgery practice. In a physician's office of this type, a professional coding specialist is likely to see many different kinds of health situations. You might think that, because most plastic surgery is considered cosmetic or elective, surgery not typically covered by insurance, and there is no need for a coder. That is not always true. The cases that you see within this chapter will, hopefully, help you gain a wider perspective.

Plastic surgeons are physicians who specialize in surgery that improves a person's appearance or functionality. Plastic surgery is not only about face-lifts and nose jobs. This health care provider performs surgery to correct congenital abnormalities, such as cleft lip and palate to enable a child to eat properly. This physician may be called in to surgically reattach a severed limb or finger, complete skin grafts to cover the scars from a severe burn, or carry out reconstruction, such as performing breast implant surgery after a mastectomy.

Plastic surgeons can subspecialize in facial reconstruction or hand surgery.

Plastic surgeons are board-certified through the Board of Plastic Surgery, which is recognized by the American Board of Medical Specialties.

You can use these cases to practice coding diagnoses, E/M, procedures, DME, or other HCPCS Level II items, as applicable; code for the physician or the facility; code inpatient and outpatient services, as applicable:

1. Code for the physician.
2. Code for the anesthesiologist, when applicable.
3. Code for the hospital, when applicable.
4. Code for the pathology and laboratory, when applicable.
5. Code HCPCS Level II codes, when applicable.